A
GLOBAL
AGENDA

Issues Before
the 46th
General Assembly
of the
United Nations

THE UNITED NATIONS ASSOCIATION of the United States of America is a national organization dedicated to strengthening the U.N. system and to enhancing U.S. participation in international institutions. UNA-USA carries out its action agenda through a unique combination of public outreach, policy analysis, and international dialogue.

Through a nationwide network of chapters, divisions, and affiliated organizations, UNA-USA reaches a broad cross-section of the American public. The Association provides information and educational services on the work of the United Nations and on other global issues for students, scholars, Congress, and the media; and each year it coordinates the observance of U.N. Day (October 24) in hundreds of communities across the nation.

UNA-USA conducts policy analysis and international dialogue through the Global Policy Project, a grass-roots national study program; the Economic Policy Council, America's premier business and labor forum; and a series of Parallel Studies programs with the Soviet Union, Japan, China, and East Central Europe.

A GLOBAL AGENDA

Issues Before
the 46th
General Assembly
of the
United Nations

An annual publication of the
United Nations Association of the
United States of America

John Tessitore and Susan Woolfson,
Editors

University Press of America
Lanham • New York • London

Copyright © 1991 by the United Nations
Association of the United States of America, Inc.

Published by
University Press of America®, Inc.
4720 Boston Way
Lanham, Maryland 20706

3 Henrietta Street
London WC2E 8LU England

ISSN: 1057-1213
ISBN: 0-934654-91-3 (cloth, alk. paper)
ISBN: 0-934654-90-5 (pbk., alk. paper)

Cover by Scott Rattray

Contents

Contributors

José E. Alvarez (Legal Issues chapter) is an Associate Professor of Law at George Washington University's National Law Center, where he teaches courses on international law and international organizations. During the spring term of 1992 he will be a visiting professor at the University of Michigan Law School.

Anindya K. Bhattaccharya (Transnational Corporations and Technology Transfer section, with David J. Dell) is an adjunct Associate Professor at Fordham University's Graduate School of Business.

Frederick Z. Brown (Indochina section) is Senior Associate at the Indochina Institute of George Mason University, Fairfax, Virginia.

David J. Dell (Transnational Corporations and the Global Economy section, with Anindya K. Bhattaccharya) is Director of Corporate Finance at the investment banking firm F. N. Wolf & Co.

Leonard Doyle (Making and Keeping the Peace and Refugees sections) is U.N. Correspondent of *The Independent* of London.

Felice Gaer (Human Rights section) has been Executive Director of the International League for Human Rights since 1982.

Thomas K. Hafen (Other Social Issues: Aging, Disabled), a UNA Communications Intern, studies English literature, German, and international relations at Brigham Young University.

Julie Jones (Other Social Issues: Youth, with Laurie Miller), a UNA Communications Intern, is a graduate of Middlebury College.

Lee A. Kimball (Antarctica section) is a Senior Associate at the World Resources Institute in Washington, D.C., examining the work of international institutions in the field.

Toby Lanzer (Drug Abuse, Production, and Trafficking section) served as a UNA Communications Intern while specializing in economic and political development at Columbia University's School of International and Public Affairs.

Craig Lasher (Population section) is a Legislative Assistant and Policy Analyst at the Population Crisis Committee, a private nonprofit organization that works to expand the availability of voluntary family planning services worldwide.

Frederick K. Lister (Finance and Administration chapter), author of *Decision-Making Strategies for International Organizations*, served the United Nations in a variety of capacities during 34 years as an international civil servant.

Martin M. McLaughlin (Food and Agriculture section) is a consultant on food and development policy.

Laurie Miller (Health section; Other Social Issues: Youth, with Julie Jones), a UNA Communications Intern, is specializing in social welfare policy at Columbia University's School of International and Public Affairs.

George H. Mitchell, Jr. (The World Economy: Retrospect and Prospect, Money and Finance, and Trade sections), is Assistant Professor of Political Science at Tufts University and the Fletcher School of Law and Diplomacy.

W. Ofuatey-Kodjoe (Africa section), Professor of Political Science at Queens College and at the City University of New York (CUNY) Graduate Center, directs the CUNY Seminar on Contemporary Africa and the fellowship program of the university's Ralph Bunche Institute.

Sharon M. Palmer (The Status of Women section), a UNA Communications Intern, is a recent graduate of Surrey University, England, with a joint degree in sociology, religious studies, and theology.

Frank Patalong (Crime section), a UNA Communications Intern, is a recent graduate of Lady Margaret Hall, Oxford University, where he studied English language and literature.

Sterett Pope (The Middle East and the Persian Gulf section) writes regularly on the Middle East for a number of publications.

Anne Rickert (International Space Year section), a recent graduate of Georgetown University, is a Public Affairs Assistant at UNA.

Carly Rogers (Environment section) is a consultant on international environment and development issues for, among others, the Natural Resources Defense Council, the National Audubon Society, and United Earth.

Benjamin N. Schiff (Arms Control and Disarmament chapter), author of *International Nuclear Technology Transfer: Dilemmas of Dissemination and Control*, is Associate Professor of Government at Oberlin College.

Ethan Schwartz (Central America, Afghanistan, Cyprus, and Other Colonial and Sovereignty Issues sections), formerly U.N. Correspondent of *The Washington Post*, now writes on international affairs from a base in Paris.

Steven K. Smith (Other Social Issues: The Homeless), a UNA Communications Intern, is completing a master's degree in international affairs at Columbia University.

John Tessitore (Co-Editor) is Director of Communications at UNA-USA.

Tullio Treves (Law of the Sea section) is a Professor of International Law at the University of Milan. Since 1984 he has served as Legal Advisor to the Permanent Mission of Italy to the United Nations in New York.

Susan Woolfson (Co-Editor) is Managing Editor of Communications at UNA-USA.

Preface

Reviewing the contents of this volume, prepared during the spring and summer of 1991, the editors find vivid evidence that this has been an extraordinary year—for the world and for the world organization.

For more than half a year, the world's attention was focused on the tiny nation of Kuwait and on a drama of war and diplomacy unlike any we have seen before. Never had the U.N. Security Council—passing 12 resolutions in response to aggression and three more subsequent to a cease-fire—played such a major and visible role in resolving international conflict. And while we do not ignore the debate about the U.S. role within the Council, few doubt the ground-breaking nature of the Council's actions during the crisis, actions that are likely to redefine U.N. peacekeeping.

But the United Nations' role in the Gulf war was by no means confined to peace and security issues. Since the very start of hostilities in August 1990—and to a far greater degree following the defeat of Iraq—nearly every organ of the vast U.N. system has been called upon to lend assistance in the region, whether for the enormous humanitarian relief effort (WHO, UNDP, UNICEF, UNDRO, UNHCR), the restabilization of the environment (UNEP), or the monitoring of Iraq's demilitarization (IAEA).

Nor has the Gulf been the only theater of turmoil. Old wars and new continue to plague the community of nations, and ethnic and factional conflicts are tearing at nations as disparate as El Salvador, Ethiopia, Indonesia, and India. Increasingly, U.N. member states are looking to the world body to take an active role in the resolution of ostensibly "internal" matters, expanding the United Nations' traditional mandate in ways that U.N. observers view with both hope and concern. Will the Organization be given the power and resources to undertake such challenges; will it successfully navigate the treacherous waters of national sovereignty; or will it be led to overreach itself and, in so doing, diminish its own credibility? Such questions will be answered in the years to come.

One area of unambiguous success for the United Nations has been the monitoring of national elections, most recently in Haiti. The presence of U.N. election and security observers during the winter of 1990–91 is largely credited with Haiti's first truly free election process and new democratic institutions—duplicating the successful transition to democracy by Nicaragua a year earlier. And in spring 1991 there is good reason to believe that the United Nations will not only supervise but conduct elections in Western Sahara later in the year as part of the long-term effort to end the war between Morocco and the Polisario independence movement. Even Cambodia—the thorniest of all sovereignty issues on the U.N. agenda—is showing signs of progress.

As one thumbs through this volume, one is likely to be struck by the extent to which the various sections overlap in terms of subject matter. Why, you might ask, do I find a discussion of population in the Environment section, of foreign debt in the Food and Agriculture section? And why does the Index listing for South Africa direct me to three different sections? The answer, of course, is that this volume is designed to reflect the work of the U.N. system in all its complexity—which is itself a reflection of the complex external world it is called upon to address.

As ever, there are many who are to be thanked for their contribution to this series. The list of talented and hard-working authors can be found in the preceding pages. There could be no *Issues/46* without their professional and personal dedication. To them, our deep thanks and respect.

In addition, we have called upon a number of men and women within the U.N. system to review the manuscripts prior to publication, and they have helped us wipe away many a sin of omission and commission. Their willingness to take on such a chore in addition to their many duties is testament to the remarkable dedication of the international civil service. Again, to each of them our thanks.

And a word of thanks, too, to our colleague Jennifer Metzger—UNA's Public Relations Coordinator—for her important assistance in the final preparation of this manuscript.

Finally, we take great pleasure in acknowledging the wonderful Communications Interns, volunteers all, who have worked hard to make this volume accurate, timely, and complete. Assisting authors, collecting documents, even drafting sections of the text—these young scholars and future diplomats were also essential to the creation of this volume. Our thanks to Thomas Hafen, Julie Jones, Toby Lanzer, Laurie Miller, Sharon Palmer, Jennifer Parkinson, Frank Patalong, Anne Rickert, and Steven Smith.

John Tessitore
Susan Woolfson

New York, 1991

I
Dispute Settlement and Decolonization

1. Making and Keeping the Peace

The conclusion of the Gulf war, which has been linked with the dawn of the "new world order" envisioned by Presidents Bush and Gorbachev, saw the stock of the United Nations reach its highest point in many years. The renaissance of the Organization had begun at the end of the Cold War as the superpowers displayed a new willingness to cooperate in the Security Council, and member states took a more practical approach to the economic and social issues on the U.N. agenda. Even before Saddam Hussein delivered a severe shock to the U.N. system by annexing Kuwait—the first time a member state had swallowed up another—the Organization was gradually reemerging as a stage on which world problems could be resolved.

The Security Council, after many arid years, has made significant progress in peacemaking and peacekeeping: the Geneva accords leading to withdrawal of the Soviet military from Afghanistan, the cease-fire ending eight years of fighting between Iran and Iraq, the establishment of Namibia as an independent state, the comprehensive plan for a settlement of the Cambodia conflict, the efforts to reach settlements throughout Central America, the progress on a referendum to decide the future of Western Sahara, and the monitoring of elections in Nicaragua and Haiti.

The Iraqi invasion of Kuwait gave the international community an opportunity to respond firmly and authoritatively to an out-and-out threat to international peace and security. The U.S.–led response—backed up in every case by the Council—was driven by at least three considerations: alarm at the prospect that the world's oil reserves, two-thirds of which are in the Gulf region, would come under Iraqi control; the need to demonstrate that aggression does not pay; and concern about the threat to Israel's security posed by the Iraqi military machine.

1

The Security Council was not at one on each of these issues, but it was concerned enough to adopt no fewer than 12 enforcement resolutions under Chapter VII of the U.N. Charter in the weeks between August 2 and November 27, 1990. The first of these, Resolution 660, was passed within hours of the invasion and was followed in short order by Resolution 661, which imposed the tightest sanctions regime in U.N. history—sanctions that were all the more effective because they were enforced by an ad hoc multinational military task force covering air, sea, and land routes to Iraq. These Council actions against Iraq culminated in Resolution 678, in which member states were given the right to use "all necessary means" to drive Iraq from Kuwait.

This was only the second time in U.N. history that military enforcement measures were approved—the Korean War in 1950 was the first—and it brought home the lesson that a new world order would be worthy of the name only if founded on the rule of law and on the principle of collective security. In the long years of superpower rivalry, the Security Council could operate merely as a sheriff's posse or fire brigade, usually arriving at the scene too late to control the situation. In the post–Gulf crisis period, the fundamental question facing the United Nations is whether member states are willing to underwrite a system based on consensus, collective action, and respect for international law. A revitalized United Nations will require financing, effort, and a commitment on the part of member states to operate multilaterally, as was demonstrated during the Gulf crisis, to defuse existing or prospective conflicts. A prominent example of a conflict at the root of regional instability is the Arab-Israeli dispute. Here, one of the parties—Israel—has said consistently that it would not welcome the Security Council's involvement.

If the new world order is to be anything more than self-serving rhetoric, it is evident that the United Nations will need new resources to establish and maintain an early-warning system about developing crises as well as the sort of political commitment that will allow the Organization to play a more prominent role in mediating conflicts, in ensuring respect for human rights, and, if need be, in dispatching aggressors or would-be aggressors by force of arms.

It is too much to say that the new world order is now locked in place. One is on surer ground in predicting that those who put much store in it will be disappointed when the Security Council turns a cold shoulder to conflict situations in which the aggression is less blatant than in the Gulf crisis. Future conflicts are as likely to be caused by environmental problems, creating special tensions and fueling mass cross-border migrations, as by old-fashioned forms of aggression. Despite growing awareness of the threat to peace and security posed by a loss of the world's natural resources, we are far from a time when that awareness will be transformed into action at the Council level. The floods that raced through Bangladesh, causing over 100,000 deaths, may be a harbinger of things to come. Certainly, they demonstrate the effects of dramatically increased population growth and increased pressure on cultivatable land—a deadly pincer movement that will one day spur mass migration. The cataclysmic floods also demonstrate the potential for conflict with neighboring countries, whose deforestation efforts at the upper reaches of the three great rivers originating in the Himalayas led to an increase in the already huge volume of water that thunders down into Bangladesh.

The State of the World Population 1991, a publication of the U.N. Population Fund, points out that projections of a "stable" world population of 10.2 billion by 2085—a population twice the size of today's—were too optimistic and that, unless fertility is reduced, the 10 billion figure may well be reached by 2050 and continue to climb for another century. The population boom, in company with environmental problems caused by ozone depletion and greenhouse gases, rain forest destruction, and industrial pollution—problems tending to cross many borders at once—contains the seeds of future conflicts that are certain to end up before the Council.

In the shorter term, the Security Council may find it difficult to respond resolutely to some of the more traditional threats to international security because big-power interests have not converged in such a way as to allow such response. This could well be the case with Cambodia, where a fitful cease-fire is in place, and the scope of the problem may prove greater than an underfunded U.N. system can handle. In the Arab-Israeli dispute, the United States has attempted to use the momentum generated by the Gulf crisis to bring both sides to the negotiating table, but it is doubtful that Washington would countenance enforcement action against Israel in any shape or form; more likely, the United States will continue to provide diplomatic cover at the Council for its close ally.

The quest for a reliable system to ensure international peace and security will be one of the main themes of the 46th General Assembly, and delegates are expected to stress what has now become obvious to many: that such security requires respect for multilateral institutions, the confidence that these institutions will be utilized, and the capacity to police and enforce the decisions of the Security Council and the rule of international law.

The use of military force by the Council to maintain international peace and security was foreseen by the founders of the United Nations nearly a half-century ago, but so far the member states have not been willing to provide a true U.N. army to aid in this effort. The General Assembly will focus on practical ways of copper-fastening the diplomatic breakthrough of the Gulf crisis, in which member states agreed to support collective action under the Charter's Chapter VII. Among the questions already being asked is whether the approach taken here is a viable model for implementing collective security in the future. In the messy aftermath of the war it became clear that although none of the 12 resolutions called for the overthrow of Saddam Hussein or the elimination of Iraq's weapons of mass destruction, these nonetheless became the goals of the coalition partners. In future operations, other member states may not be as willing to provide individual states with carte blanche to "take all necessary action" to reverse an aggression but may, instead, insist that military action come under the direct authority of the moribund U.N. Military Staff Committee.

The Committee was established 46 years ago to "advise and assist the Security Council on all questions relating to military requirements," but it never has been put to proper use and, despite an attempt by the Soviet Union to resurrect it, was given no particular role during the Gulf crisis. Pressure is certain to grow for a more soundly based U.N. military deterrent force. One proposal would give the Secretary-General the authority—not subject to the veto—to send an armed observer corps to any international border at any time [*Foreign Affairs*, Spring 1991]. Under Article 99 of the Charter, the Secretary-General "may bring to the attention of the Security Council any matter which in his opinion may threaten the maintenance of international peace and security."

2. The Middle East and the Persian Gulf

The Gulf Crisis

Iraq's invasion of Kuwait in August 1990 and the ensuing Gulf war of February–March 1991, involving nearly a million troops, thrust the Security Council—and the United Nations—into a dynamic role in which it showed energy and dispatch unequaled since the start of the Korean War more than 40 years earlier. In the wake of the Secretary-General's successful negotiation of the Iran-Iraq cease-fire in 1987 and the U.N.-led decolonization of Namibia in 1989, the authority, prestige, and sheer necessity of the United Nations as a forum for international conflict resolution have never been greater.

But the scale and speed of U.N. actions during the Gulf crisis demanded much more of the Organization than these other recent successes. In the four months following the invasion, the Security Council passed **12 resolutions condemning the invasion,** imposing a total trade boycott on Iraq, dealing with such ramifications as hostage-taking and aid to refugees, and finally authorizing "all necessary means" [S/Res/678] to reverse the invasion and restore the proper borders—i.e., a massive multinational military action, led by the 350,000-troop U.S. expeditionary force. After the quick and decisive (and astonishingly costly in terms of Iraqi lives and allied matériel) victory in March 1991, the Council passed three further resolutions, most notably Resolution 687, which set forth the terms of a full military settlement, with provisions for the cease-fire, the establishment of a demilitarized zone along the Iraq-Kuwait border to be patrolled by U.N. peacekeeping forces, and the eventual lifting of U.N. sanctions against Iraq. Resolution 687 demanded Iraq's recognition of the Iraq-Kuwait border prior to Iraq's invasion, as well as the principle of reparations resulting from Iraq's occupation of Kuwait and its conduct during the war. It also mandated the partial demilitarization of Iraq, including the destruction of Iraq's nuclear, chemical, and biological weapons capabilities.

Above and beyond the permanent restoration of borders and the normalization of relations between Iraq and Kuwait, and within the entire region, Resolution 687 imposes new and challenging responsibilities on the United Nations and the Secretary-General: most notably, the supervision and maintenance of Iraqi demilitarization. A second resolution, 686, directs the Secretary-General to examine the Kurdish problem and to supervise assistance to over a million Kurdish refugees fleeing the civil war that followed Iraq's defeat by the coalition forces. In April, allied troops were airlifted to an Iraqi enclave on the Turkish border to protect and assist these refugees and to facilitate their repatriation. In May, U.N. supervision of this zone began with the gradual replacement of allied troops with U.N. forces. The plight of the Kurds under Saddam Hussein, and after him, remains precarious; and the U.N. role, involving a controversial intrusion onto Iraqi sovereignty, is particularly problematic. This consequence of the Gulf war, like so many others, will command the attention of the United Nations for years to come.

On August 2, 1990, Iraqi President Saddam Hussein invaded Kuwait with over 100,000 troops, which he had massed along the border during the previous week. Wielding tremendous force against a completely unprepared and sporadic Kuwaiti defense, Iraq secured control of the small Gulf emirate within 48 hours. Initially Iraq announced that it would transfer power to a bogus Kuwaiti resistance front and then promised to withdraw its army from Kuwait if the invasion was not condemned. However, Iraqi troops quickly dug in and, on August 8, Saddam Hussein announced "the comprehensive and eternal merger" of Kuwait and Iraq, formally annexing the emirate as Iraq's "Province No. 19" [*The New York Times*, 8/9/90].

Launched less than two years after the end of the eight-year Iran-Iraq War, which had left Iraq victorious at the cost of 400,000 casualties and hundreds of billions of dollars, Hussein's invasion took the world by complete surprise and seemed to astonish almost all the heads of state most immediately concerned. In retrospect, it seems clear that, starting in the spring of 1990, Hussein had prepared his coup with a propaganda campaign carefully designed to strengthen his hand in the Arab arena, press his grievances against Kuwait, and simultaneously disguise his intention to invade.

Having achieved total surprise, Hussein expected his timid Arab neighbors, and the cynical and distant superpowers as well, to grudgingly accept the invasion as just another exercise in regional *realpolitik* too costly in blood and treasure to fight. He could then sell Kuwait's oil as his own and, equally important, intimidate the rest of the Arab Gulf oil-producing states, themselves vulnerable to invasion, into following his lead on oil policy. In effect, Hussein hoped to **dominate world oil markets,** and maximize his own oil sales, by commandeering the third of world oil production and the two-thirds of global strategic reserves collectively controlled by the Arab Gulf states.

What Hussein didn't count on was the universal condemnation his invasion provoked, and the Soviet Union's decision to join the consensus and permit the mobilization of the Security Council. Nor did he foresee U.S. President George Bush's determination to contain and ultimately reverse the invasion by force. Global condemnation and U.S. determination persuaded Iraq's non-Arab neighbors **Turkey and Iran** to support the alliance or at least to stay neutral, while key Arab countries, including Saudi Arabia, Egypt, and Syria, rallied to the alliance against Iraq. Throughout the Gulf crisis, Saddam Hussein stood virtually alone.

In April, four months before the invasion, Hussein had alarmed the West with an oblique but inflammatory threat to launch missiles against Israel: "By God, we will devour half of Israel in fire if it tries anything against Iraq," he announced in a long speech. In May, at an emergency Arab summit in Baghdad, Hussein seized control of the Arab agenda by stridently championing the Palestinian cause. Playing on growing Palestinian and Arab fears of Soviet Jewish immigration to Israel, and disillusionment with Yasser Arafat's failed rapprochement with the United States, Hussein called for the liberation of Jerusalem and held the United States accountable for "Israel's aggressive, expansionist, terrorist policies" [*Middle East International*, 6/8/90]. Behind closed doors, he reviled Kuwait's oil strategy and its cross-drilling of Iraqi border fields as "economic warfare" and demanded $27 billion from the emirate as an ad hoc settlement [Judith Miller and Laurie Mylroie, *Saddam Hussein and the Gulf Crisis* (New York: Times Books/Random House, 1990), p. 15].

In early July, Iraqi officials repeated these grievances openly, blasting Kuwait and its corrupt rulers as American puppets pursuing U.S.–inspired "theft tantamount to military aggression" against Iraq, and Hussein himself spoke of resorting to military action. In mid-July, the **Gulf Cooperation Council** (GCC, a regional security organization representing the six Arab emirates and kingdoms of the Persian Gulf: Kuwait, Saudi Arabia, Bahrain, Qatar, United Arab Emirates, and Oman) sent the Saudi foreign minister to Baghdad, but the next day Hussein sent 30,000 Iraqi troops to the Kuwaiti border. Several days and many Arab demarches later, Egyptian President Hosni Mubarak announced that he had arranged a face-to-face meeting between Saddam Hussein and Kuwait's Emir As–Sabah in Jeddah, but when this meeting finally took place on July 31, Iraq had moved another 70,000 troops to the border [*Middle East International*, 8/3/90]. Iraq retired from negotiations the next day, and 18 hours later the invasion began.

The reaction of the U.N. Security Council was swift and decisive. On the day of the invasion the Council unanimously passed Resolution 660 "condemn[ing] the invasion of Kuwait," "demand[ing] that Iraq withdraw immediately and unconditionally all its forces to [their] positions [of] August 1, 1990," and "call[ing] upon Iraq and Kuwait to begin immediately intensive negotiations." (The vote was 14–0; Yemen, the only Arab country of the Council's ten rotating members, abstained.) On August 6, acting under Article 51 of the U.N. Charter, the Council again voted unanimously (Cuba and Yemen abstained) to impose **mandatory sanctions on Iraq**—notably a full trade embargo barring all imports from and exports to Iraq, excepting only "supplies intended strictly for medical purposes, and in humanitarian circumstances, foodstuffs"—and to establish a special Committee of the Security Council to monitor these sanctions and report on their progress [S/Res/661]. On August 9, the Council unanimously (and without abstentions) "decide[d] that annexation of Kuwait by Iraq under any form and whatever pretext has no legal validity, and is considered null and void" [S/Res/662].

Washington's reaction was equally energetic and decisive. On August

3, the United States secured a joint U.S.–Soviet communiqué condemning the invasion and suspending Soviet arms shipments to Baghdad, signed by Soviet Foreign Minister Eduard Shevardnadze and U.S. Secretary of State James Baker in Siberia, where they were holding talks. On August 5, President Bush declared that Iraq's "brutal, naked aggression . . . will not stand" and dispatched Secretary of Defense Richard Cheney to the Gulf to confer with Saudi officials [The New York Times, 8/6/90]. On August 7 the U.S. Defense Department announced that King Fahd of Saudi Arabia had agreed to host a U.S. expeditionary force to defend the kingdom and that American troops were already landing on Saudi shores. (Initially estimated at up to 15,000, American forces in Saudi Arabia would grow to 150,000 by late September.) The Saudis also agreed to raise their oil production sharply to help meet the shortfall of lost Iraqi and Kuwaiti exports caused by the U.N.–mandated embargo. (At the end of the month the Organization of Petroleum Exporting Countries (OPEC) reached a decision in Vienna to increase oil output by 4 million barrels a day to ensure "adequate global energy supply" for the rest of the year [The New York Times, 8/30/90].) American officials further noted that Egypt agreed to send troops to Saudi Arabia and that the United States had also contacted Morocco and Pakistan for this purpose [The New York Times, 8/8/90, 8/9/90].

In New York, the U.S. delegation to the United Nations, brooking initial Soviet resistance, pushed for a new Security Council resolution approving the use of force to press trade sanctions on Iraq, a policy the U.S. Navy was pursuing publicly as of August 12 [The New York Times, 8/13/90]. On August 25, the Council unanimously passed (with Cuba and Yemen abstaining) Resolution 665, "call[ing] on Member States co-operating with the Government of Kuwait which are deploying maritime forces to the area to use such measures commensurate to the specific circumstances . . . to halt all inward and outward shipping . . . to ensure strict implementation of the provisions . . . laid down in Resolution 661." A major victory for Washington, Resolution 665 marked the first time in U.N. history that the Council had authorized military action without U.N. command and control to enforce its own sanctions [The Washington Post, 8/26/90]. On September 25, the Council closed the circle with Resolution 670, which mandated a full air transport blockade of Iraq. (The vote was 14–1, with Cuba voting against.)

By the end of August, the main lines of U.S. strategy were already clear: President Bush was determined to dispatch troops, including a huge land force and a naval armada, to enforce a trade embargo, to defend Saudi Arabia from further Iraqi aggression, and to press Iraq to withdraw from Kuwait. U.S. forces would provide both the bulk and the vanguard of a U.N.–sanctioned multinational force that would include European Community (EC) units, principally British, French, and Italian, and Arab-Islamic forces, eventually including those of the GCC countries, Morocco, Egypt, Syria, and Pakistan, which provided all-important protective regional coloration. (The dispatch of U.S. and later multilateral forces was rationalized under Article 51 of the U.N. Charter, which reads in part: "Nothing in the present Charter shall impair the inherent right of individual or collective self-defense if an armed attack occurs against a Member of the United Nations, until the Security Council has taken measures necessary to maintain international peace and security.")

Although the United States fully intended to lead this alliance, it sought multilateral advice and consent for its actions on two levels: at the U.N. Security Council, which it lobbied sedulously throughout the Gulf crisis, and within the region, by conferring with its principal Arab allies—Saudi Arabia, Egypt, and Syria—three states whose views and interests often differed. At the Security Council, the United States wielded the club of moral obloquy and global authority against Iraq; in the Middle East, it sought to ratify its actions with regional consensus and also to isolate Iraq completely. Isolation required Washington to court and confer with both its North Atlantic Treaty Organization (NATO) ally Turkey and its erstwhile enemy Iran.

President Bush's determination to defend U.S. interests against aggression through forceful leadership tempered by multilateralism contrasted sharply with the fitful unilateralism of his predecessor Ronald Reagan, who often gave the United Nations short shrift. George Bush's consistent and dynamic recourse to the Security Council, together with the Soviet cooperation that made it possible, have cast the Council and the United Nations into a new and powerful prominence, a development that must be counted among the more significant aspects of what President Bush calls a new world order.

Facing nearly universal condemnation and the decisive dispatch of U.S. and Egyptian troops, Saddam Hussein was not without weapons— or surprises. Days after the invasion, Hussein offered to retreat from Kuwait if Israel would also withdraw from the territories it has occupied since the Six-Day War of June 1967. This ploy seemed a gross non sequitur to most Westerners, but it touched a raw nerve among Arabs, especially the Palestinians and their champions, revolted by the cynical double standard that allowed the great powers to condemn and punish

Iraq's occupation of Kuwait in a matter of days while refusing to reverse Israel's occupation of Arab lands in the course of decades.

Hussein's "linkage" intended not so much to justify his own actions before the world as to rally Arab populations against the West and those Arab governments "in their pay." Donning the mantle of Saladin, Hussein posed as an Arab hero leading them against the West and the poor against the rich (the "corrupt" Kuwaiti emirs). In this way, he succeeded in dividing the Arab peoples and states. All notions of Arab unity dissolved as the GCC states together with Egypt, Syria, and Morocco confronted Jordan, the Palestine Liberation Organization (PLO), Sudan, and most of the states of Arab North Africa. (The latter group condemned the invasion, but opposed the "foreign" military presence in the Gulf and supported an elusive "Arab solution" to the problem.) While the emergency Arab Summit of August 4 condemned the invasion, it ended in embittered chaos, which defeated all further attempts to achieve an Arab consensus or even meet to discuss one. The Arab League collapsed under the strain, its top officials resigning in the following weeks. Those Arab governments that sided with the United States and sent troops to the Gulf—especially Syria and to a lesser extent Egypt—found their own populations growing increasingly restive. In the months that followed, demonstrations from Jordan to Morocco rocked the Arab world, with a reported 200,000 demonstrating in distant Casablanca.

Next, on August 15, Saddam Hussein publicly accepted Iran's conditions for a peace treaty by renouncing Iraqi claims to full sovereignty over the Shatt-al-Arab waterway dividing Iran and Iraq. One of Baghdad's primary goals during its eight-year, one-million-casualty war with Iran, Iraqi claims to full sovereignty over the Shatt had also been the primary obstacle to a peace treaty in the two years following the August 1988 cease-fire. This astonishing demarche freed Iraqi troops from duty on the Iranian border; it also prompted speculation that Iran might break the embargo or, worse, that Hussein might woo Tehran's radicals into an anti-American alliance [*The Economist*, 8/18/90].

Hussein's next move was less astonishing. On August 18 the Speaker of the Iraqi Parliament announced that the nearly 10,000 Western nationals trapped in Iraq and Kuwait, including nearly 4,000 British citizens and 3,100 Americans, would be detained as "guests of the Iraqi people" as long as Iraq remained under the threat of aggression. Two days later Iraqi officials confirmed rumors that these "guests" would be housed at military facilities as "human shields" [*The New York Times*, 8/19/90, 8/21/90]. Portending a reprise of the Iranian hostage crisis, this time en masse,

Hussein's new tack produced outrage in Western capitals and across the world. It was condemned forthwith, on August 18, by the Security Council, which unanimously "demand[ed] that Iraq permit and facilitate the immediate departure from Kuwait and Iraq of the nationals of third countries" and "that Iraq take no action to jeopardize the safety, security and health of such nationals" [S/Res/664]. During the next three months a succession of peace missions to Baghdad by elder statesmen, primarily from EC countries, resulted in the piecemeal release of small groups of hostages. Increasingly aware that this process of detention was more inflammatory than productive, Hussein released all Western hostages in December.

In September and October, the United States pursued its strategy of coalition-building to isolate Iraq. On September 9, U.S. and Soviet Presidents Bush and Gorbachev issued a joint statement on the Gulf crisis, repeating their determination to fully implement the relevant Security Council resolutions. The text allowed that should these measures fail to produce results, "additional ones consistent with the U.N. Charter" might be required [*The New York Times*, 9/10/90]. On September 13, U.S. Secretary of State James Baker visited **Syria**—a state Washington had long accused of harboring and dispatching terrorists, particularly in connection with the downing of Pan Am Flight 103 over Lockerbie, Scotland, in December 1989—to confer with Syrian President Hafez el-Assad. President Assad had already sent 2,000 troops to join the growing multinational force in Saudi Arabia and had rejected Iraq's linkage of the Gulf and Arab-Israeli questions, despite Syria's long-standing grievances against Israel. Assad was concerned about U.S. talk of a post-crisis "security structure" in the Gulf, and Baker told reporters that America had "no intention or desire to keep a permanent ground presence in the Gulf" [*The Christian Science Monitor*, 9/13/90]. At the end of the month, Assad again proved his usefulness to Washington by visiting Iran for the first time in 11 years. Syria, Iran's only Arab ally during its war with Iraq, sought to allay Iranian suspicions of U.S. activities in the Gulf and to ensure Iranian compliance with U.S. sanctions against Iraq. "We have common positions [in all contingencies of the Gulf crisis]," Iranian President Hashemi Rafsanjani told reporters after four days of talks. He and President Assad declared themselves "in full agreement" in their opposition to Iraq's invasion [*The New York Times*, 9/26/90].

On November 2, President Bush ordered a further, more massive mobilization of U.S. troops to be sent to the Gulf. Announcing his intention to station up to 400,000 soldiers in Saudi Arabia, the President acknowledged that this further mobilization—which involved calling up reserve troops and suspending troop rotation in the Gulf—constituted a switch from a strictly defensive posture to an offensive one. The President said he could not be certain that U.N. sanctions were working and that, given constraints of time, offensive action, or at least the threat of it, was needed to get Iraq out of Kuwait. Within four days the Saudis publicly approved the new mobilization and Syria announced plans to send more troops of its own [*The New York Times,* 11/2/90, 11/7/90]. The President's announcement took the American public by surprise and sparked intense debate in the press and Congress over the merits of sanctions versus those of war. Lawmakers assailed the President's "rush to war" and asked why he refused to give sanctions the time necessary to work [ibid., 11/10/90].

Once again, President Bush eagerly sought the approval of the Security Council for his new initiative. The notion of mandating the use of military force against Iraq had been under discussion at the Council for several months. As early as September 25, Soviet Foreign Minister Shevardnadze had told the U.N. General Assembly that "the United Nations has the power to suppress acts of aggression. There is ample evidence that this right can be exercised. It will be, if the illegal occupation of Kuwait continues" [*The Christian Science Monitor,* 9/27/90]. However, in October and November, as the United States lobbied the Security Council for specific language authorizing force, they found the Chinese and the Soviets, together with "the Gang of Four" (rotating Council members Colombia, Cuba, Malaysia, and Yemen), resisting the idea of a hasty and intemperate resort to war before the weapons of peace, i.e., U.N. sanctions against Iraq, were exhausted [*The Christian Science Monitor,* 11/16/90, 11/20/90, 11/29/90]. At home, U.S. senators from both parties called on the President to convene a special session on the Gulf crisis [*The New York Times,* 11/14/90].

Throughout the debate, the Security Council continued to pass new resolutions on the crisis. Resolution 666 of September 13 directed the special Security Council Committee established by Resolution 661 to monitor humanitarian needs inside Iraq and Kuwait and to report to the Council. Cuba and Yemen voted against the resolution, which granted the Council sole authority to approve humanitarian assistance in light of its own embargo on Iraqi trade [ibid., 9/14/90]. Resolution 667 of September 16 condemned "aggressive acts perpetrated by Iraq against diplomatic premises and personnel in Kuwait, including the abduction of foreign nationals" and demanded the release of those nationals. Resolution 669 of September 24 directed the Committee to study the needs of states suffering hardships as a result of Resolution 661's implementation and to report to the Council. Resolution 674 of October 29 demanded "that

Iraqi authorities and occupying forces immediately cease and desist from taking third-State nationals hostage and oppressing Kuwaiti and third-State nationals." Finally, Resolution 677 of November 28 "condemn[ed] the attempts by Iraq to alter the demographic composition of the population of Kuwait and to destroy the civil records maintained by the legitimate Government of Kuwait."

On November 29, after three weeks of close debate, the Security Council voted 12–2–1 (Cuba and Yemen voted against, China abstained) to pass **Resolution 678** "authoriz[ing] Member States co-operating with the Government of Kuwait, unless Iraq on or before January 15, 1991, fully implements . . . the foregoing resolutions, to use *all necessary means* [emphasis added] to implement Security Council Resolution 660 and all subsequent relevant resolutions to restore international peace and security in the area." All parties read this language to mean recourse to military force, marking only the second time—the Korean War was the first—that the Council had invoked its power to sanction such force to counter armed aggression. In the closing speeches before the Council, U.S. Secretary of State Baker said, "If Iraq does not reverse course peacefully, then . . . the use of force should be authorized. We must put the choice to Saddam Hussein in unmistakable terms." Soviet Foreign Minister Shevardnadze declared that those "who break the peace must know all available means will be used against them" [ibid., 11/30/90].

On January 12, after an emotional debate, the U.S. Senate voted 52–47 to support President Bush's policy in the Gulf, thus freeing him to liberate Kuwait by force should the Iraqis fail to evacuate the emirate by the January 15 Security Council deadline. As expected, the deadline stimulated a series of 11th-hour peace initiatives to forestall what Saddam Hussein had long been touting as "the mother of all battles." On December 1, two days after the passage of Resolution 678, President Bush had announced that he would send Secretary of State Baker to meet Saddam Hussein in Baghdad and would receive Iraqi Foreign Minister Tarik Aziz personally. This initiative faltered when the Iraqis proposed January 12 as the date for the Baghdad meeting, and the United States denounced this move as a transparent play for time and a show of bad faith. Secretary Baker did meet his counterpart in Geneva on January 9, but there was no meeting of the minds, and Baker later commented that Aziz had shocked him by refusing even to mention the word "Kuwait." A "last chance" mission to Baghdad by Secretary-General Pérez de Cuéllar, who met with Hussein on January 14, also went nowhere, and a French plan involving Iraqi withdrawal in tandem with the convening of an international peace conference to resolve all regional issues, including the Arab-Israeli conflict, was scrapped on January 15. With American officials estimating a total of 680,000 allied troops, including 410,000 Americans, facing 545,000 Iraqi soldiers dug into Kuwait and southern Iraq, the President was anxious to proceed [ibid., 1/16/91].

Hostilities began on January 16 as the allies initiated a nearly six-week-long aerial bombardment of Kuwait and Iraq, executed primarily by U.S. sea- and land-based warplanes and missiles. This bombardment, pursued relentlessly and with an intensity unprecedented in military history, sought to prepare a massive land attack on Kuwait by destroying Baghdad's unconventional (nuclear, chemical, and biological) weapons capability as well as its command-and-control structure, reducing Iraq's extensive tank and artillery forces, and destroying the morale of the hundreds of thousands of Iraqi troops dug into fortifications in Kuwait. Touting the revolutionary precision of "SMART bombs" and other new-generation guided missiles and aerial ordnance, U.S. military authorities insisted they were systematically avoiding civilian casualties while pursuing their legitimate war aims. Nevertheless, civilian casualties in Baghdad, and elsewhere in Iraq, mounted. The bombing of a Baghdad air raid shelter, which the U.S. military insisted was a command-and-control center, killed over 300 civilians on February 15, while the bombing of a bridge at Falluja killed another 50 in a nearby market [*Middle East International*, 2/22/91].

Baghdad responded by launching modified Soviet-made Scud missiles, 12 at Israel and one at Saudi Arabia, causing only minor damage and 30 injuries, in the first three days of hostilities. Most Iraqi Scud attacks against Israel fell wide of populated areas or were downed by U.S.–supplied Patriot antimissile batteries, but one Scud hit an apartment building in Tel Aviv on January 23, killing 3 and wounding 70 [*The New York Times*, 1/20/91, 1/24/91]. Despite Israeli fears that the Scuds might carry chemical or biological weapons, such threats never materialized. These attacks, continuing sporadically throughout the war, were primarily political in intent: Hussein hoped to provoke Israeli retaliation, which might have discredited the Arab governments allied with the United States against him. However, at the urging of the United States, Israel did not respond. Iraqi Scud attacks on Saudi Arabia were also largely ineffective, with the exception of a single hit upon a Marine barracks, resulting in 28 killed and 97 wounded.

On February 15, after four weeks of devastating bombardment, Iraq's Revolutionary Command Council issued a vague statement allowing for the possibility of an Iraqi withdrawal from Kuwait. A week later, Moscow tabled a peace plan, endorsed by Soviet President Gorbachev and Iraqi Foreign Minister Aziz, providing for a phased Iraqi withdrawal from Kuwait two days after a cease-fire. After two-thirds of Iraqi troops had withdrawn from Kuwait, the United Nations would lift its trade embargo on Iraq and then, following the withdrawal of the remaining third, suspend all other Security Council resolutions. Poised for an all-out land offensive and piqued by Moscow's last-minute meddling, Washington rejected the initiative after two days of feelers [ibid., 2/22–24/91].

The land war began in earnest on February 25. In 12 days, allied forces decisively defeated Iraq's army of occupation, decimating it in the field and pushing surviving units back into Iraq. While allied infantry, including large Arab contingents, stormed and quickly overran Iraqi fortifications along the Kuwaiti border, a huge armored force composed of U.S., British, and French units flanked Iraqi positions to the west, cutting off the emirate from the rear, engaging and decimating elite Iraqi armored reserve forces, and driving deep into Iraq to sever Iraqi supply lines along the Euphrates River. Contrary to expectations, the frontal assault encountered little resistance and the Iraqi infantry quickly retreated, while a major tank battle developed between allied and Iraqi columns along the Kuwait-Iraq border. Refusing to pursue surviving Iraqi armor across the border, President Bush ordered a halt to hostilities and declared a provisional cease-fire on March 2, leaving allied armies in control of a large swath of Iraqi territory south of the Euphrates. Allied casualties were astonishingly low. The United States lost 309 lives, with 230 of them resulting from pre-combat incidents; wounded totaled some 213 [Center for Defense Information]. In contrast, Iraqi casualties were appallingly high. The U.S. Defense Department has estimated "tentatively" that in the 43 days of the war, 100,000 Iraqi soldiers died and 300,000 were wounded [*The New York Times*, 6/5/91], taking a higher toll on Iraqi soldiers than did the eight-year Iran-Iraq war. Experts have further estimated that between 5,000 and 15,000 civilians died during the air war and that up to 86,000 more have died since the cease-fire, due to disease, malnutrition, and civil war [ibid., 6/22/91].

Most observers assumed that a defeat of this magnitude would quickly—and finally—end the tumultuous career of Saddam Hussein. Instead, the Iraqi President rode out the storm, surviving the cease-fire and rallying his battered tank legions to ruthlessly repress two rebellions that threatened both his rule and the survival of Iraq as a single nation-state. Within a week of the cease-fire, **Iraqi Shiites,** the majority sect living in southern Iraq, had launched a spontaneous and poorly armed rebellion against Hussein, while in the hills and mountains of northeast Iraq, **Iraqi Kurds,** a minority with a long and tragic history of armed struggle against Baghdad, mounted a more disciplined revolt. Aware of the limits of the U.N. mandate and anxious to preserve the territorial integrity of Iraq, Washington and its Arab allies refused to intervene. By the end of March, the Iraqi army had dealt harshly with the Shiite threat in the south; Hussein's repression of the Kurds lasted into April and produced the flight of nearly a million Kurdish refugees into neighboring Turkey and Iran.

On March 2 the Security Council passed Resolution 686 which, inter alia, reaffirmed all previous resolutions pertaining to the Iraqi invasion and demanded that Iraq accept the principle of reparations, immediately release the thousands of Kuwaiti and third-country nationals held by Baghdad, and arrange for the immediate release of prisoners of war. A month later, on April 3, the Council set forth its unconditional terms for an official cease-fire in Resolution 687, which demands that "Iraq shall unconditionally accept the destruction, removal or rendering harmless of . . . all chemical and biological weapons and stocks of agents and all ballistic missiles with a range greater than 150 kilometers . . . ," "Iraq shall submit to the Secretary General within 15 days . . . a declaration of locations, amounts. and types" of these materials, "Iraq shall unconditionally undertake not to use, develop, construct or acquire" such materials, "Iraq . . . is liable under international law for any direct loss, damage, including environmental damage and the depletion of natural resources, or injury to foreign Governments, nationals and corporations, as a result of Iraq's unlawful invasion and occupation of Kuwait." Resolution 687 further declared that the full trade embargo against Iraq, mandated by Resolution 661, is still in place, pending review of the above provisions and Iraqi cooperation every 60 days.

Resolution 687 also established a 200-kilometer-long demilitarized zone along the Iraq-Kuwait border, extending 10 kilometers into Iraq and 5 kilometers into Kuwait, to be patrolled by the **U.N. Iraq-Kuwait Observer Mission (UNIKOM)**—up to 1,400 U.N. troops from 36 countries, at an estimated cost of $83 million for the first six months. On May 9 the Secretary-General announced that UNIKOM had completed its deployment along the border [The InterDependent 17, no. 3, 1991].

Resolution 687 tasks the Secretary-General with (1) the submission, within 45 days, of a Special Commission plan to carry out the on-site inspection and demilitarization of Iraq specified above, to be implemented within another 45 days, in cooperation with the relevant U.N. agencies, (2) the approval of a plan for the immediate dispatch of a U.N. peacekeeping force along the demilitarized zone between Iraq and Kuwait, and (3) the development within 30 days of recommendations for a fund for the payment of claims relating to Iraqi debts incurred before the crisis and reparations incurred during it. In addition to the stringent demands this "mother of all resolutions" places on Iraq, the related tasks it places before the Secretary-General are the most complex and demanding in the history of the Organization. Many experts feel the demands placed on the Secretary-General, and the relevant U.N. agencies, are unrealistic, especially with respect to their timetables.

Security Council Resolution 688, passed on April 5, "condemn[ed] the repression of the Iraqi civilian population . . . most recently in Kurdish populated areas," and "demand[ed] that Iraq . . . immediately end this repression and express[ed] the hope that an open dialogue will take place to ensure that the human and political rights of all Iraqi citizens are respected." Further burdening the Secretary-General, it asks him to pursue humanitarian efforts "with all the resources at his disposal" and "to address urgently the critical needs of the refugees."

On April 6, following a vote of the Iraqi Parliament, Iraq accepted the "unjust" terms mandated by 687, making the truce official. Two days later, the United States announced that 100,000 troops were starting to evacuate the region, with the remaining 330,000 U.S. forces scheduled to leave during the summer. On April 7, U.S. forces began to airlift nonmilitary supplies to the Kurds in northern Iraq. In the wake of the Iraqi civil war, there were more than 500,000 Kurdish refugees in Turkey and some 1.4 million in Iran [ibid.]. On April 20, 500 U.S. Marines entered the Iraqi border town of Zakhlo from Turkey, the vanguard of an allied emergency force assigned to build refugee camps to assist the protection and repatriation of Kurdish refugees. Baghdad quickly protested the allies' decision to occupy a buffer zone along the Turkish border for this purpose. The allied relief effort, undertaken in consultation with the U.N. High Commissioner for Refugees (UNHCR), was commandeered in May by U.N. forces, who replaced their allied counterparts. On April 24, Kurdish leaders and Saddam Hussein signed an agreement guaranteeing democratic rule and limited autonomy for Iraqi Kurdistan along with the right of peaceful return of all Iraqi Kurdish refugees [*The New York Times*, 4/25/91].

The Arab-Israeli Conflict and the Occupied Territories

Forty-three years after the establishment of the state of Israel, the Arab-Israeli conflict persists. During the 1980s various U.S. peace plans and inter-Arab initiatives failed to bridge the enormous differences separating Israel and the PLO, two parties that had long refused to recognize or even address each other. In December 1987 this diplomatic stalemate was shaken by a massive and **sustained Palestinian uprising,** or *intifadah,* in the Occupied Territories, forcing Israelis to confront Palestinian demands for self-determination and pushing the Palestine National Council (PNC)—the PLO's parliament in exile—to recognize Israel formally. Since then, however, Israel's government has declined to reciprocate or even devise a unified negotiating posture capable of advancing the long moribund "peace process."

In late May 1990, responding to a resurgence of violence in the Occupied Territories following the shooting of seven Palestinians by a purported mentally unstable Israeli, Yasser Arafat asked to address an emergency session of the U.N. Security Council. In order to avoid the possibility that the PLO leader might be denied a U.S. visa, the Council moved its deliberations to Geneva. There the United States vetoed the dispatch of a U.N. mission to the West Bank to monitor the treatment of Palestinians by Israeli security forces [*The New York Times,* 6/1/90]. At the same time, Arab states and the PLO began to stridently protest increasing immigration by Soviet Jews to Israel, where they might be settled in the Occupied Territories. Soviet President Gorbachev warned that he would curtail this exodus (facilitated by a recent change in U.S. immigration law that sharply curtailed quotas for the direct immigration of Soviet Jews to the United States) if Israel did not pledge to bar the newcomers from the territories. The United States also opposed such settlement. In June, Israeli Housing Minister Ariel Sharon announced that Israel would not move Soviet Jews to the West Bank and Gaza, but this announcement begged the question of whether he would allow immigrants to settle there of their own free will [ibid., 6/25/90]. Also in June, the United States suspended its dialogue with the PLO, citing the organization's failure to properly condemn an abortive amphibious raid on Israel by a radical PLO faction and to censure its leader, Abul Abbas [ibid., 6/21/90].

Secretary Baker's unsuccessful attempt to revive the Arab-Israeli peace process in early 1990 was eclipsed by Iraq's invasion of Kuwait on August 2. While Iraqi President Saddam Hussein quickly offered to withdraw from Kuwait if the Israelis withdrew from the Occupied Territories, his linkage of the Gulf crisis and the Arab-Israeli conflict was rejected out of hand by Washington and its Arab allies, whose attention remained firmly fixed on the Gulf throughout the fall and winter of 1990.

With the decisive victory of U.S.–led allied armies over Iraq in March 1991, U.S. diplomats returned to the Arab-Israeli conflict with new hopes. They saw the Gulf war as the kind of sea change, like the October War of 1973, that might recast the dynamics of the Arab-Israeli conflict and its moribund "peace process." With U.S. military power and diplomatic prestige cresting in the region, President Bush and Secretary Baker spoke of "a window of opportunity," a limited period of time following the Gulf war during which they might impose themselves on the "peace process" and prevail. A new round of Arab-Israeli diplomacy under U.S. auspices was therefore in the offing.

The war had changed much in the region, but not necessarily for the better where the Arab-Israeli conflict was concerned. The Riyadh-Cairo-Damascus axis, the heart of the anti-Iraq regional alliance that the United States had successfully promoted, held some hope that Saudi Arabia, Egypt, and Syria might cooperate on negotiations with Israel. Further, the prestige of the PLO, which had taken Hussein's linkage to heart and supported him during the crisis, was at an all-time low, making the organization perhaps more amenable to persuasion. However, the war had also divided the Arab world and left much bitterness in its wake, especially between the Gulf Arabs and the Palestinians, who found themselves isolated within the Arab camp as a whole. Saudi Arabia cut its financial support to the PLO, rechanneling it to the more radical Islamic group Hamas; several Gulf countries expelled Palestinian residents; and the liberation of Kuwait led to reprisals by "resistance" vigilantes that left at least 30 Palestinians dead and many more tortured and detained, according to the human rights group Middle East Watch [ibid., 4/10/91]. The Israelis, who had seen the Arabs' largest army decimated in the war and watched Palestinians cheer Iraqi Scud missile attacks on Tel Aviv, seemed less amenable than ever to making concessions on the Palestine question.

From August 1990 through April 1991, the Gulf crisis naturally preoccupied the Security Council, although the Council did pass several resolutions—with U.S. support—critical of Israel during this time. On October 8, Israeli security forces killed 21 Palestinians and wounded up to 150 others during a riot on the Temple Mount in Jerusalem [*Middle East International,* 8/21/90]. Resolution 672 of October 12 "condemn[ed] especially the acts of violence committed by Israeli security forces resulting in injuries and loss of human life" and asked the Secretary-General to send a mission to investigate the killings at the Temple Mount. Resolution 673 of October 24 "deplore[d] the refusal of the Israeli government to receive the mission." Resolution 681 of December 20 "call[ed] upon the high contracting parties of the Fourth Geneva Convention, of 1949, to ensure respect by Israel, the occupying Power, for its obligations under the Convention, under Article 1 thereof," and "deplore[d] the decision by . . . Israel . . . to resume the deportation of Palestinian civilians in the occupied territories." These votes came at a time when the United States was eager to placate its Arab allies; nevertheless, the content of these resolutions differed little from those passed in 1987 and 1988, and they used language far less severe than that of Resolution 465 of 1980. Indeed, Resolution 681 was passed after two months of debate during which the United States refused to endorse an international conference on the Middle East in the framework of the resolution [ibid., 1/11/91].

Starting in late March and ending in May 1991, Secretary of State Baker made four trips to the Middle East, directed primarily at jump-starting a new round of Arab-Israeli diplomacy. He found that many of the obstacles and differences that had defeated his predecessors remained. Canvassing the various parties for "confidence-building measures," he found the Israelis willing to release more than 1,000 of the over 10,000 Palestinians detained as a result of the *intifadah;* but on the day of his second visit, Tel Aviv insisted on establishing two more settlements on the West Bank, the first since the new Shamir government had been formed in the spring of 1990 [*The New York Times,* 4/9/91, 4/26/91]. On his third trip Secretary Baker secured Soviet sponsorship for a regional conference to be launched under U.S.–Soviet auspices [ibid., 4/26/91].

At the end of his fourth visit to the region, Baker was able to report some results, though minor. "I'm not disappointed, because I do think we are making progress. There are many, many more areas of agreement with respect to this process on the part of Israel, and indeed on the part of many Arab governments, than there are areas of disagreement," he remarked. As he left Tel Aviv on May 16, Baker could point to at least one achievement. The previous year's negotiations had collapsed over the question of how Palestinian representatives would be chosen, with Israel insisting that an Arab resident of East Jerusalem could not represent the Palestinians. This time, Baker and Israeli Prime Minister Shamir agreed that a former resident of Jerusalem might be acceptable to Israel. Upon hearing this, Faisal Husseini, the leading PLO representative on the West Bank, commented that "the formation of the Palestinian delegation is solely the concern of the Palestinian people" [ibid., 5/17/91].

The Secretary was unable to bridge important gaps between Arab governments and Israel regarding the convening of a regional conference. Harking back to the old "international conference" formula, Syria insisted that the United Nations or the Security Council play an "important" role in any conference as an ongoing presence to which negotiations could be referred at difficult points. Israel refused any U.N. role at all; it was comfortable with U.S.–Soviet sponsorship and might accept the involvement of other powers, but only as a cover to convene the conference before it split into a series of bilateral negotiations over which the "sponsors" could exert no influence. Sticking to traditional, deeply felt positions, Jordan and Syria said they would enter into negotiations only if Israel recognized the principle of land for peace, but the Shamir government remained adamantly opposed to this notion [ibid., 4/13/91]. The linkage between the Gulf crisis and the Arab-Israeli conflict, first bruited by Saddam Hussein in August 1990 and given quite a different reading by President Bush and Secretary Baker in March 1991, again seemed entirely beside the point.

More than 13 years of rebellion in the Occupied Territories, together with the PNC declarations in Algiers, have very much changed the terms of the Palestine question, but these developments have brought the parties no closer to peace. In Israel, the *intifadah* has shattered the complacent illusion that peaceful coexistence between Arabs and Israelis under the present occupation is still possible. The uprising has vindicated many moderates, both Israeli and Palestinian, who have long felt that peace must be made before Israel's annexation of the Occupied Territories becomes irreversible. As of 1986, Israel controlled, directly or indirectly, 50 percent of the West Bank, where more than 140,000 Israelis lived in some 110 settlements, and East Jerusalem [ibid., 1/26/86]. Israel has also confiscated a third of the Gaza Strip, which Israeli demographer Meron Benvenisti has called the "Soweto of the state of Israel." Benvenisti's figures suggest that the Gaza Strip is now as crowded as Hong Kong and will grow in population to 900,000 by 1999 [*The Jerusalem Post*, 6/7/86].

The uprising has accelerated the grim logic of Israeli occupation and settlement of the territories, whereby the Jewish state must eventually evacuate them or expel their Arab population. Both scenarios, endorsed by marginal Israeli factions, represent extreme choices that the Jewish state has so far refused to contemplate. The *intifadah* has not arrested the rightward movement of Israeli politics; indeed, it would be easy to argue that it has assisted this trend. The current Shamir government, the most militant in Israeli history, appears confident of its ability and its mandate to contain the *intifadah* by force.

The 45th Session of the General Assembly passed a number of resolutions condemning Israel's occupation of the West Bank and the Gaza Strip. The Assembly's resolution on "The Situation in the Middle East" [A/Res/45/54] repeated the body's conviction that "the question of Palestine is at the core of the conflict" and that a just solution to the Arab-Israeli conflict must include the PLO. The resolution demanded "the total and unconditional withdrawal by Israel from all the Palestinian and other Arab lands occupied since 1967, including Jerusalem." It also reaffirmed its call to convene an international peace conference under the auspices of the United Nations. Following Yasser Arafat's address to the General Assembly in Geneva, the Assembly acknowledged the proclamation of the state of Palestine and changed the name of the PLO's U.N. Observer Mission to the Palestine Observer Mission [43/177]. Forty-four countries voted against the resolution, including Israel, the United States, and the entire NATO bloc.

The 46th Session of the General Assembly will again address these issues and will very likely adopt more resolutions condemning Israel for unlawful occupation of Arab lands.

Lebanon

Persistent sectarian strife and public disorder have kept Lebanon in a state of virtual anarchy since the outbreak of the Lebanese civil war in 1975. In the past year, however, the government of Lebanese President Elias Hrawi, assisted by the Syrian army and Arab mediation efforts, has made unprecedented progress in extending the central government's rule and restoring order to Lebanon. Hrawi's success remains preliminary and tenuous, and further momentum toward the reintegration of Lebanon will depend on the wishes of outside powers, principally Syria and Israel, and most of all on the will of the country's many fractious militias to sacrifice their hard-won positions of influence for an elusive greater good.

The power vacuum created by the civil war led to the occupation of large parts of the country by Syria, which invaded in 1976 at the behest of beleaguered Christian forces. Syrian occupation saved the Christians from defeat and ruin, but only dampened the ferocity of intra-Lebanese strife. The situation was further complicated by Israel's invasion of Lebanon in 1982. Israel's 1985 withdrawal from southern Lebanon to a six-mile-wide "security zone" north of the Israeli border raised new hopes that Lebanese internal disputes might be peacefully resolved. However, without a functioning central government or a national consensus on how to restore one, Lebanon's many private armies continued their bloody turf battles.

Since the start of the civil war, Lebanon has faced the growing threat that the country might be partitioned into two (or more) ministates, Christian and Muslim. The process of partition was further advanced in September 1988, when the election of a new Lebanese president was deadlocked, splitting the country into two rival regimes: a Christian government under General Michel Aoun, who had been appointed acting president by outgoing President Amin Gemayel, and a Muslim government under former Prime Minister Selim al-Hoss. In March 1989, "President" Aoun launched a new round of civil war by blockading Muslim ports outside Beirut and declaring his intention to chase Syria's 40,000 troops from Lebanon. Artillery duels and several pitched battles between Aoun's Christian forces and his Syrian foes killed 835 and wounded some 4,000 people before an Arab League–sponsored truce took hold in September 1989. Meanwhile, as many as 500,000 residents had fled predominantly Muslim West Beirut, and 175,000 had left East Beirut [*The New York Times*, 9/22/89; *The Christian Science Monitor*, 9/11/89].

In May 1989 the Arab League met in Casablanca and created the **Arab Tripartite Commission,** composed of Saudi King Fahd, Algerian President Chadli Benjedid, and Moroccan King Hassan II, to mediate the crisis. After numerous shuttles between Arab capitals, the foreign ministers of Saudi Arabia, Algeria, and Morocco announced that they had reached a dead end. In a report prepared for the Arab League, the Tripartite Commission later blamed its failure on Syria, which had refused to pull its troops out of Beirut and the northern coast of Lebanon and redeploy them in the Bekaa Valley in return for Arab and international guarantees to embargo arms deliveries to the warring Lebanese militias [*The New York Times*, 8/2/89, 9/1/89].

A second effort at mediation was more successful. In late September the Tripartite Commission invited the 73 surviving members of Lebanon's parliament, last elected in 1972, to Taif, Saudi Arabia. Sixty-three attended, and 59 approved a new peace plan, which combined a phased redeployment of Syrian troops over two years with reform of the Lebanese National Charter. A new constitution would divide power more evenly between Christians and Muslims, reducing the prerogatives of the Christian presidency and reallocating seats in parliament from the previous 54–45 Christian-Muslim split to an even 54–54. Syria quickly approved the **Taif Agreement,** but Aoun and several Muslim groups rejected it.

In November, 52 Lebanese M.P.s met in northern Lebanon to ratify the new Tripartite peace plan and to elect Ren Moawad as the new President of Lebanon. After just 17 days in office, Moawad was assassinated by a car bomb and replaced by Elias Hrawi, another pro-Syrian politician.

The Taif Agreement and the new constitution it had created remained stillborn without the approval of the captious General Aoun. The new national charter hammered out at Taif had gained the support of many Christian leaders, including Samir Geagea, commander of the

Lebanese Forces (LF) militia. Eager to unify Christian ranks, Aoun's 15,000 troops attacked the 10,000-man LF in January 1990. By April, the intra-Christian fighting had killed over 900, wounded some 3,000, and driven some 300,000 Lebanese Christians abroad [ibid., 4/9/90]. Aoun's *coup de main* ultimately failed. In the end he lost valuable territory, including the port of Beirut and its revenues, to Geagea, and he forfeited considerable power and prestige as well. In October 1990, after a year-long siege by Syrian troops, Aoun fled from his presidential palace at Baabda to the French embassy when Syrian warplanes began bombing the presidential residence. Hours after Aoun's flight, Syrian troops overran and pillaged Aoun's palace and his enclave. (The Syrian move was widely interpreted as the result of a "green light" from Washington, contingent on Syrian participation in the U.S.–led multinational forces deployed in the Gulf following Iraq's invasion of Kuwait [*Middle East International*, 10/26/90].)

Soon thereafter, President Hrawi announced his "Greater Beirut" plan, which called for the disarming of militias in and around the capital by mid-November and for the reestablishment of Lebanese sovereignty over the area. The next step in the Taif process called for the dissolution of all militias throughout the country, the full restoration of Lebanese internal sovereignty, and the full implementation of the reformed national charter mandated at Taif. To the astonishment of many, the Greater Beirut plan was achieved in mid-December, when Samir Geagea withdrew his Lebanese Forces from the capital to his Christian enclave north of the city. However, Geagea was deeply disillusioned when President Hrawi announced a 30-man reconciliation cabinet packed with pro-Syrian Lebanese politicians [ibid., 10/26/90, 12/7/90, 1/11/91].

In the spring of 1991 the Lebanese government succeeded in disarming all militias operating in the southern region between Beirut and Sidon; and in early July, with support from Syrian units, the Lebanese army inflicted a decisive defeat on PLO forces south of Sidon. At the same time, the Lebanese parliament approved, and Presidents Hrawi and Assad signed in May, the first Syrian-Lebanese treaty since Lebanon's independence in 1943. The treaty recognized Lebanon's "sovereignty and independence," while mandating "close cooperation" between the two states "in all spheres," including the establishment of a joint Military Affairs Committee. This committee would decide the terms and timetable of a full withdrawal of Syrian troops from Lebanon—an event that the treaty postponed until 1992. The Israeli government denounced the treaty, calling it a document of "annexation [of Lebanon by Syria] pure and simple," and launched a series of punishing aerial raids into southern

Lebanon the day after its signing. Israeli officials declared that they would not consider evacuating Israel's "security zone" in Lebanon "as long as there are foreign forces and a foreign presence in Lebanon" [*The New York Times*, 7/8/91].

Violence in the south has abated over the last five years, but it shows no sign of resolution. During this period the fiercest fighting has been the **"war of the camps,"** which started in May 1985 when the Shiite Amal, supported by elements of the Syrian and Lebanese armies, stormed three Palestinian refugee camps in Beirut and southern Lebanon in an effort to impose Shiite hegemony in the area and forestall the return of PLO guerrillas. This campaign did not drive armed Palestinian defenders from their homes, and Amal has renewed its "war of the camps" several times, bringing Palestinian settlements to the brink of starvation and epidemic by February 1987, when Amal lifted its siege and allowed shipments of food and emergency supplies into the Palestinian camps [*Time*, 2/23/87]. The brutal battles between the Shiite Amal and the Palestinians, and also the Hizbollah, have underscored Amal's fierce determination to control southern Lebanon, moving other factions in the country to oppose Amal's drive for hegemony and to support a steady revival of PLO power in Lebanon. While 8,000 Palestinian fedayeen fled Lebanon in 1982 during the Israeli invasion, up to 11,000, including 5,000 members of Yasser Arafat's moderate Fatah faction, have returned to south Lebanon [*The New York Times*, 4/2/90]. In June 1990 an inter-Shiite battle, pitting Amal against the Hizbollah but also involving PLO fighters, claimed almost 200 lives in two weeks in a contest to control the southern district of Iqlim al-Tuffah [*Middle East International*, 8/2/90].

Meanwhile, fighting along Israel's security zone continues in the south. The Hizbollah, whose power and influence has grown rapidly since its formation in the wake of the Israeli invasion, has fired rockets on settlements in northern Israel and attacked Israeli and South Lebanon Army (SLA) positions in southern Lebanon, prompting retaliation in force by Israeli warplanes. Various PLO factions have continued to stage raids across the border, although Yasser Arafat's Fatah group has suspended raids into Israel since the start of the U.S.–PLO dialogue in December 1988 [*The Economist*, 3/4/89]. All of these actions have drawn Israeli reprisals in the form of air and land raids against PLO and Hizbollah positions in southern Lebanon. In December 1988, Israel launched a combined air, land, and sea raid just ten miles south of Beirut. The United States later vetoed a Security Council draft resolution deploring the Israeli attack and demanding that Israel withdraw from Lebanon to internationally recognized boundaries [SC/5052]. In January the United

States had vetoed a similar Security Council resolution that "strongly deplore[d] repeated Israeli attacks against Lebanese territory and all other measures and practices against the civilian population." The United Kingdom abstained [PR SC/4977/88]. More recently, in January 1991, Israel bombarded a 100-square-mile area of Palestinian villages and positions after the PLO fired dozens of rockets toward Israel and sent infiltrators into Israel's security zone [The New York Times, 2/1/91]. In early June, Israeli jets again bombed PLO and Lebanese leftist strongholds in southern Lebanon, reportedly killing 22 and wounding 82 [ibid., 6/6/91].

The mandate of the U.N. Interim Force in Lebanon (UNIFIL), which was sent to restore Lebanese sovereignty in southern Lebanon in 1978 after an Israeli incursion, has been thwarted by Israel's refusal to evacuate its security zone and also by the harassment of UNIFIL by local militias, including the Israeli-backed SLA. UNIFIL has also had to contend with the violence of the Hizbollah, which was not appeased by Israel's withdrawal from most of southern Lebanon in 1985 and remains committed to the "liberation" of Jerusalem and the destruction of Israel.

Another war between Syria and Israel in Lebanon is unlikely. In April 1986 allegations that Syria was behind a failed attempt to blow up an Israeli airliner spurred rumors of a new war, but tensions between Syria and Israel quickly subsided. Israel's withdrawal to its security zone in southern Lebanon in 1985 has eased friction between the two countries, restoring Lebanon as a buffer zone separating the Syrian and Israeli armies. At present, Israel, Syria, and the Shiite Amal all have an interest in checking the growth of PLO and Hizbollah influence in southern Lebanon. Both insurgent groups threaten to upset the delicate strategic balance that Israel and Syria have struck.

UNIFIL, which has nearly 6,000 troops in southern Lebanon, continues to play its peacekeeping role, although its U.N. mandate proscribes the use of force to stop guerrilla attacks or Israeli countermeasures. Since the establishment of UNIFIL, 156 members of the force have died, 60 as a result of hostile fire and bomb or mine explosions. During the last six months of 1988, 5 UNIFIL soldiers lost their lives in accidents and 17 were wounded, 10 of those from hostile fire or explosions. In February 1988 a U.S. Marine colonel attached to UNIFIL was kidnapped, and in December three UNIFIL soldiers were kidnapped by armed elements before being rescued by Amal forces two days later [S/20416].

In his semiannual report of January 1989, the Secretary-General noted that UNIFIL's finances "have continued to deteriorate," owing to the failure of some U.N. members to meet their UNIFIL obligations. As of June 1991, unpaid contributions to UNIFIL totaled $231.9 million, against an authorized gross annual budget of $144 million [A/45/802]. The United States, whose annual UNIFIL assessment is between $45 and $47 million, began to withhold part of that assessment in 1988, paying only $18.7 million. Since then it has paid $18.2 million (1989), $28.3 million (1990), and $40.1 million (1991). For 1992 the President has requested full payment of $45.6 million. As of June 1991 the request awaited congressional approval.

The Soviet Union has also been delinquent, but in 1987 it announced it would start paying its assessed share.

UNRWA

The United Nations Relief and Works Agency for Palestine Refugees in the Near East (UNRWA) was created in 1949 to provide humanitarian assistance to some 700,000 Palestine refugees. Today, the agency extends a wide range of quasi-governmental services to over 2.4 million eligible refugees in the Middle East. It provides education to 358,000 Palestine refugee children in Jordan, Lebanon, Syria, and the Occupied Territories and vocational and teacher training to some 5,000 students. It maintains a primary health care service for all refugees through a network of some 100 health centers concentrating on vulnerable groups, especially mothers and children. Under its relief program it provides food, as well as other forms of assistance, to more than 150,000 refugees it classes as "special hardship cases," runs special programs for women and the disabled, and assists in promoting economic self-sufficiency through small income-generating projects.

In addition, UNRWA has mounted emergency relief operations in Lebanon since 1987 and in the Occupied Territories since 1988. A longer-term special program to improve infrastructure in the Occupied Territories, at an estimated cost of $65 million, is in the process of implementation, with over $30 million pledged or contributed. UNRWA has also launched an appeal for $35 million to construct a 200-bed hospital in Gaza and maintain it for three years.

UNRWA's regular operations for 1991 were budgeted at $254.6 million, the largest contributions coming from the United States ($62 million) and the European Economic Community ($53.2 million). In 1990 the emergency operations in Lebanon and the Occupied Territories cost some $23 million, with a similar level of expenditure envisaged for 1991.

As in past years, the anarchy and violence of Lebanon have imperiled both UNRWA clients and personnel, making the agency's work extremely difficult and dangerous. Since June 1982, 26 UNRWA workers have been killed in Lebanon, out of a total staff of 2,500. The recent indications of a return to normality have lessened the pressure on the refugees and on the agency serving them. It remains to be seen, however, whether this trend will continue.

Since the start of the Palestinian uprising in the Occupied Territories in December 1987, UNRWA has faced difficulties in delivering emergency food, water, and medical care in the refugee camps and villages due to curfews and interference by Israeli armed forces. Beatings of refugees and restrictive economic policies imposed by the Israeli occupation authorities have also led to increased demands for UNRWA medical and emergency relief services [PR DH/85/88]. Increasingly, UNRWA workers are risking their lives in the pursuit of their duties. Since the *intifadah* began, seven UNRWA staffers alleged to be Israeli collaborators have been killed by unidentified assailants, three of these on UNRWA premises [*UNRWA News*, 4/30/91].

UNRWA's largest program, education, has been hit by Israel's closing of schools in the Occupied Territories. The agency's 98 schools for 40,000 students in the West Bank remained closed for most of the 1987–88 school year. Schools were reopened in December 1988 and shut down again in February 1989. During the six-month teaching period starting in the fall of 1990, UNRWA schools lost about half of their teaching days to closure, orders, strikes, curfews, and other *intifadah*-related causes. Closures by military order were by far the largest cause, accounting for two-thirds of days lost on the Gaza Strip and three-quarters on the West Bank [*UNRWA News*, 4/17/91].

3. Africa

The agenda of the 46th Session of the U.N. General Assembly will feature two major categories of African issues. One is the persistent economic crisis in sub-Saharan Africa; the other is the continuing struggle against apartheid in the Republic of South Africa and the peace and security issues associated with its attempt to destabilize and dominate the region. A number of sub-issues fall under each category. Related to the economic crisis, for example, are matters affecting humanitarian and emergency assistance to refugees and others who have been displaced by regional conflicts and ecological failures. Under the category of southern Africa, the General Assembly will be reviewing its own role in liquidating

South Africa's illegal occupation of Namibia, and it will also be attempting to discourage South Africa from mounting any further attacks on the Frontline states, especially Mozambique and Angola.

The African Economic Crisis

Africa is in the throes of an economic crisis of devastating proportions characterized by a precipitous decline in growth rates and real incomes, falling rates of production, internal and external deficits, declining agricultural production, and serious failures in the organization of industrial and agricultural management [John Ravenhill, *Africa in Economic Crisis* (New York: Columbia University Press, 1986), p. 36]. A 1983 assessment of the situation by the **U.N. Economic Commission for Africa (ECA)** offered a disturbing prognosis:

> The picture that emerges from the analysis of the perspective of the African region by the year 2008 under the historical trend scenario is almost a nightmare. Poverty would reach unimaginable dimensions since rural incomes would become almost negligible relative to the costs of physical goods and services. The conditions in the urban centres would also worsen with more shanty towns, more congested roads, more beggars and more delinquents. The level of the unemployed searching desperately for the means to survive would imply increased crime rates and misery. Against such a background of misery and social injustice, the political situation would inevitably be difficult. The very consequence of extreme poverty would be social tensions and unrest which, in turn, would result in political instability [*ECA and Africa's Development, 1983–2008* (Addis Ababa: ECA, 1983), p. 93].

As late as 1989 most observers were agreed that for all the efforts of the African countries and the various international agencies, the economic crisis had worsened appreciably. In his appeal to the international community at the 45th General Assembly, Uganda's President Yoweri Museveni, current head of the Organization of African Unity (OAU), stated that, rather than abating, the crisis in Africa has become worse [*Africa Recovery* 4, no. 3–4, 10–12/90, p. 3].

The crisis in Africa is the result of a combination of external and internal factors. Entering the world capitalist system with a legacy of colonial exploitation that placed them on unequal terms with other actors and forced to depend upon an international political economy that continues to reduce the terms of trade for the continent's export commodities, the states of Africa have been severely limited in their ability to acquire sufficient resources for development. This problem is exacerbated by the internal policies of most African governments, whose attempts to control prices and exchange rates and subsidize some sectors of the economy have contributed to the generally dismal economic performance.

In 1980 the OAU adopted as a blueprint for development the **Lagos Plan of Action for the Economic Development of Africa, 1980–2000 (LPA),** based on the concept of collective self-reliance and regional economic integration. The plan concentrated on the development of some nine sectors in order to attain self-sufficiency in food production, eliminate illiteracy, develop indigenous technical manpower, preserve the environment, and integrate development with African sociocultural values. A year later came the **World Bank's own blueprint, Accelerated Development in Sub-Saharan Africa: An Agenda for Action (AD).** According to the analysis that informed AD, while external factors play a role in the African economic crisis, the main causes are domestic policy deficiencies—specifically, overvalued exchange rates, inappropriate agricultural policies, and excessive government interference in the economy. AD's prescription for economic growth included the eradication of the exchange rate problem (through devaluations), renewed priority on agricultural development, and improvement in economic management.

For the past decade the LPA and AD were thought to represent two opposing tendencies in the search for appropriate strategies to overcome the African economic crisis. Today many observers agree that these tendencies are far from incompatible and that the World Bank's blueprint can be viewed as a statement of "what should be done now and during the next few years to achieve the longer-term objectives of the Lagos Plan of Action" [S. Please and K. Y. Amoako in J. Ravenhill, *Africa in Economic Crisis*, p. 132]. There is also agreement that, whatever strategies are adopted, African economic recovery will require massive transfers of resources in the form of investments and official assistance.

As the discussion continues, Africa has been sinking into almost total economic collapse. Contributing to the situation is a **debt crisis** fueled by increasing interest rates and other costs of paying off the huge sums that were borrowed to implement development programs. This debt servicing leaves the African countries with even less revenue for domestic consumption or investment.

One of the issues with which the 46th Session will deal is African industrial development. In 1980 the General Assembly proclaimed the 1980s as the **Industrial Development Decade for Africa** [A/Res/35/66B] to spur the development of industry through mobilization of domestic resources by the African governments, with the technical and financial assistance of the U.N. system, especially the U.N. Industrial Development Organization and the Economic Commission for Africa. A mid-term evaluation in 1988 concluded that the program has been hampered by the scarcity of foreign exchange. Nevertheless, the 44th General Assembly proclaimed a **Second Industrial Development Decade for Africa** [A/Res/44/237]. Among the areas for which technical and financial assistance will be provided to aid country programs are the rehabilitation and expansion of existing industries, development of factory inputs, standardization and manufacture of spare parts, and subregional industrial cooperation. A progress report on preparations for the Second Industrial Development Decade for Africa [A/45/257] will be presented to the 46th General Assembly for further action. Another question to be considered by the 46th General Assembly will be the Secretary-General's report on the Preparation of the Programme for the **Second United Nations Transport and Communications Decade in Africa** [A/45/185], on the basis of which the General Assembly is expected to launch the Decade in September of 1991.

The **13th Special Session of the General Assembly** in May 1986 was an important milestone in the General Assembly's involvement in the issue of African economic recovery. It was here that the Assembly adopted the **U.N. Programme of Action for African Economic Recovery and Development 1986–1990 (UNPAAERD),** which made specific policy recommendations for governments and established the levels of capital assistance to be provided by the international community. The Secretary-General then set up an interagency committee under the chairmanship of the Director-General of Development and International Economic Cooperation to monitor the implementation of UNPAAERD. In April 1987 the Secretary-General also appointed a 13-member **Advisory Group on Financial Flows for Africa,** chaired by Douglas Wass (former head of the United Kingdom's treasury), to offer advice on finding the capital assistance called for by UNPAAERD. Despite these efforts, the Secretary-General reported in October 1987 that as a result of debt service and the serious **drop in commodity prices,** $16 billion more was flowing out of Africa than was being brought in through development assistance and private lending combined. He went on to note that Northern protectionism and global economic contraction were among the causes of Africa's worsening economic situation [A/42/560].

By the end of 1987, 33 African countries had embarked on **International Monetary Fund–mandated structural adjustment programs (SAPs),** representing the orthodox view of the causes of the economic crisis in Africa as outlined in the Accelerated Development report. These involved currency devaluation, reduction of government deficits, and privatization of government industrial and agricultural enterprises. While most observers agree that the African countries are in need of some form of internal policy reforms, the SAPs have been criticized for their tendency to benefit the commercial elites at the expense of poorer classes, leading to appeals for "adjustment with a human face" [*Africa Recovery* 3, no. 1–2, 10/89].

In September 1988, the Ad Hoc Committee of the General Assembly undertook a midterm review of the progress made by UNPAAERD. This report [A/43/664] and the Secretary-General's own report to the 43rd Session of the General Assembly [A/43/500] noted that the **international community's financial assistance** was substantially less than was called for by UNPAAERD. On the basis of these reports the 43rd Session noted that the goals of the Programme of Action were not being met and also expressed doubt that meeting these goals would, in fact, lead to development. The Assembly nonetheless called for a redoubling of efforts to implement UNPAAERD and for structural adjustment programs that would go beyond mere adjustment of the African economies by working toward the sort of fundamental structural transformation that is conducive to long-term development. Its resolution asked for a final review of UNPAAERD during the General Assembly's 46th Session in 1991 [A/Res/ 43/27].

On March 8, 1989, the World Bank and the U.N. Development Programme (UNDP) undertook a study of "Africa's Adjustment and Growth in the 1980s." The main thrust of their report was to defend SAPs on the grounds that African countries pursuing SAPs were showing better signs of economic recovery than were others. One month later the ECA Council of Ministers commissioned a study of the World Bank report. **Statistics and Policies: ECA Preliminary Observations on the World Bank Report** "Africa's Adjustment and Growth in the 1980s" [Addis Ababa: ECA, 1989] took issue with a number of the conclusions of the World Bank report. The most serious objection was that, in its eagerness to make SAPs attractive, the Bank had made selective and inconsistent use of its data to arrive at the conclusions of its own earlier report, "Adjustment Lending: An Evaluation of Ten Years of Experience" (1989), and the General Assembly's midterm review of UNPAAERD. Further, the Bank's study had paid no attention to the devastating social consequences of the SAPs.

As a result of this review, the ECA developed its own **"African Alternative Framework to Structural Adjustment Programmes for Socio-Economic Recovery and Transformation"** (AAF-SAP), which called on "African governments to move beyond a narrow preoccupation with short-term adjustment to embrace a range of far-reaching policy reforms that seek to transform the very structures of their economies" [Addis Ababa: ECA, 6/6/89]. At its 44th Session, the General Assembly adopted a resolution urging the international community and international financial and development institutions to consider the **"African Charter"** adopted at the February 1990 International Conference on Popular Participation in the Recovery and Development Process in Africa, held at Arusha, Tanzania, under the auspices of the Secretary-General's Interagency Task Force on African Recovery. The charter sought recognition of the benefits of popular participation in Africa's economic recovery and recommended measures that governments, the United Nations, and donor agencies could take to encourage such participation. In addition to the "African Charter," the 45th General Assembly considered the report of the Secretary-General's Expert Group on African Commodity Problems [A/45/51 and Add. 1] and set up a committee of the whole to prepare a final review of UNPAAERD, to be reported to the 46th General Assembly pursuant to the 43rd General Assembly's Resolution 27. In the meantime the debate on African development continues with the **World Bank's latest study "Sub-Saharan Africa: From Crisis to Sustainable Growth,"** which was described by ECA Executive Secretary Adebayo Adedeji as a report that would "contribute towards building a consensus on the vital policy issues that confront Africa."

In addition to the general problem of economic recovery, the General Assembly has considered a variety of specific problems that affect the economic situation in sub-Saharan Africa. Among the most serious is that of **desertification**—the result of such natural disasters as locust and grasshopper infestations and persistent drought but frequently compounded by such man-made catastrophes as deforestation and armed conflict. The invariable consequences of these occurrences are famine, migrations, and the creation of refugees. At its 44th Session, the General Assembly adopted a number of resolutions urging donors to provide humanitarian and emergency assistance to refugees and displaced persons in **Angola, Chad, Djibouti, Ethiopia, Malawi, Somalia,** and **Sudan.** At the same session the Assembly authorized **"Operation Lifeline Sudan,"** which coordinated emergency humanitarian assistance—some 120,000 metric tons of food and other supplies at a cost of $78 million—to help alleviate the suffering of those displaced by civil war in Sudan and adjacent countries [A/Res/44/12]. Pledges totaling $106.4 million (U.S.) made as a result of an appeal by the General Assembly in April 1990, under the auspices of the World Food Programme and the Food and Agricultural Organization, have yet to be tapped. Relief efforts have been hampered by drought as well as inaccessibility of the affected areas due to **continued armed conflict in Sudan, Ethiopia, Angola, Mozambique, and lately Somalia and Liberia.**

In Ethiopia, for example, ongoing civil war resulted in a yearlong closing of the port at Massawa, but in the face of the most severe famine in Ethiopia's history, occupying Eritrean rebel forces reopened the port in spring 1991 to allow U.N. relief supplies to enter the country. The entry of the rebels into Addis Ababa and the toppling of the government increased the need for emergency humanitarian assistance. Meeting these needs was rendered even more difficult by the obstruction of major transit routes. In this same period, three World Food Programme employees were abducted and two more were murdered. In early June, the U.N. Secretary-General dispatched an interagency team to facilitate access to relief supplies and survey current assistance requirements [U.N. press release DH/903, 6/4/91]. The Assembly will continue to monitor the situation in Ethiopia and elsewhere in the sub-Saharan region during its 46th Session.

Southern Africa

As in years past, the Assembly's attention will be directed to several issues that fall under the general heading of southern Africa: apartheid in the Republic of South Africa, developments relating to the independence of Namibia, and relations between South Africa and its neighbors.

Apartheid

Apartheid became the official policy of South Africa in 1948, when the **Afrikaner-dominated National party** came to power. It was the culmination and formalization of policies from the turn of the century aimed at creating a completely segregated society based on the domination and exploitation of the black population by the minority of whites. This racist policy was met by the opposition of the **General Assembly** almost immediately. In 1952 the Assembly established the U.N. Commission on the Racial Situation in the Union of South Africa and during the rest of the decade adopted a number of resolutions condemning apartheid. These resolutions went unheeded by the Republic of South Africa, which maintained, often with the support of the major Western powers, that apartheid was an internal matter and that General Assembly discussions of the matter were in violation of Article 2(7) of the U.N. Charter.

In the aftermath of the Sharpeville massacre of 1960, in which 67 people were killed by police during a demonstration, the General Assembly, energized by a group of new African members, began to urge more drastic actions against South Africa. These included requests for member states to take specific unilateral or collective measures to help dismantle apartheid and calls to the Security Council to take some measures of its own, including sanctions against South Africa. In 1962 the General Assembly established an 18-member **Special Committee against Apartheid,** which became the source of most of the resolutions condemning South Africa. In the two decades that followed, the Assembly took even more drastic actions against apartheid. Among these actions were the adoption of a resolution expressing solidarity with the opponents of apartheid [A/Res/2054 (XX)], the adoption of an International Convention on the Suppression and Punishment of the Crime of Apartheid [A/Res/3068 (XXVIII)], a Declaration of the U.N. Decade of Action to Combat Racism and Racial Discrimination [A/Res/3380 (XXX)], and the many endorsements of "armed struggle" against apartheid. The **Security Council,** for its part, imposed a voluntary arms embargo on South Africa in 1963 and a mandatory embargo in 1977. Throughout this period South Africa remained defiant, generally ignoring the hundreds of resolutions deploring apartheid.

In 1982 the Republic began introducing measures that it claimed were reforms of the system, among them the establishment of a tricameral legislature for whites, Indians, and coloreds. The General Assembly condemned these reforms because they maintained power exclusively in the hands of the white minority and failed to offer any political rights to black South Africans [A/Res/39/2]. In 1985 the South African government introduced a **state of emergency,** banning many opponents of apartheid or detaining them without trial. Reactions to the state of emergency were almost universally negative. In 1986 the U.S. Congress, overriding a presidential veto, voted to adopt unilateral economic sanctions against the Republic. As international pressure increased, the General Assembly stepped up its anti-apartheid activities.

At the 44th Session, the Assembly adopted several resolutions directed against South Africa. Among these were a bid to exclude the "racist apartheid régime" from participating in meetings of the Antarctic Treaty Consultative Parties [A/Res/44/124A]; a call for a Special Session on Apartheid and Its Destructive Consequences [A/Res/44/408]; and a catchall resolution that expressed solidarity with the two black anti-apartheid organizations in South Africa—the African National Congress (ANC) and the Pan-Africanist Congress (PAC). The resolution called for comprehensive, **mandatory sanctions and an oil embargo against South Africa** and condemned South Africa's internal and external terrorist policies, including its aggressive actions to destabilize its neighbors [A/Res/ 44/27A–L]. The Secretary-General was asked to prepare a report on progress in implementing this resolution for the 45th Session [A/Res/44/27K].

At the **16th Special Session** (December 12–14, 1989), devoted to the question of apartheid, the General Assembly approved specific guidelines for the peaceful dismantling of apartheid in South Africa. The guide-lines—recommendations of the international community for the Pretoria regime—were contained in the **"Declaration on Apartheid and Its Destructive Consequences in Southern Africa"** and adopted without a vote [A/Res/S-16/1]. After reaffirming its duty to support all those in South Africa seeking to eradicate the crime of apartheid, the declaration cited a "conjuncture of circumstances" that "could create the possibility" of ending apartheid through negotiation, "if there is a demonstrable readi-ness on the part of the South African regime to engage in negotiations." These negotiations, it said, should be based on acceptance of the funda-mental principles that South Africa should be a "united, non-racial and democratic" state, where the rights of all citizens will be equally pro-tected through an "entrenched bill of rights," a "legal system that will guarantee equality of all before the law," and an "independent and non-racial judiciary."

To pave the way for negotiation, the Special Session urged the present government to release unconditionally all political prisoners and detain-ees, lift the bans and restrictions on all proscribed and restricted organi-zations and persons, remove all troops from the townships, end the state of emergency, and cease all political trials and political executions. Before relaxing existing sanctions, the Assembly said, it would have to have "clear evidence of profound and irreversible charges" in the Republic. As requested by Resolution S-16/1, the Secretary-General sent a **high-level U.S. mission to South Africa** in June 1990 to investigate the progress that had been made toward the dismantling of apartheid. On the basis of the Secretary-General's report, the 45th General Assembly adopted a resolution that inter alia called for the maintenance of the oil embargo and the sanctions against South Africa and requested the Secretary-General to prepare a report on the implementation of the resolution for the 46th General Assembly.

Events in South Africa have given the anti-apartheid forces some hope. In a speech at the opening of parliament two months after the Special Session, **South African President F. W. de Klerk** lifted the ban on the ANC and other anti-apartheid movements. Even more dramatic was the release of ANC leader **Nelson Mandela** on February 11, 1990, after 27 years of imprisonment. Talks between de Klerk and Mandela, scheduled for April, had to be postponed after police fired upon and killed several anti-apartheid demonstrators.

Representatives of **the South African government and the ANC** met at Cape Town from May 2 to May 4. After the meeting they released a **joint statement** in which they expressed a commitment "toward the resolution of the existing climate of violence and intimidation from whatever quarter as well as a commitment to stability and to a peaceful process toward negotiations." The statement also announced the temporary immunity from prosecution of the National Executive Committee members of the ANC and set up a joint working committee to determine the modalities for the release of political prisoners and the granting of immunity with respect to political offenses. In addition, the government promised to work toward lifting the state of emergency. After several inconclusive meetings, the South African government and the ANC met on February 7, 1991, and concluded an accord involving the **renunciation by the ANC of armed struggle within the country in return for the government's recognition of the ANC's right to engage in mass political action.** This agreement led to the feeling on both sides that, as Mr. de Klerk put it, "we will be moving rapidly toward the commencement of multi-party negotiations" [*The Washington Post*, 2/16/91]. The accords were made possible by the actions of the government in the autumn of 1990 to **dismantle apartheid,** including the lifting of the state of emergency in Natal and Transvaal, an agreement on the phased release of ANC political prisoners, and the repeal of the Separate Amenities Act, the Population Registration Act, the Land Act, and the Group Areas Act, leaving only the **Internal Security Act** as the remaining major piece of apartheid legislation. One major result of the Pretoria/ANC accords was the February 21, 1991, formation of a nine-member ANC/Government Joint Working Committee to work toward the establishment of a single educational system.

The progress toward the dismantling of apartheid has not been without setbacks. Complicating the process have been a number of occurrences that have tended to undermine the ability of the two sides to trust each other. One obstacle has been the **bloody confrontations between the supporters of the ANC and the Zulu-based Inkatha,** whose leader, **Mangosuthu Buthelezi,** has vowed to make it impossible for the ANC to act as the sole representative of the black people. Even with a January 29, 1991, peace agreement between Buthelezi and Mandela, the bloodletting has continued intermittently at the cost of an estimated 5,000 lives. Apart from the instability that this violence has caused, it has led to widespread suspicion that some conservative whites, and the government, have been supporting the Inkatha and using the situation to perpetrate acts of violence against ANC supporters. This suspicion is increased by the fact that the report of the **Harms Commission,** set up to investigate acts of terrorism against anti-apartheid leaders by the secret military Civil Cooperation Bureau, has been widely regarded as a whitewash. Another obstacle to the negotiation process has been the intransigence of the **Pan-Africanist Congress** and the nationalist right-wing **Afrikaner Resistance Movement,** which have declared their intention to boycott any negotiations.

In spite of these difficulties, on June 5, 1991, the South African government adopted new legislation repealing the Land Acts of 1913 and 1936 and the Group Areas Act, which had allocated 87 percent of the land to the whites, who make up 14 percent of the population, and dictated residence on the basis of race. As a result of this—and of new initiatives by the South African government aimed at combating the violence between Inkatha and ANC elements—there is new hope of constitutional discussions in the near future.

Namibia

The United Nations has been dealing with the problem of South West Africa since 1946, when the then Union of South Africa attempted to annex the territory it administered under a League of Nations mandate, claiming that the mandate had lapsed with the demise of the League. Internal opposition to the occupation began with the formation of the **South-West Africa People's Organization (SWAPO)** in 1960, and by 1966, SWAPO had become a guerrilla force engaged in armed struggle in the territory and in adjoining Angola.

In the mid-1960s the **General Assembly** stepped up its challenge to South Africa on the Namibian issue. In 1966 it declared South Africa's occupation illegal, terminated the League mandate, gave the U.N. direct responsibility for the territory, set up the **U.N. Council for Namibia** to administer it [A/Res/2145 (XXI), A/Res/2248S–V], changed the territory's name to Namibia in accordance with the wishes of the majority of the population, and recognized SWAPO as the "authentic representative of the Namibian people" [A/Res/3111 (XXVIII)].

In 1975 the Republic of South Africa responded to the challenge by attempting to establish an "independent" Namibia under the leadership of the **Turnhalle Conference,** to which it gave the responsibility of drafting a new constitution. In an effort to break this impasse, the "**Western Contact Group**," made up of five Western governments with seats on the U.N. Security Council at the time, proposed a plan for a cease-fire in Namibia and tried to work out the basis of a compromise. The world body's response to the South African maneuverings was the now-famous **Security Council Resolution 435 of 1978,** setting out provisions for the movement toward Namibian independence. The resolution called for a cease-fire in Namibia, the abolition of apartheid laws in Namibia, the withdrawal of South Africa from Namibia, the election of a constituent assembly, and establishment of the **United Nations Transitional Assistance Group (UNTAG)** to oversee free and fair elections under U.N. supervision. The mandate of this force went far beyond anything ever assigned to previous U.N. peacekeeping missions. It called for UNTAG to participate in nearly every aspect of Namibia's path to independence: monitoring elections, helping the former colony draft a constitution, and overseeing the transition to independence.

The implementation of Security Council Resolution 435 was resisted by South Africa with the support of the United States, which proposed in 1980 that implementation be **linked with the withdrawal of Cuban troops stationed in Angola.** The General Assembly accepted Angola's response that this linkage was fraudulent, since the Cuban troops had been invited by the Angolan government to assist it in its war against the U.S.–supported resistance forces of the **National Union for the Total Independence of Angola** and, at the same time, declared its intention of establishing a Multi-Party Conference (excluding SWAPO) as a prelude to a South African–sponsored form of Namibian independence. Between 1985 and 1987, using as a basis Security Council Resolutions 566 and 601, the U.N. Secretary-General made several attempts to start up negotiations with a view to placing UNTAG in Namibia.

In 1988 several factors combined to create conditions that led to some movement toward the independence of Namibia: the war weariness of Angola and SWAPO, Angolan fears about a reduction in Soviet assistance, South Africa's unwillingness to accept more casualties, and the development of a new U.S.–Soviet understanding about the need for a peaceful settlement of the conflict. A series of diplomatic meetings with vigorous U.S. participation produced a set of **Principles for a Peaceful Settlement in South Africa** in July; and at a U.S.–Soviet summit, Washington and Moscow set a target date of September 29, which coincided with the tenth anniversary of the adoption of Resolution 435, for reaching an agreement on the independence of Namibia. In December 1988 a protocol on the independence of Namibia was signed. Cuba began its troop withdrawal, and the way was paved for the deployment of UNTAG.

In spite of the problem of armed SWAPO guerrillas crossing into Namibia within hours of the official beginning of the transition period on April 1, 1989, and the controversial decision of U.N. Special Representative in Namibia Martti Ahtisaari to allow elements of the South African Defence Forces to interdict them, and despite sporadic activity by the South African counterinsurgency group Koevoet, plans went smoothly for the election of a constituent assembly in November. An estimated 97 percent of registered voters turned out at the polls, and the constituent assembly went on to approve a constitution for Namibia. On March 21, 1990, Namibia joined the ranks of independent states, with SWAPO leader Sam Nujoma as its first president, and on April 23 it became a member of the United Nations. Having completed their mission, the **UNTAG forces were withdrawn from Namibia at the end of March 1990.** The mission had involved 7,900 military, police, and civilian personnel from 109 countries at a cost of $373.4 million. The 44th General Assembly dissolved the United Nations Council on Namibia [A/Res/44/234]. However, as the Secretary-General was quick to point out, "this does not mean that our commitment to Namibia has diminished." The United Nations has already begun to orient its activities and cooperation to the task of helping the Namibian people consolidate their newly won freedom through social and economic development [A/44/PV 96, p. 40]. Activities that will be reported to the 46th General Assembly are a **pledging conference** organized for Namibia under the auspices of the U.N. Development Programme, **emergency relief for refugees,** and the progress of negotiations with South Africa on the issue of **Walvis Bay.**

With the transition to independence of the last major non-self-governing territory, an important chapter in the history of the United Nations comes to a close. The Namibian experience was unique—the first time that the United Nations has taken on the role of administering authority in a territory and provided the machinery for its transition to independence.

The Frontline States

South Africa's **strategy for the survival of apartheid** has involved a foreign policy of sub-imperialism for the past 20 years. In 1977, P. W. Botha, then Minister of Defense, presented a white paper in which he introduced the "total strategy" for reaching South Africa's foreign policy objectives. The aim was to keep the Republic's neighbors economically dependent, politically unbalanced, and militarily unstable so as to provide a *cordon sanitaire* against any international opposition to apartheid. The strategy involved coordinated efforts to destroy the regional transportation routes of neighboring states, to control regional trade, to mount a massive diplomatic offensive to gain some legitimacy for a cosmeticized version of apartheid, and to pursue a "strike Kommando" tactic, involving the use of surrogates as well as South African forces in overt and covert warfare, sabotage, and terror [Reginald Green and Carol Thomson, "Political Economies in Conflict: SADCC, South Africa and Sanctions," in Phyllis Johnson and David Martin, eds., *Destructive Engagement: Southern Africa at War* (Harare: Zimbabwe Publishing House, 1986)].

To reduce their economic dependence on and military vulnerability to the Republic, South Africa's neighbors formed the **Frontline States** (Angola, Botswana, Mozambique, Tanzania, and Zimbabwe) and, in April 1980, the **Southern Africa Development Coordinating Conference** (Angola, Botswana, Lesotho, Malawi, Mozambique, Swaziland, Tanzania, Zambia, and Zimbabwe) [R. Green, "The SADCC on the Frontline: Breakdown or Breakthrough?" in Colin Legum, *Africa Contemporary Record* (New York: Africana Publishing Corp., 1988)]. South Africa reacted by stepping up its strategy of destabilization, and this pattern of terror continued until 1988. It is estimated that 1.5 million people, two-thirds of them children, have lost their lives as a result of South African aggression and that the SADCC countries have lost $62.6 billion in revenue [U.N. Interagency Task Force, Africa Recovery Program/Economic Commission for Africa, *South African Destabilization: The Economic Cost of Frontline Resistance to Apartheid*, 10/89].

The two countries that have borne the brunt of South Africa's aggression are **Mozambique and Angola,** due to their strategic location on the Atlantic and Pacific coastal flanks of South Africa and their importance to the communications and transportation systems of the region. In addition, both countries have been supportive of the ANC and SWAPO, providing sanctuary to the organizations' members.

South Africa's efforts to destabilize the two countries have included not only direct military attack but support for the Mozambique National Resistance (RENAMO) and the forces of the National Union for the Total Independence of Angola (UNITA). As a result of this pressure, Mozambique accepted the **Nkomati Accords** of 1984, according to which the government would expel the ANC from its territory as a condition for withdrawal of South African support for RENAMO. In the same year, Angola accepted the **Lusaka Accords** in an attempt to get South African assurances of nonintervention, but South Africa continued its actions against the Frontline states, and Mozambique and Angola in particular. In Angola it saw justification for such actions in the continued presence of 40,000 Cuban troops, which had been helping the government conduct its war against UNITA. The interest of the United States in removing these troops and the introduction of linkage between their removal and negotiations toward the independence of Namibia further complicated the Angolan situation.

By 1987 the devastating effects of war, evidence of the withdrawal of Soviet support, and movement toward an understanding between Moscow and Washington had put the governments of Mozambique and Angola in a mood to negotiate with their enemies and attempt a reconciliation. With regard to Angola, aggressive diplomacy on the part of the United States produced the New York agreement of 1988, which arranged for the **withdrawal of Cuban troops** within a 30-month period and peace talks between the Angolan government and UNITA. Lending support to this agreement, the U.N. Security Council established the **United Nations Angola Verification Mission (UNAVEM)** to monitor the pullout of Cuban troops, one-half of which were scheduled to leave by November 1, 1989 [S/Res/626 (1989)]. These developments paved the way for a meeting between Angolan President Edoardo dos Santos and UNITA leader Jonas Savimbi on June 22, 1989. The **Gbadolite Accords** signed at this meeting were intended to form a transitional government, but these plans fell through. On January 27, 1991, the ruling party (the Popular Liberation Movement of Angola, or MPLA) accepted peace plans presented by Portugal, the United States, and the Soviet Union to end the 15-year war, but a month later the sixth round of talks between the MPLA and UNITA broke down on the issue of a cease-fire.

By May, however, the hurdles had been cleared. Angola and Cuba announced late in the month the departure of the last of the Cuban troops 36 days ahead of deadline [S/22644 Annex], and the U.N. Secretary-General headed for Lisbon to witness the signing of **Peace Accords between the Angolan government and UNITA** [S/22609] on June 1. On May 30, the Security Council agreed to enlarge and prolong the mandate of UNAVEM, newly dubbed **UNAVEM II,** to carry out verification tasks associated with the accords, with the intention of withdrawing the mission after completion of general elections on November 30, 1992 [S/Res/696]. A preliminary estimate for the intervening 18 months placed the cost at $132.3 million [U.N. press release SC/5279, 5/30/91].

Hopes for peace in Mozambique continue to run into obstacles. On November 30, 1990, the government of Mozambique accepted a new constitution clearing the way for a multiparty political system and a free-market economic system. Following this development a cease-fire agreement was signed to cover the Beira and Limpopo corridor between the Mozambique government and RENAMO in December 1990, followed by the formation of a **Joint Verification Commission** to oversee the cease-fire. Since then, however, the agreement was broken by a RENAMO attack on the Zimbabwe-Maputo rail line in February 1991.

On April 26, 1990, the U.N. Secretary-General convened a conference of donors to secure emergency food aid and logistical support for Mozambique, and a thorough in-country review of Mozambique's requirements was conducted between July and August 1990. The 45th General Assembly adopted a resolution that called for international assistance to aid in the economic rehabilitation of Angola and requested the Secretary-General to consult with the Angolan government to ascertain the level of aid required and report his findings to member states, international agencies, and the 46th General Assembly. Also on the agenda of the 46th Session is the issue of cooperation between SADCC and the U.N. system and the Secretary-General's Report on U.N. Assistance to the Frontline States.

4. Central America

The situation in Central America has brightened somewhat due to the landmark U.N. monitoring of elections and the demobilization of Nicaraguan rebels in spring 1990. But the deep social and economic problems that underlie regional insurgencies and tensions remain, proving that political agreement is just the first step on the road to stability.

The region remains mired in deep poverty, with two-thirds of its 30 million people destitute, and the five nations saddled with $20 billion in regional debt [*International Herald Tribune*, 6/19/90]. The Secretary-General's report on Central America of November 8, 1990 [S/21931, A/45/706], highlighted the myriad problems still faced by Central Americans, and stated that there could be "no peace" without "reconstruction and reconciliation."

The installation of Nicaragua's democratically elected government and the demobilization of the Nicaraguan rebels—completed on June 28, 1990—ended that nation's civil war. By the end of 1990, 28,700 refugees and 17,500 demobilized resistance leaders had been brought back to the nation under the auspices of the U.N. High Commissioner for Refugees (UNHCR) [*Refugees*, 12/90]. However, repatriation and the end to the insurgency have not brought true political stability or economic growth. **President Violeta Barrios de Chamorro** is under constant pressure on the left from entrenched Sandinista elements in the army, unions, and civil service, and on the right from embittered former rebels and hard-line factions of the opposition coalition, UNO, which she led in her campaign against the Sandinistas. The Sandinistas used up one-half of the country's annual budget during their last days in power, leaving the nation destitute and facing $11 billion in foreign debt, with inflation running at 50 percent per month [*U.S. News & World Report*, 7/2/90]. U.N. plans called for the world body to assist only 90,000 Nicaraguans per year [S/21931].

Chamarro moved rapidly to consolidate her new government's hold on power. In June 1990 she announced plans to end the military draft and cut the Sandinista-controlled army by a third, reducing it to 40,000 soldiers. However, Sandinista-dominated unions prevented her from imposing harsh economic measures. A ten-day Sandinista-backed strike crippled the nation in July, forcing Chamarro to back off plans to reclaim land allotted by the Sandinistas. She also granted government employees a steep wage increase [*U.S. News & World Report*, 7/23/90].

Meanwhile, the former rebels were growing restive over Chamorro's perceived weaknesses and government delays in granting them land. Complaints arose over her failure to oust some former Sandinista officials from key posts. In October 1990 former contras and several mayors launched a series of strikes and attacks, seizing government buildings and key roads [*The Economist*, 11/24/90]. The government used the Sandinista-dominated army to thwart the protests. On February 16, 1991, rebel leader and former national guardsman Enrique Bermudez was gunned down.

Civil unrest has continued amidst charges that Chamorro has failed to back her promises both to the contras and to right-wing members of her opposition group loyal to Vice President Godoy. Yet she has continued to move gingerly toward economic reform. In March 1991 she imposed a 400 percent devaluation, announcing plans to cut many Sandinista-held government jobs and to privatize much of the property taken by the Sandinistas while they were in power [*Le Monde*, 4/2/91]. This action drew more scathing attacks from the Sandinista-allied National Workers Front, which promised to increase its struggle against the government. So far, the government has prevailed.

El Salvador remains in a far bleaker state, with the civil war now in its 12th year. One in four Salvadorans has fled the country [*Le Journal de Genève*, 2/25/91], and 70,000 people have died in the fighting. U.N. efforts have centered on bringing the two sides—the government and the Farabundo Martí National Liberation Front (FMLN) rebels—to the negotiating table.

Fresh from the successful elections in Nicaragua, **Secretary-General Javier Pérez de Cuéllar** launched a new Salvadoran diplomatic effort on April 4, 1990, in Geneva, where he oversaw a meeting between government and rebel officials. The two sides agreed to begin talks under U.N. auspices, with the aim of "reinserting the FMLN into Salvadoran society." Pérez de Cuéllar named his chief aide, Alvaro de Soto, as his personal representative to the talks.

On May 21, 1990, de Soto oversaw talks between the two parties in Caracas, Venezuela. They agreed to seek an end to hostilities by mid-September. However, de Soto later agreed to a rebel demand that the deadline be lifted, drawing U.S. criticism for not pressing the insurgents [*The New York Times*, 2/1/91].

At first the talks seemed to make progress. In late July 1990, meeting in San José, Costa Rica, the two sides agreed to a plan to end human rights violations in the country, subject to U.N. verification [*Le Monde*, 7/26/90]. Talks in August failed, however, due to a disagreement over what to do with El Salvador's army [*The New York Times*, 8/21/90]. The rebels want the army disbanded, and this has remained the main sticking point to date, with February and March 1991 negotiations failing to forge an agreement on the issue [*Le Monde*, 3/2/91]. By mid-March the United Nations was circulating a "secret plan" under which it would nominate a commission of five notables to clean up the army by examining officers' pasts, to investigate human rights violations, and to disband the national police, the national guard, and the treasury policy [*The New York Times*, 3/13/91]. In addition, a "truth commission" would be appointed to study past human rights abuses. On May 20, 1991, the U.N. Security Council voted to establish a **U.N. Observer Mission in El Salvador** to monitor compliance with the human rights provisions of the San José plan agreed to in July of 1990 [S/Res/693].

During three weeks of Mexico City negotiations in April 1991, de Soto tried a new tack, getting the two sides to place military questions on the back burner and focus instead on constitutional reforms. This led to an important April 28 agreement under which the army would be subject to greater civilian control, the judiciary would become independent of military and political circles, police and intelligence units would be removed from the military, and the National Assembly would approve judicial and electoral board appointments by majority vote [*International Herald Tribune*, 4/29/91]. Both sides agreed to the appointment of the "truth commission" but not yet to a cease-fire. An accord must first be reached on the status of the army and, more broadly, on the rebels' reintegration into society. The two sides continued their negotiations in Caraballeda, Venezuela, in late May and early June, then recessed for a week of "internal consultations" [U.N. press release CA/44, 6/3/91].

The FMLN stepped up attacks on military and civilian targets throughout the autumn of 1990, downing government and U.S. aircraft with new missiles provided by Sandinista army officers [*The Economist*, 10/27/ 90]. The January 2, 1991, rebel downing of a U.S. helicopter led President Bush to free $42.5 million in military aid previously denied to the Salvadoran government because of its failure to investigate the murder of six Jesuit priests in 1989. Meanwhile, there were numerous accusations that the United States was itself protecting army officers implicated in the assassination [*Le Monde*, 12/18/90].

March 1991 regional and legislative elections in El Salvador saw the first entry of guerrilla-allied leftists into the parliament [*Reuters*, 3/13/91]. The governing nationalist Republican Alliance, or Arena, took 39 of the 83 seats; the opposition Christian Democrats took 26 seats; and Democratic Convergence, a leftist coalition, received 12 percent of the vote. Convergence leader Ruben Zamora accused the government of perpetrating massive fraud and warned that this would harden the rebels' stance [*The New York Times*, 3/13/91].

Both sides involved in the fighting continue to kill civilians, persecute opponents, and violate human rights. On December 18, 1990, the General Assembly adopted by consensus a resolution expressing "deep concern about the persistence of politically motivated violations of human rights in El Salvador, such as summary executions, torture, and abductions." It also noted the "unsatisfactory judicial system" and the "irregularities" in the government's investigation of the Jesuit killings. The Assembly voted to keep El Salvador's human rights situation on its own agenda as well as on the agenda of the U.N. Commission on Human Rights.

Guatemala has made some progress toward ending a low-scale guerrilla war and eliminating human rights violations. On March 30, 1990, the Commission for Guatemalan National Reconciliation, a government-appointed group, and the National Revolutionary Union of Guatemala held talks in Oslo, during which they agreed to seek peace. On June 1, 1990, in Madrid, the government and rebels signed an agreement to negotiate. The Secretary-General's report of November 8, 1990, noted these efforts.

There have been several regional efforts to normalize the situation in Central America. On June 19, 1990, the **five nations' presidents** met in

Guatemala and proposed to establish a regional common market and a unified approach to development. In a July 31 accord, the five proposed a plan to eliminate offensive military capability, promote disarmament, come up with new security arrangements, agree on the role of foreign forces, and draw up an inventory of arms and new arms limits. They proposed permanent U.N. verification of any disarmament accords, but the Secretary-General judged a U.N. role on that score "premature" in a report of October 26, 1990. Nevertheless, he did propose extending through May 1991 the presence of the over 400-man **military observer group for Central America,** known by the Spanish acronym **ONUCA,** originally placed in the region to implement the Esquipulas II accords. The Security Council approved that request in November 1990 and again in May 1991.

The General Assembly voted on several resolutions dealing with the regional situation. On November 20, 1990, the Assembly adopted by consensus a draft requesting Pérez de Cuéllar to "continue to afford the fullest possible support to the Central American governments in their efforts to consolidate peace." It also called for continued FMLN-government negotiations in El Salvador and asked the international community and international organizations to "increase their technical, economic, and financial cooperation with the Central American countries."

A December 14 resolution adopted without a vote endorsed the goals of the International Conference on Central American Refugees, held from May 29 to 31, 1989. It said "voluntary repatriation of refugees and the return of displaced persons to their countries or communities of origin is one of the most positive signs of progress of peace in the region." The resolution also pledged to protect the role of women and the development of children, to preserve ethnic and cultural values, and to protect the environment [A/Res/45/141]. A December 21, 1990, draft adopted without vote endorsed a Special Plan of Economic Co-operation for Central America and urged "immediate measures" to implement the plan's goals.

The United Nations' success in monitoring Nicaragua's elections has encouraged other nations in the region to turn to the world body for such help. Haiti asked the United Nations to monitor its December 17, 1990, elections, and the General Assembly granted that request in an October 10 resolution setting up the **U.N. Observer Group for Verification of Elections in Haiti,** known by its French acronym **ONUVEH.** The elections went off well, though some dissidents attempted a January coup against the winner, Jean-Bertrand Aristide. This coup attempt was put down by the army [*The New York Times*, 1/9/91].

In short, there are many hopeful signs in the region. As the situation in Nicaragua and elsewhere demonstrates, U.N. member states are quick to back efforts to end insurgencies when such action coincides with their interests. However, they are much tighter with their pocketbooks when the new democratic governments seek the funds to restore social and economic stability.

5. Afghanistan

It has now been over three years since the April 1988 signing of the U.N.–brokered **Geneva accords,** under which the United States, the Soviet Union, and Pakistan pledged not to interfere in Afghanistan's civil war, and more than two years since Moscow completed the withdrawal of its troops from the country. When the accords were signed it was hoped that the superpowers would leave the Afghans to their own devices, forcing a settlement of the country's decade-old internal conflict.

If anything, the prospects for a peaceful solution have deteriorated over the past three years. Despite the Geneva agreement's noninterference pledges, U.S., Pakistani, and other aid to rebel forces continues, while the Soviet Union still pays about $300 million per month to keep the Marxist government in Kabul in power [*Far Eastern Economic Review*, 1/24/91]. The bombings that killed 1.5 million Afghans and destroyed 22,000 villages during the heat of the Soviet-led fighting have waned, but civilian deaths continue, and more than 5 million refugees in Pakistan and Iran show few signs of returning to their homeland [Secretary-General's report on the Situation in Afghanistan, S/21879]. International attention has turned to other regions, meaning that "both the conflict and the people seem to have become a 'forgotten war' and a 'forgotten people' " [Situation of Human Rights in Afghanistan, A/45/664].

In his most recent report on the conflict in Afghanistan, the Secretary-General declared that "only an international consensus will solve the problem" [S/21879]. Not all analysts share that assessment. There are disturbing signs that both the government and rebel forces are becoming increasingly independent of their respective Soviet and American supporters, which means that the superpowers are losing their ability to broker a solution between opposing forces [*Le Monde*, 6/29/90]. The two opposing sides have themselves become fractured and confused.

A government split between the dominant Partcham faction and the more radical Khalq supporters in the army has worsened; the latter are believed to have led some attacks on pro-Kabul forces to inflame tensions

[*Est-Ouest*, 2/91]. Meanwhile, **opposition forces** are split along many lines. Some moderate factions are believed to be in contact with the Afghan government; a seven-militia "provisional government" led by Sibghatullah Mojadedi is bent on President Najibullah's departure before any settlement with the government, and a still more radical Islamic faction led by Gulbuddin Hekmatyar is intent on evicting the Marxists through warfare. Each faction has its own backers in Moscow, Kabul, Islamabad, Tehran, Riyadh, and Washington, and efforts to reach a settlement remain stuck as the factions try to outmaneuver one another [ibid.].

More disturbing, some analysts believe that fighting could continue almost indefinitely, even if all outside supporters halted military aid and observed the Geneva accords. The **Afghan army** appears to have hardened its resolve in the face of guerrilla assaults and is believed to have enough weapon reserves to fight on for several years, even if Soviet aid is cut. Meanwhile, the guerrillas could continue a low-scale civil war for decades. **Opium production** has become a lucrative source of cash for many militia elements; the chaotic situation in the country has allowed Afghanistan to increase its crop to three times the size of Mexico's, producing 800 tons of raw opium per year [*Far Eastern Economic Review*, 6/14/90]. Much of it passes across the border into Pakistan, where it is processed into heroin for export. Heroin sales now equal about a quarter of Pakistan's gross national product, according to some sources [*Le Figaro*, 7/25/90]. Almost all involved in the fighting get a cut of that revenue, so there is plenty of cash to finance the conflict.

U.S. and Soviet efforts to bring about a settlement of the conflict made some halting steps forward over the past year but failed to make any great strides in the face of Afghan government and rebel opposition. On March 15, 1990, the mandate of the 40-man **U.N. Good Offices Mission in Afghanistan and Pakistan (UNGOMAP)** ran out. UNGOMAP was created under Security Council auspices in May 1988 to monitor compliance with the Geneva accords; all sides accused it of ignoring the others' blatant violations of the accords. In its place the Secretary-General placed a smaller ten-man team, supporting a high-level political Office of the Secretary-General in Afghanistan and Pakistan, to be paid out of the U.N. regular budget. The function of this office is to advise the Secretary-General on the military and political situation in order to assist him with the task of finding a settlement.

Soviet and U.S. negotiators began forming new proposals for a settlement in May 1990 [*Le Monde*, 5/11/90]. The issue remained what to do with President Najibullah's government if a cease-fire were to be called and elections organized. At first it looked as if the United States and rebel forces might allow Najibullah to remain in the country and run in any elections following a settlement [ibid.]. The moderate Islamic National Front, led by Pir Gaylani, appeared receptive to that solution.

The June 1990 superpower summit failed to advance any peace plans. Then in July, the Soviets offered a new plan under which Najibullah would retain symbolic power as president before and during the election process but would hand real power over the administration and security forces to a broad-based electoral commission that would govern the country before any vote [*The New York Times*, 7/15/90]. If agreed to, the plan would have the United States and the Soviet Union end arms supplies to the nations, impose a cease-fire, and allow U.N.–sponsored elections [*Le Figaro*, 7/26/90]. However, the agreement failed to make any progress. Najibullah rejected his demotion to a puppet ruler [*Le Monde*, 7/24/90]. The United States, under rebel pressure, hardened its position and called for Najibullah's full ouster [ibid., 9/4/90]. The opposition groups also rejected any power-sharing with the President [ibid., 10/23/90].

Najibullah has made some attempts to reform the appearance, if not the substance, of his totalitarian regime. In May 1990 he convened a Loya Jirgah, or council of tribal and community leaders, and lifted Afghanistan's state of emergency. The change has had little practical impact [A/45/664]. In June the Loya Jirgah adopted several reforms of the constitution, deleting references to the ruling People's Democratic party, installing pluralism—at least in theory—and adding a new clause allowing free elections. The ruling party changed its name to the Watan party but continues to control the government [ibid.]. In September 1990, Najibullah met the Secretary-General in Paris. One month later he claimed to have met some opposition representatives, as well as representatives of Afghanistan's former king, in Geneva. The **ex-king, Zaher Shah,** put forward his own **peace plan,** to be based on the convocation of a representative Loya Jirgah, the creation of an interim government, the drafting of a new constitution, and the holding of free elections in November 1990.

None of these proposals has made much progress. The rebels continue to reject Najibullah's Loya Jirgah. In October 1990 about 400 Afghan commanders, including Shiite and Sunni commanders, held a Shura in northeast Afghanistan and agreed to create a unified military strategy. They agreed to establish nine administrative zones with administrators who would be elected by the commanders, religious leaders, and elders in each zone. They also agreed to set up a security system to maintain law and order and to protect supply routes in *mojahedin*-controlled areas. The commanders established a government administration center to coordinate activities and programs approved by all the commanders and demanded the regime in Kabul to transfer power to the "Muslim Nation of Afghanistan" in order to avoid further bloodshed. The commanders emphasized that, should the Kabul regime continue to deny these requests, the armed struggle would continue [conversations with *A Global Agenda: Issues Before the 46th General Assembly of the United Nations*].

In January 1991, Washington and Moscow failed to agree on the role of the king, or on whether a cease-fire should precede a cut in military aid, as Moscow wants, or the aid should be cut before a cease-fire, as Washington wants [*Far Eastern Economic Review*, 1/24/91]. The *mojahedin* continued to reject any retention of power by Najibullah, even during an interim period [ibid.].

Meanwhile, there have been signs of increasing radicalization and division among the rebels. The radicals, led by Hekmatyar, have upped the ante, launching a new offensive in September 1990 that was condemned by the seven-party opposition alliance presided over by Mojadedi [*International Herald Tribune*, 9/17/90]. One month later, Hekmatyar and another rebel leader, Ahmad Shah Masud, reached a cooperation agreement, but that too was rejected by the seven-member alliance [*Le Monde*, 10/24/90]. While some moderate rebel groups backed the U.S. attack on Iraq and sent forces to help, Hekmatyar's radicals reacted furiously, calling it "zionist" and "imperialist" plotting against an Islamic state [ibid., 3/7/91]. Finally, rebel forces launched a spring offensive and took the city of Khost in early April [*The Economist*, 4/6/91]. Government forces retaliated with renewed attacks, including one Scud missile attack that killed 500 civilians in the border town of Asadabad in late April [*Le Monde*, 9/24/91].

All of this has made the task of aiding Afghan refugees and civilians so difficult that the U.N. Special Rapporteur for human rights in Afghanistan, Felix Ermacora, says that the human rights, refugee, and general humanitarian situations "have not changed much" since the signing of the Geneva accords [E/CN.4/1991/31].

The situation in **refugee camps** has now deteriorated to such a point that they are run like little fiefdoms by competing militia forces. Bribes, special agreements, and politicking are now required of humanitarian workers wishing to enter the camps [*Le Figaro*, 7/11/90; *Libération*, 7/19/90]. Throughout the spring and summer of 1990 there were reports of radical militia forces harassing Western aid workers—and accusing them of spreading anti-Islamic doctrines [*The New York Times*, 6/24/90].

The Secretary-General's report on the situation in Afghanistan, released October 17, 1990 [A/45/635, S/21879], said the world body had raised over $1 billion to aid those trapped by the fighting since a special appeal was launched in October 1988. Over 400 U.N. projects are now under way inside the country.

Ermacora's human rights report of October 31, 1990 [A/45/664], said that few of the 3.7 million refugees in Pakistan or the 2.3 million refugees in Iran have shown any signs of wanting to return. Only 11,000 families participated in a U.N. pilot project to encourage repatriation in the Chitral province. Many of those seeking to go home have been forced back by militia forces, who accuse those willing to live in government-controlled Afghanistan of betraying the rebel cause. "As long as refugees cannot return safely and freely to their homes, the exercise of the right to self-determination will not be fully realized," Ermacora stated in his report.

The October report, as well as a later version released on January 28, 1991 [E/CN.4/1991], showed some improvement in the situation when compared to reports Ermacora wrote during the heaviest fighting, in which he described almost genocidal attacks on civilian populations. Attacks on civilians continue, however, particularly rebel rocket attacks on populated areas under government control. The government claimed that 4,771 civilians died during the first ten months of 1990 from these bombardments. Ermacora saw no signs of political progress toward a solution. "No real dialogue between the parties involved has taken place," he wrote.

In another blow to the U.N. effort, Sadruddin Aga Khan resigned in December 1990 as head of **Operation Salaam,** the U.N.–coordinated effort for aid from U.N.–affiliated agencies to Afghan civilians. The Operation had been accused of poor management and of overstating its effectiveness.

The General Assembly adopted two resolutions on Afghanistan at its 45th Session. On November 7, 1990, the Assembly adopted by consensus a resolution calling for an intra-Afghan dialogue, for the right of Afghans to determine their own form of government free of outside intervention, subversion, coercion, or restraints, and for strict compliance with the Geneva accords. This despite the fact that it is an open secret that a half-dozen countries are aiding one fighting force or another.

On December 18, 1990, the Assembly adopted without vote a human rights resolution urging all parties to respect the Geneva Conventions of 1949. It noted atrocities committed against government soldiers and civilians and called upon Afghan government authorities to investigate the disappearance of opponents of the regime.

On May 21, 1991, the Secretary-General made a public statement outlining the elements that could serve as a basis for a political settlement in Afghanistan. He stressed the need for a credible transition mechanism that would lead to a broad-based, democratically elected government, through free and fair elections based on Afghan traditions. He called further for a cessation of hostilities during this transition period and an end to the supply of arms to all sides. The statement met with positive reactions, most notably from the United States, the Soviet Union, Pakistan, and Iran.

6. Indochina

The question of Cambodia continued to occupy much of the 45th General Assembly's attention, as well as that of the Security Council. The search for a political solution to Cambodia's 11-year-old civil war evolved in several respects. The most significant development was the decision by the five Permanent Members of the Security Council—the Perm Five—to play a more active role in the peace process. This was triggered by the indefinite suspension of the Paris International Conference on Cambodia (PICC) in late August 1989. Attention then turned toward more direct involvement of the United Nations in Cambodia. The Perm Five assumed the lead in negotiating first the framework and then the specific provisions of a blueprint for a settlement. The Secretary-General's special representative, Under-Secretary Rafeeuddin Ahmed, played an essential role in this process [see "Towards Peace in Cambodia," U.N. DPI/ 1091, 9/90].

Thanks to these external pressures, the four Cambodian parties in mid-1991 finally agreed to talk in concrete terms about political compromise. As the 46th General Assembly convenes, there are solid grounds for optimism that the endgame leading to a settlement in Cambodia, probably within a U.N. framework, is actually beginning.

On the military front, activity continued sporadically throughout 1990, characterized by increased Khmer Rouge efforts to infiltrate cadres and supplies into the interior, build communications networks, and lay the groundwork for future operations away from their border sanctuaries. Sharp military engagements continued in the western provinces of Siem Reap, Banteay Mean Chey, and Battambang, particularly around the gem-mining center of Pailin. Khmer Rouge attacks, occasionally in coordination with noncommunist groups, were stepped up in areas closer to Phnom Penh, placing further demands on the government's resources. Fighting during the rainy season produced about 150,000 internal refugees in nine provinces—some fleeing, others forced by the government to vacate their homes rather than come under Khmer Rouge influence. By September 1990 some 50,000–60,000 refugees in Thai camps had been moved into Cambodian areas under the control of resistance forces, mainly the Khmer Rouge.

Some names in the Cambodia game have changed and these should be noted, even though the fundamental character of the political problems persist (see box on page 55).

Vietnam's protégé government, the State of Cambodia (SOC)—called the People's Republic of Kampuchea (PRK) until April 1989—remains in power in Phnom Penh and has influence over the majority of Cambodia's population and geography. The Socialist Republic of Vietnam (SRV), which deposed Pol Pot's Khmer Rouge and installed the PRK in January 1979, continues to support the SOC, describing it as sovereign and independent.

Opposing the SOC is the anti-Vietnamese resistance, which consists of three factions associated loosely in what is now called the National Government of Cambodia (NGC). The NGC replaced the Coalition Government of Democratic Kampuchea (CGDK), which withered away in early 1990. One faction, the communist Khmer Rouge, uses the Democratic Kampuchea label as it did during its years in power, 1975–78. The Democratic Kampuchea party is the Khmer Rouge's political wing; the National Army of Democratic Kampuchea is its military designation.

The coalition's two noncommunist resistance (NCR) groups are the National United Front for an Independent, Neutral, Peaceful and Cooperative Cambodia (FUNCINPEC), headed by Prince Norodom Sihanouk, and the Khmer People's National Liberation Front (KPNLF), headed by a former Sihanouk prime minister, Son Sann. These groups are supported by the Association of Southeast Asian Nations (ASEAN), the United States, some of the European Community states, and to some degree the People's Republic of China.

Cambodia's U.N. seat was previously occupied by the CGDK's three factions. At the 46th General Assembly, the Supreme National Council (see below) is expected to represent Cambodia. On July 19, 1990, U.S. Secretary of State James Baker announced that the United States would no longer lend its political support to the coalition and that it would open direct negotiations with Vietnam (and, later, the SOC) on Cambodia [The New York Times, 7/19/90]. The **"Baker shift"** was caused by anxiety in the international community over the growing power of the Khmer Rouge and by the U.S. Congress's refusal to continue aid to the two noncommunist groups as long as they were associated effectively

A Guide to Cambodian Acronyms

The Phnom Penh government

PRK — People's Republic of Kampuchea, regime's name, 1979–89.
SOC — State of Cambodia, its current name.
KPRP — Khmer People's Revolutionary Party, ruling political party.

The Resistance: Terms commonly used

CGDK — Coalition Government of Democratic Kampuchea, 1982–90.
NGC — National Government of Cambodia (also "Cambodia"), since February 1990.
CNR — Cambodian National Resistance, NGC military coordinating body.

The Resistance: Terms applied to the individual factions

KR — Khmer Rouge.
DK — Democratic Kampuchea, KR regime in power 1975–78.
DKP — Democratic Kampuchea Party, KR political party.
NADK — National Army of Democratic Kampuchea, KR military.
FUNCINPEC — National United Front for an Independent, Neutral, Peaceful and Co-operative Cambodia, pro-Sihanouk political party.
ANS — Armée Nationale Sihanoukiste, its military arm.
KPNLF — Khmer People's National Liberation Front, party of Son Sann.
NCR — Noncommunist resistance, generic term for the Sihanouk and Son Sann groups.

The United Nations Perm Five Plan

UNTAC — United Nations Transitional Authority in Cambodia.
SNC — Supreme National Council, planned repository of Cambodian sovereignty.
PICC — Paris International Conference on Cambodia.

with the Khmer Rouge. Since 1979, the United States has given political and material support to the NCR. In view of the evolution of U.S. Indochina policy during 1991, discussed below, the nature, extent, and duration of U.S. support for the NCR is uncertain.

Although the Cambodia conflict's two communist great-power patrons—**China and the Soviet Union**—are less directly involved in 1991, they must be reckoned with because of their positions on the Security Council and because they still provide significant political and material assistance to the Cambodian protagonists, particularly China's assistance to the Khmer Rouge.

ASEAN (Thailand Malaysia, Singapore, Indonesia, the Philippines, and Brunei) continues to oppose Vietnam for purposes of arriving at a political solution to a problem that, in truth, all the regional powers would like to see disappear. At the same time, the ASEAN countries have pursued their own national policies toward both Phnom Penh and Hanoi, including lively commercial relationships. More than ever, it is difficult to speak of an "ASEAN policy" when addressing Indochina affairs, the Cambodia problem, or relations with Vietnam. Moreover, Australia, Canada, Great Britain, France, and Germany, among others, are according de facto legitimacy to the SOC bilaterally (and developing fuller relations with Vietnam) even though the Cambodia situation remains unresolved.

During six formal meetings held in New York and Paris between January and August 1990, the five permanent members of the Security Council produced a "framework document" defining **"the key elements of a comprehensive political settlement of the Cambodia conflict based on an enhanced UN role"** [A/45/472; S/21689, 8/31/90]. The five sections of this document address what the Perm Five described as "the indispensable requirements for such a settlement":

- Transitional arrangements for administering Cambodia during the pre-election period;
- Military arrangements during the transitional period;
- Elections under U.N. auspices;
- Human rights protection;
- International guarantees.

This framework document was drafted by the Perm Five with only the indirect participation of the concerned parties. The Cambodian factions were consulted throughout, of course, as were Vietnam and ASEAN, one of whose members, Indonesia, was cochairman of the PICC's Co-ordinating Committee. In reality, the agreement had to be sold to those who would have to implement it. Initially, both the SOC and Vietnam accepted the principles of the document [A/45/477; S/21702, 9/4/90]. In a press statement released in Beijing, Prince Sihanouk, on behalf of the three resistance factions, gave full support to the framework document in his capacity as President of Cambodia and of the CNR [A/45/471; S/21687, 8/31/90].

Neither the SOC nor Vietnam, however, had forgotten the U.N. position regarding Vietnamese actions in Cambodia since 1979, namely, the annual votes of disapproval in the General Assembly and the 1981 U.N. International Conference on Kampuchea (ICK), not to mention Democratic Kampuchea's presence in the General Assembly.

In mid-September at an "informal meeting on Cambodia" in Jakarta, the PICC's two cochairmen presented the framework document to the Cambodian factions and then acted as midwives to the birth of Cambodia's Supreme National Council, a key element of the plan [A/45/490; S/21732, 9/17/90]. The three resistance factions—especially the Khmer Rouge, whose political legitimacy was now enhanced—reiterated their approval. Still expressing agreement "in principle," the SOC continued to refer to the August framework document as a "basis for further negotiation."

On September 20, 1990, the U.N. Security Council adopted a resolution endorsing the framework and indicated that it would welcome the Supreme National Council as Cambodia's representative at the United Nations [S/Res/668 (1990)].

However, at the first full-fledged meeting of the SNC in Bangkok, the differences between the SOC and the resistance resurfaced and caused the meeting to break up in disarray. The argument centered on whether Prince Sihanouk should be invited to chair the SNC and, if so, whether he should become its 13th member or replace one of the Sihanouk delegation's two members [see the CNR's denunciation of the SOC, conveyed to the U.N. in A/45/620; S/21866, 10/10/90]. Despite these obvious problems, the General Assembly adopted without a vote a draft resolution endorsing Security Council Resolution 668 (1990) [A/45/L.5, 10/15/90].

During the succeeding months, the Cambodian parties, under the guidance of the PICC's cochairmen and U.N. special representative Rafeeuddin Ahmed, negotiated the specific elements of the draft framework document. It became apparent that practical elements of the "agreement in principle" that existed immediately following publication of the Perm Five framework in August were not acceptable to the SOC. Vietnam increasingly assumed a hands-off attitude, out of respect for the SOC's presumed "sovereignty," and stated that it could do little more than communicate the position of the United Nations and PICC cochairmen to its Phnom Penh ally [*Far Eastern Economic Review*, 11/22/90, 12/6/90, 1/31/91].

Among the SOC's objections were crucial aspects of the Perm Five plan's implementation under the **U.N. Transitional Authority in Cambodia (UNTAC)**, which would supervise the peace process in-country for many months. It had become clear by this time that the reservations of the SOC were based not only on principles but on the realization that the Phnom Penh regime's hold on political power would be challenged by the proposed peace process.

In Phnom Penh the draft framework had taken on domestic political ramifications. Prime Minister Hun Sen, the SOC's chief negotiator, had come under sharp criticism from conservative elements in the Khmer People's Revolutionary Party (KPRP) for having yielded too much. Another factor was the cloud of Sino-Vietnamese disagreement that continued to hang over Cambodia negotiations throughout late 1990, despite the top-level meeting of Vietnamese and Chinese government and Communist party leaders in September in Chengdu, Sichuan province, reportedly held to seek an understanding on Cambodia. Beijing, it seemed, had concluded that Hanoi had gone back on its pledge to induce the SOC to cooperate with the Perm Five plan—in Chinese eyes, yet another case of "Vietnamese perfidy" [ibid., 10/4/90].

These negotiations by the PICC cochairmen culminated in the December 21–23, 1990, meeting of the Cambodian parties in Paris. At that time, it was apparently believed by some PICC members that the clarifications provided to Phnom Penh and Hanoi by U.N. Under-Secretary Ahmed might be sufficient to gain the SOC's and Vietnam's agreement. On January 8, 1991, the PICC chairmen's final statement laid out the details of the U.N. plan, together with an "explanatory note concerning certain provisions of the drafts" by Under-Secretary Ahmed [A/46/61; S/22059, 1/11/91].

The **U.N. plan** stipulates a two-stage cease-fire and then a transitional period beginning with the entry into force of an agreement signed by all the Cambodian parties. This period terminates when a constituent assembly is elected and a constitution drawn up and approved, after which the constituent assembly becomes a legislative body and a new government is created [Part I, Article 1].

Some of the agreement's major principles are:

• The Supreme National Council with 12 members representing all factions—six from the SOC and two from each of the three opposition groups—is formed. The SNC is the "unique legitimate body and source of authority in which, throughout the transitional period, the sovereignty, independence, and unity of Cambodia are enshrined" [Part I, Article 3]. It represents Cambodia at the United Nations and internationally. The

SNC commits itself to holding "free and fair elections organized and conducted by the United Nations as the basis for forming a new and legitimate government" [Part I, Article 4].

• UNTAC, having civilian and military components and under the direct responsibility of the U.N. Secretary-General, is put into place. The SNC delegates to UNTAC "all powers necessary to ensure the implementation of the agreement. . . . In order to ensure a neutral political environment conducive to free and fair general elections, administrative agencies, bodies, and offices which could directly influence the outcome of elections will be placed under direct United Nations control." Special attention will be paid to five SOC ministries: foreign affairs, national defense, finance, public security, and information. Other SOC government entities continue to operate normally, but under certain circumstances they can come under UNTAC "control," "supervision," or "investigation" [Part I, Article 6].

• Any foreign forces, advisors, and military personnel still in Cambodia are withdrawn under UNTAC verification [Part I, Article 8].

• A cease-fire then takes effect, with all forces disengaging and refraining from hostilities and "deployment, movement or action that would extend the territory they control or that might lead to renewed fighting." The U.N. Secretary-General is asked to provide good offices to assist in the cease-fire process until UNTAC's military component can supervise, monitor, and verify it [Part I, Article 9].

• All outside military assistance to all Cambodian parties ceases [Part I, Article 10].

• Elections are held "under United Nations auspices in a neutral political environment with full respect for the national sovereignty" and "all Signatories commit themselves to respect the results of these elections once certified as free and fair by the United Nations" [Part II, Articles 12–14].

• All Cambodians, inside the country or living outside as refugees or displaced persons, enjoy the rights and freedoms embodied in the Universal Declaration of Human Rights. Other signatories agree to respect these rights and (in an oblique reference to the Khmer Rouge period) are encouraged "to prevent the recurrence of human rights abuses" [Part III, Article 15].

• Cambodian refugees and displaced persons outside Cambodia have the right to return and "to live in safety, security and dignity, free of intimidation or coercion of any kind." The United Nations facilitates their repatriation "as an integral part of the comprehensive political settlement" [Part IV, Article 20].

"The Devil is in the details"—this is surely the case in a Cambodia settlement. The annexes that elaborate the principles set forth in the main agreement and detail the modalities of their implementation are extremely important. They take up 22 of the document's 37 pages. The annexes address the proposed mandate for UNTAC regarding civil administration, military functions, elections, and human rights; withdrawal, cease-fire, and related measures; repatriation of refugees and displaced persons; and principles for a new constitution for Cambodia.

The "**explanatory note**" appended to the main agreement as Annex III attempts to clarify UNTAC's relationship to the SNC, and it too is critically important. It reemphasizes inter alia that the SNC is the sovereign power in Cambodia and that it delegates to UNTAC only those functions necessary to ensure fair and free elections. The note explains how the United Nations sees these powers being exercised, how consultation is performed with the SNC, and how differences of opinion between the two might be handled. The note says UNTAC would exercise "certain personnel powers" in civil administration only if "certain individuals have acted in a manner inconsistent with the objectives of the settlement agreement." These clarifications are designed to allay the SOC's fear of the "dismantlement" of its administrative structure, something the NGC has demanded.

The explanatory note also describes the two-phased cease-fire plan. It states that each step of the phased disarmament and demobilization will be taken only after the previous step has been completed to the satisfaction of all parties.

During the autumn months of 1990, there was considerable optimism among PICC members, including the cochairmen and the United States, that the Perm Five plan could be explained and amplified sufficiently to the SOC and Vietnam to render it acceptable. In November, there were hopes that at the Jakarta meeting in December the document would actually be signed and that a full-fledged PICC could reconvene in early 1991 to ratify it. The plan would then be returned to the United Nations for final approval, and implementation could begin during the first half of 1991. So went the hopeful scenario.

It was not to be. Soon after Jakarta, peace negotiations lapsed into a stalemate once again [*Far Eastern Economic Review*, 1/3/91]. This stalemate continued well into 1991. The three resistance factions were prepared to sign the Perm Five agreement as it is currently written. Their reaction to the implications of the "explanatory note," however, was ambiguous. The SOC, on the other hand, refused to sign the agreement and was therefore seen as the intransigent party [*Asian Wall Street Journal Weekly*, 2/25/91]. The Cambodian parties' inability to make functional the essential first step in the

Perm Five plan—the Supreme National Council—because of their disagreement on the chairmanship question was a major roadblock to progress. The Perm Five and the PICC cochairmen made three formal demarches on this point during October and November alone, but to no avail [A/45/671; S/21908, 10/25/90; A/45/719; S/21940, 11/13/90; and A/45/829; S/21985, 12/6/90].

There were other fundamental points of disagreement. Sovereignty and genocide are issues of principle that have a practical impact on peace negotiations. Regarding the first, the SOC claims that it has the great majority of Cambodia's geography and population under its control or significant influence. Although it appears to endorse the idea of U.N. supervision in a settlement, it has objected to "an unacceptable degree of intrusiveness" into the five key ministries the U.N. plan envisions, saying that UNTAC should be restricted to supervising elections. The SOC maintains that UNTAC should not become involved in governance to an extent that amounts to the "dismantlement" of the SOC. As of July 1991, it was still unclear whether the plan's "explanatory note," and negotiations among the Cambodian parties themselves, had resolved this issue.

Genocide refers to the Pol Pot era, during which a million or more Cambodians died. From the early days of peace talks, the Phnom Penh regime sought to make the nonrecurrence of genocide a prominent feature of any settlement document. In any election, it would expect to use this issue against the Khmer Rouge, who would be running as the DKP. For obvious reasons, the latter refuses to accept any language that would block senior Khmer Rouge cadres from participating in Cambodia's political life and could even lay the groundwork for eventual trials for "crimes against humanity."

Other unresolved issues are the conditions under which cantonment (or regroupment), disarmament, and demobilization of the armed forces of the Cambodian factions will take place. While the three resistance groups have accepted the current language, the SOC has not, citing what it claims are vague provisions for enforcement, supervision, and control. It makes the point that while the SOC's military units are conventional and for the most part stationed in fixed, easily identifiable positions, the Khmer Rouge guerrilla units are based mainly in jungle, forest, and mountain areas, and thus not susceptible to international control. The SOC evidently seeks a more detailed UNTAC plan, including comprehensive on-site measures in Khmer Rouge zones so that precise verification and supervision become possible.

The SOC has stated that it might agree to national elections after cantonment but before full disarmament; that is, when arms are stacked under U.N. supervision but are not yet irretrievable. This has been rejected by the resistance, since the SOC could gain an advantage in much of the country. For the peacemakers, the dilemma is to find a realistic formula under which the Cambodian parties would be willing to lay down their arms before an election—and not take up arms again after. With regard to demobilization, the SOC fears that the Khmer Rouge might demobilize partially or cosmetically but, owing to its disciplined cadre organization, would regroup rapidly and conduct politico-military warfare out of uniform. The resistance factions, of course, have similar suspicions of the SOC and KPRP. To date, the United Nations, the Cambodian parties, and the PICC cochairmen have not been able to achieve a satisfactory formula on these contentious points.

U.S. policy regarding Cambodia continued to evolve during the period following the "Baker shift" of July 1990 [see Robert G. Sutter, *The Cambodian Crisis and U.S. Policy Dilemmas* (Boulder, Colo.: Westview Press, 1991)]. In April 1991 the **Bush administration** attempted to get the U.N. process moving again by laying out a "road map" for **normalization of relations between the United States and Vietnam.** It offered a four-step timetable for reciprocal actions concerning a peace settlement in Cambodia and U.S.– Vietnam bilateral problems. In testimony before the House Foreign Affairs Committee (HFAC) and Senate Foreign Relations Committee (SFRC)—and in formal presentations to the Vietnamese and SOC authorities in New York and Vientiane, respectively—the administration also sought to overcome Hanoi's and Phnom Penh's objections on the issues of sovereignty, genocide, and dismantlement ["Cambodia and Vietnam: Time for Peace and Normalization," testimony of Department of State Assistant Secretary for East Asian and Pacific Affairs Richard H. Solomon before the HFAC Asia and Pacific Affairs Subcommittee, April 10, 1991. Mr. Solomon's April 11, 1991, testimony before the SFRC is identical in substance. See also *The New York Times, The Washington Post,* and *The Wall Street Journal,* 4/12/91].

Arguing that the Perm Five documents could not be renegotiated because this "would be an endless exercise likely to undermine the settlement process," the administration cited the plan's "explanatory note." By so doing, the administration signaled its explicit acceptance of certain key assurances by the U.N. negotiators and thus attempted to remove some of the ambiguities that the SOC has used as justification for rejecting the Perm Five plan.

Disavowing any intention to dismantle the Phnom Penh administrative structure during the pre-election period, the administration stated that UNTAC's role would be to bring about free and fair elections in a neutral political environment and thus establish a "legitimate government." The administration emphasized UNTAC's peacekeeping functions in all areas of Cambodia (that is, Khmer Rouge as well as SOC) and its monitoring functions to encourage compliance with the settlement agreement, including cross-border resupply of any faction. It pointed out that the disarmament and demobilization would occur in stages, with verification by all parties at each stage to ensure compliance.

On genocide, the Bush administration went slightly beyond previous formulations, pledging to state at the time of signing a settlement—unilaterally, if necessary—its "strong support for those elements of the settlement agreement designed to protect the human rights of the Cambodian people and to ensure that such genocidal violence never again occurs."

A high-level U.S. mission led by General John Vessey, President Bush's special emissary to **Vietnam** for humanitarian affairs, visited Hanoi, April 19–21, 1991. The visit yielded the announcement of the opening of a temporary U.S. POW/MIA office in Hanoi to investigate unresolved cases of American servicemen still listed as missing from the war. The United States also announced a "humanitarian" grant of $1 million to Vietnam for prosthetics assistance, the first official U.S. aid to that country since 1975 [*The Asian Wall Street Journal Weekly*, 4/15/91; *The New York Times*, 4/21/91, 4/26/91].

Vietnam's overall reaction to the U.S. "road map" was subdued, no doubt because the United States had again clearly linked normalization to a Cambodia political settlement based upon the Perm Five plan as now written [*Far Eastern Economic Review*, 4/25/91]. Vietnam reiterated its support for the Perm Five framework and a U.N. role in implementing an agreement but emphasized the need to respect Cambodia's sovereignty. On linkage, Vietnam said that it sought normalized relations with the United States on its own merits, regardless of Cambodia [press release, SRV Permanent Mission to the U.N., 4/16/91].

Pressure to get the peace process moving again came from other sources as well. In late April, France and Indonesia, the PICC cochairmen, noting "with concern the recent reports of intensified fighting in Cambodia," appealed to all parties "to exercise maximum restraint" and to observe a cease-fire beginning May 1, 1991 [SG/SM/4559, 4/22/91]. Their purpose was to create favorable conditions for another—and, it was hoped, more productive—meeting of the SNC in Jakarta. To the surprise of many observers, all four Cambodian parties eventually accepted the call for a voluntary cease-fire, and on May 1 it entered into force.

Although the parties charged one another with violations and with using the cease-fire as cover for reinforcement, it held sufficiently well to allow the U.N. Secretary-General to announce that the PICC cochairmen would send a three-man military team to make an on-the-spot review of the situation [SG/SM/4565, 5/6/91]. Headed by Major-General Timothy Dibuama, the Secretary-General's Military Advisor, the team began by visiting resistance camps along the Thai-Cambodian border, and planned to visit Phnom Penh subsequently [UPI, AP, Reuters, 5/13/91].

In a cautiously hopeful atmosphere, the SNC met again in Jakarta, June 2–4. Familiar problems continued to elude resolution. The Khmer Rouge insisted that there be no changes in the U.N. Perm Five plan, while the SOC demanded that some provision be made for a war crimes tribunal for persons accused of genocide. The cochairmen of the PICC—Indonesia's Foreign Minister Alatas and France's Deputy Foreign Minister Vivien—accepted a Phnom Penh proposal that the plan stipulate that Cambodia's new constitution be "consistent with the provisions . . . of the UN Convention on the Prevention and Punishment of Crimes of Genocide." This was the first time a reference to genocide had been accepted in official documents related to the U.N. peace plan. The cochairmen said that although progress had not been as great as desired, there were grounds for hope. They announced at the conclusion of the SNC meeting that the PICC would be convened at an unspecified later date.

It was on the question of SNC leadership that the June Jakarta meeting made significant headway. Prior to the last meeting, Prince Sihanouk (not then an SNC member) and SOC Prime Minister Hun Sen had agreed on a formula in which Sihanouk would be added to the SNC as chairman, Hun Sen would serve as vice-chairman, and another member would be added from the Phnom Penh side to replace Hun Sen, thus raising the membership to 14. The Khmer Rouge did not agree to this arrangement, which had been rejected by them in October 1990. Following the SNC meeting, however, Sihanouk announced his decision "to join the SNC as one of its 12 members, a simple member," replacing one of the ANS representatives. This move, which was endorsed by Hun Sen, would give Sihanouk de facto primacy in the SNC yet allow Hun Sen equal status formally. It would also tend to marginalize the political capacity of the Khmer Rouge (which announced on June 6 that it would no longer honor the cease-fire).

On June 8 the Cambodian parties announced that the SNC would reconvene in Thailand on June 24. Even more surprising was Sihanouk's invitation to Hun Sen to visit him in Pyongyang during the summer, and the announcement that the Prince would go to Phnom Penh for two months beginning in November, his first visit to that city since January 1979. In a separate meeting in Jakarta immediately after the SNC talks,

China's Foreign Minister, Qian Qichen, affirmed Chinese support for the Sihanouk-Hun Sen agreement and expressed the hope that the SNC would become operational quickly.

At the June 24 SNC meeting held in Pattaya, Thailand, and presided over by Prince Sihanouk, there was further progress on key issues. The Cambodian parties agreed to continue the cease-fire and to implement a ban on foreign military aid. They agreed to set up the SNC's headquarters in Phnom Penh, thus permitting the accreditation of diplomatic missions to the SNC. (Australia immediately announced its intention to open a mission; Japan, Thailand, and France appeared ready to follow suit.) The three resistance factions would be allowed to open and operate their own offices—a remarkable development, given the past decade's bitter hostilities. And Sihanouk declared his desire to take up residence in Phnom Penh once more to help guide the reconciliation process.

The next meeting of the SNC, scheduled for Beijing in July, was to continue discussions on a peace settlement and on Sihanouk's role. Still to come were Perm Five consultations later in the summer, and eventually a reconvened PICC—assuming that the Cambodian parties were able to sustain the momentum achieved during the first half of 1991.

7. Cyprus

The division of the little Mediterranean inland of Cyprus into Turkish-occupied and Greek Cypriot–governed zones is a running wound on Europe's southern border, one that poses problems as the continent attempts to draft new security arrangements. The conflict pits two members of the North Atlantic Treaty Organization (NATO)—Greece and Turkey—against one another; it complicates arms and strategic negotiations in the region and will have to be dealt with as the big European agencies—NATO, the European Community, the West European Union, the Conference on Security and Cooperation in Europe (CSCE), and the Council of Europe—move toward a new post–Cold War structure.

Despite the issue's importance, little progress was made toward resolving the conflict this year. World attention was focused on the Gulf crisis, and negotiations on Cyprus have not yet recovered from their crashing collapse in March 1990.

Cyprus has been a divided island since 1974, when Turkish forces invaded following stepped-up persecution of Turks by Greek Cypriots and a coup d'état by Greek Cypriot militarists who favored Greece's

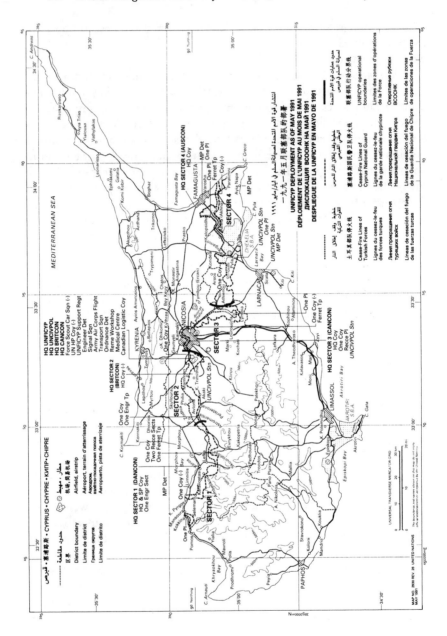

annexation of the island. Roughly 200,000 Greek Cypriots are said to have fled the occupied portion of the island following the invasion, leaving roughly 100,000 Turkish Cypriots, about 18 percent of the population, in control of 40 percent of the territory. There have been allegations that up to 80,000 settlers from mainland Turkey have moved to the island since the invasion [*Le Soir*, 10/5/90].

The Turkish-controlled part is secured by an estimated 35,000 troops. It is governed by Rauf Denktash, the Turkish Cypriot leader who unilaterally declared an independent Turkish Republic of Northern Cyprus on November 15, 1983. Only Turkey recognizes this entity; the United Nations and all of its members other than Turkey recognize only the Greek Cypriot government based in Nicosia. Nevertheless, the Secretary-General has negotiated in the past with Denktash in his capacity as representative of the Turkish Cypriot community, according to the mandate given to him by the Security Council.

The world body's presence in Cyprus dates back to March 4, 1964, when the Security Council established the **U.N. Peacekeeping Force in Cyprus (UNFICYP)** because the situation at the time presented a threat to international security. Since the invasion, UNFICYP has maintained a buffer zone between the two regions that extends about 180 kilometers across the island. The U.N. High Commissioner for Refugees (UNHCR) and the World Food Programme (WFP) run efforts to assist those harmed by the conflict.

For 16 years the United Nations has tried to win both sides' agreement to reunify the island under a federal government. Both the General Assembly and the Security Council have affirmed numerous times their recognition of the Republic of Cyprus and their opposition to a permanent division of the island. The Security Council formally condemned the unilateral declaration of independence three days after Denktash declared it.

Most plans put forth by the United Nations have centered on the creation of some form of "bizonal, bicommunal, and federal" Republic of Cyprus under which both halves of the island would be largely autonomous. On March 12, 1990, Security Council Resolution 649 reaffirmed the Council's wish to see a settlement along those lines.

Secretary-General Javier Pérez de Cuéllar offered a **unification plan,** accepted by the Turkish side but rejected by the Greeks, in January 1985. Four months later Denktash rejected a revised peace plan that took Greek Cypriot views into account. In March 1986 the Greek side rejected a third version of the U.N. peace proposal and demanded that Greek Cypriots be accorded "three freedoms": the right to move around the island freely, settle anywhere, and own property anywhere. The Turkish side accepted the U.N. proposal but equivocated on the three freedoms. Pérez de Cuéllar tried once more to solve this difficult conflict in late 1989 and early 1990.

Efforts to forge a settlement suffered a major blow in early March 1990, after a round of talks in New York betweeen Pérez de Cuéllar, Denktash, and Greek Cypriot President George Vassiliou. Pérez de Cuéllar made some concessions to Denktash, describing the Turkish Cypriot side as participating in the talks on an equal footing—a key Turkish Cypriot demand. The Greek side also appeared willing to accept some temporary restrictions on the three freedoms in order to prevent Turkish Cypriots from being swamped by returning Greek settlers. The talks collapsed when Denktash demanded that his people be granted the right to "self-determination" and that this right be enshrined in any future Cypriot constitution. This demand stoked Greek Cypriot fears that the Turks might choose secession [*The Washington Post*, 3/3/90]. The Greek side balked, and the Secretary-General also criticized Denktash's demand, claiming it was outside the framework for a settlement approved by the Security Council and the General Assembly.

Security Council Resolution 649 reaffirmed the framework, speaking of "two communities" while supporting earlier resolutions and agreements calling for a settlement that would retain the island's independence, territorial integrity, and sovereignty, and that would not allow for secession or union with another nation.

There has been little progress since then, other than a March meeting between Denktash and a group of Greek politicians [*Le Monde*, 3/21/91]. NATO members want the issue resolved to eliminate conflicts between Greece and Turkey. The Soviet Union remains nervous about an island state allied to a NATO member (Turkey) but not covered by arms control agreements. Cyprus's recognized Greek government has said it wants to join the European Community. Turkey has also indicated a desire to join the Community, but Greece, already an EC member, could veto that application if the Cyprus question is not resolved.

8. Other Colonial and Sovereignty Issues

The scenes this year of millions of Kurds fleeing Saddam Hussein's troops while allied forces sat on the sidelines, or of Baltic and Armenian protesters being shot down by Soviet soldiers, revealed once again a paradox in the idea of "colonialization." The notion of a "colony," as enshrined in myriad U.N. documents and in international law, has been used over the past 40 years to free dozens of territories from outside control. However, as often as not, it has also been used to uphold the status quo, to ignore the claims of clearly indigenous and distinct peoples who seek independence or self-government. International law recognizes as a colony only what various U.N. or other international forums, for whatever political reasons, declare to be colonies; the rest fall outside the boundaries of the present international power structure.

Thus, Palestinians are a distinct people with a right to "self-determination" according to various nonbinding General Assembly and binding Security Council resolutions; Kurds, though they have their own language and distinct, ancient culture, have no land of their own because it suited neither the Middle East's ex-colonial powers nor their Arab allies to recognize the Kurds when they drew up a map of the region 70 years ago.

More recently, Namibia was, until its independence, Africa's last colony, according to the United Nations, while Eritrea remains a nonissue and the Western Sahara something in between. The Western Saharan Berbers' strongest ally, Algeria, itself faces internal strife from its own Berber minority in the Kabyle, some of whom want independence. Puerto Rico is a territory deprived of the right to self-determination, according to various votes of the Special Committee on Decolonization [GA/COL/2706, 8/17/89]. Yet Guadeloupe, Tahiti, Lithuania, Sikkim, Tibet, and a long list of clearly distinct regions seized by U.N. member states are not.

The official list identifies approximately 18 territories—located mainly in the Atlantic and Pacific Oceans—as non-self-governing, affecting approximately 3 million people. Two major problem areas—**Namibia and the Falkland Islands (Malvinas)**—slid off the hot-spot list in 1990, with the former winning independence from South Africa and holding U.N.–sponsored elections and the latter dispute moving to the back burner after Great Britain and Argentina resumed relations in February 1990.

A third source of conflict, the **Western Sahara,** may be on the road to resolution. Morocco seized the territory from Spain in 1975 and has since colonized it with hundreds of thousands of troops and settlers. Since then the small Frente Popular para la Liberación de Gaguia el-Hamra y de Rio de Oro (Polisario) has battled Moroccan troops. It claims to represent 200,000 Sahraoui nomads, who do not recognize the Moroccan King Hassan II's right to rule over the land; the last Spanish census in 1974 placed the number of Sahraouis in the 110,000-square-mile territory at only 76,000 [The New York Times, 4/22/91].

For years Hassan II refused to recognize the Polisario; he finally did so in August 1988, under pressure from the OAU. Numerous Security Council resolutions have called on Morocco to negotiate with the rebels. Talks toward a settlement foundered as Algeria backed the rebels and Moroccan forces constructed huge walls of sand across the territory to isolate the guerrillas. However, the restoration of Moroccan-Algerian ties in 1989, the rebels' increasing military weakness, and growing international pressure on King Hassan to improve his human rights record appear to have unstuck the peace process.

Talks throughout 1990 and early 1991 have centered on the holding of a territorial referendum under U.N. auspices, through which natives will be able to choose between independence and annexation. Hassan II accepted the idea in principle at an OAU summit in 1981 [Le Monde, 4/12/91]. Pérez de Cuéllar, confident enough that he had won both Polisario and Moroccan approval, finally presented firm plans for a referendum to the Security Council in April 1991 [S/22464]. His report, based on an earlier proposal of June 1990 [S/21360], recommends the emplacement in the territory of the U.N. Mission for the Referendum in Western Sahara (MINURSO), a 1,700-man U.N. peacekeeping force that would monitor a cease-fire to be declared on an agreed "D-Day." Over an 11-week period following a cease-fire, Morocco would reduce its troops in the territory to 65,000, confining those that remain to defensive positions along the sand wall and in bases. The Polisario would do the same. Political prisoners and prisoners of war would be exchanged.

In one key proposal, a special Identification Commission would take 11 weeks to register voters eligible to participate in the referendum, based on the last Spanish census of the colony. Moroccans who have settled in the region since the invasion would be excluded, leaving only native Sahraouis to decide on the region's fate.

About 285 civilian personnel would then oversee the return of refugees, with UNHCR support, and the holding of the referendum 20 weeks after D-Day. All for a cost of $200 million.

It now remains up to the parties to agree on a D-Day, but last-minute hitches could arise. Most Moroccans support their nation's continued possession of the Western Sahara as a matter of national pride; losing it would be a strong blow to Hassan II's esteem. Given his already shaky domestic situation, the monarch probably will not allow a referendum unless he is sure of winning.

East Timor is a particularly grave case of colonialism—some might say genocide—against an indigenous people. Indonesia annexed the Portuguese colony in 1976. Since then, Indonesian forces have murdered or allowed to die 100,000 to 200,000 people, as a result of torture, disease, malnutrition, and forced deportation [*The Financial Times*, 11/7/90]. The 600,000 Timorese are Catholic and seek independence from predominantly Muslim Indonesia; the United Nations still regards Portugal as the administering power. While the Special Committee on the Situation with Regard to the Implementation of the Declaration on the Granting of Independence to Colonial Countries and People—a committee whose long name some say masks its short list of accomplishments—continues to hold brief hearings on East Timor, both it and the General Assembly defer action on the situation each year as a result of pressure from Indonesia's friends.

Portugal and Indonesia agreed on May 9, 1989, to resume talks under U.N. auspices on East Timor's future. But the situation has gotten worse since then. In October 1990, Indonesian forces began a crackdown on Timorese opposed to their own deportation from the region as well as to the influx of Indonesian colonists [Agence France Presse, 10/28/90]. Up to 50 people disappeared and 90 more were executed, according to Portuguese relief agencies [*Le Monde*, 1/30/91]. Numerous witnesses testified to continued Indonesian human rights abuses in the Special Committee's summer hearings [A/45/23, 9/27/90]. Twelve thousand government forces have largely smashed the FRETELIN rebel group; it now has only 200 guerrillas [*The Financial Times*, 11/7/90].

In an uncharacteristic move, **Australia,** usually quick to defend human rights, signed in December 1990 a pact with Indonesia dividing up the oil reserves in the Timor Gap, East Timor's territorial waters. Portugal contends that this is a clear violation of international law, as Indonesia's control over East Timor and its water and resources has never been recognized. Thus, Australia is in effect negotiating with a thief over stolen goods. In March 1991, Lisbon filed a suit against Australia in the International Court of Justice over the matter [*Le Journal de Genève*, 3/13/91].

The **International Trusteeship System,** supervised by the Trusteeship Council, was created under the U.N. Charter to oversee trust territories administered by colonial powers. The goal was to move the trust territories toward independence, if they so chose, or toward permanent association with other nations. Of the original 11 trust territories, ten have become independent or joined neighboring countries. On December 22, 1990, the Security Council—which has final say on strategic territories—just missed terminating the system when it voted to end trusteeship over three of four Pacific island groups belonging to the 11th territory, the Trust Territory of the Pacific Islands. That Trust, composed of the Federated States of Micronesia, the Marshall Islands, the Northern Mariana Islands, and Palau, has been under U.N.–authorized U.S.–administered trusteeship since 1947. The first two island groups have drawn up compacts of free association with the United States; the Mariana Islands have agreed to become an American commonwealth. The Security Council voted, therefore, 14 to 1—with only Cuba against—to recognize the agreements and to end U.N.–trusteeship over the islands [S/Res/683].

The final island state, Palau, has drafted a compact of free association with the United States. However, the compact has not come into force because it would allow the United States to place nuclear weapons on the territory, in violation of the Palauan constitution. Several referendums have failed to garner the 75 percent majority needed to alter the constitution in favor of the compact's nuclear agreement. Thus, Palau remains the final Trusteeship territory, until it works out an agreement with the United States that matches its constitution.

Finally, there are over 12 other territories that the Special Committee considers each year, recommending resolutions to the General Assembly. Among the resolutions adopted by the General Assembly are:

• A resolution on the French Pacific territory of **New Caledonia,** acknowledging the "positive measures" France has taken to promote progress toward self-determination.

• Resolutions on the **Cayman Islands, Bermuda, the Turks and Caicos Islands, Anguilla, Montserrat, and the British Virgin Islands**— all administered by the United Kingdom—that raised several issues, including the need to protect these lands from drug traffickers, the requirements of development, the problems posed by military bases, and the region's "right to self-determination and independence," to be ensured by the British.

• Similar resolutions on **American Samoa, Guam, and the U.S. Virgin Islands,** all belonging to the United States. Guam remains in limbo because of a 1987 Commonwealth Act endorsed by the islanders. It must be approved by the U.S. Congress, but Congress believes portions of the Act recognizing rights of native Guamians, the Chamorros, are unconstitutional and discriminate against other U.S. citizens. The Assembly urged speedy resolution of that issue.

• A consensus on **Pitcairn,** the rocky Pacific outcrop peopled by the mutineers from the famous HMS *Bounty,* that urged Britain to "respect the very individual lifestyle that the people of the Territory have chosen" and to "promote the economic and social development" of the territory.

• A resolution on **Tokelau,** administered by New Zealand, that noted the Tokelauans' opposition to regional nuclear testing, their fears of toxic waste dumping and global climate change, and their rights to self-determination and independence.

• A resolution on the French territory of **Mayotte** [A/45/I.13] that again urged France to accelerate negotiations with the Islamic Republic of the Comoros over the territory's fate. One hundred eighteen countries voted in favor; only France voted against.

Every year there are additional resolutions and programs for funding development projects, social and cultural plans, and other U.N. programs to aid newly decolonized peoples or those still under foreign control. The General Assembly has named the **1990s the International Decade for the Eradication of Colonialism;** a report on the Decade from the Secretary-General [A/45/624] listed member countries' activities. The report from Iraq did not mention the Kurds, India's did not mention Sikkim, and China's ignored Tibet.

On what some, but not all, might consider a more humorous note, there are signs that other organizations are adopting the vocabulary of official U.N. functions on colonialism. From May 26 to 28, 1990, Barcelona saw the convening of the first Conference of West European Nations Without a State. At the conference, representatives of Corsican, Catalan, Northern Irish, Breton, Welsh, Basque, and other European groups who seek their regions' independence discussed and passed U.N.-style resolutions. The groups' distinct native tongues made up the conference's "official languages" [*Imprecor*, 7/13–26/90]. Just one more reminder that the difference between colonized peoples recognized under international law and those who are not owes much to historical luck and political circumstance.

II
Arms Control and Disarmament

By the end of 1990, East-West confrontation had practically disappeared. The idea of a "peace dividend" attracted wide discussion within Western governments and internationally. It looked as if reduced military budgets might free resources for assistance to emerging Eastern European countries, Third World states, and social spending in the West. The "peace dividend" discussion sputtered out, however, as Iraq's invasion of Kuwait on August 2 led to a massive military response and reinforced the arguments of those who believed that security threats abounded even in the wake of East-West accommodation. A U.N. Security Council unhampered by superpower confrontation voted to impose sanctions on Iraq and permitted military action against it, underscoring the reality that even as the Cold War ended, serious threats of armed conflict remained in much of the world.

Following the "four plus two" negotiations that established major power agreement over German reunification, and assurances to Poland that current borders would be respected, East and West Germany officially unified on October 3, 1990. In November the members of the Warsaw Treaty Organization (WTO) and the North Atlantic Treaty Organization (NATO) agreed in principle in Paris to limit the deployed military equipment of **Conventional Forces in Europe** (CFE) at equal levels, requiring significant cuts by the Eastern bloc. By the time the agreement was reached, the WTO was disintegrating as a military alliance. On July 1, 1991, members of the WTO formally dissolved the organization.

A **U.S.–Soviet summit** conference had been planned for February 1991 as the final session for negotiating the **Strategic Arms Reduction Treaty (START)** and for signing the treaty. The summit was postponed indefinitely due to the ongoing war in the Gulf, because of U.S. concerns that instability in the Soviet Union made it an unpropitious time to conclude the agreement, and because of U.S. uncertainties about **Soviet**

CFE compliance. Some issues of verification, definitions, and counting rules also remained to be worked out to complete the START treaty.

Despite increasing confidence that East-West relations would not return to armed confrontation, the United States and Britain remained convinced that military strength in general, and nuclear deterrence in particular, preserved international stability. Citing remaining uncertainties about the future of the Soviet Union, the threat of global weapons proliferation, and the need to continue testing in order to maintain the safety and reliability of existing nuclear weapons, the two states resisted calls for a nuclear **Comprehensive Test Ban (CTB)**. They sought to insulate the upcoming **Fourth Review Conference of the Parties to the Treaty on the Non-Proliferation of Nuclear Weapons (NPT)** from demands of non-nuclear countries for prompt negotiation of a CTB. States seeking a CTB had called for the **Amendment Conference of the Parties to the Treaty Banning Nuclear Weapon Tests in the Atmosphere, in Outer Space and under Water** (or Partial Test-Ban Treaty, **PTBT**). In the summer of 1990 they agreed to hold the PTBT conference after the conclusion of the NPT review. The NPT review ended without a consensus document because Mexico and other leading CTB proponents were unable to reach agreement with the United States and United Kingdom on wording dealing with the test ban issue. In major steps forward for the NPT in June 1991, **France** announced that it would reverse long-standing policy and sign the Treaty; and on July 8, South Africa signed it.

In the **Conference on Disarmament (CD)**, negotiations in the ad hoc committee on a **chemical weapons (CW) treaty** were slowed by U.S. and Soviet reluctance to dispose of their CW stockpiles prior to multilateral acceptance of a control regime. The desire of Arab states to link CW limits to Israeli denuclearization complicated the negotiations. General fears about CW proliferation were underscored by Iraqi threats to use such weapons during the Gulf war. In May the United States renounced the use of CW for any purpose, including retaliation against chemical attack, and said it would destroy its CW stockpile once a treaty was signed [*The New York Times*, 5/14/91].

During the coalition's six weeks of aerial bombardment of Iraq, Iraq responded with more than 70 Scud missile attacks against Saudi Arabia and Israel, but apparently all of these were armed with conventional explosives. Coalition bombings targeted Iraqi chemical, biological, nuclear, and other military production installations, as well as a wide array of infrastructure, communications, and industrial targets. Following a brief period of ground combat, coalition sources reported finding Iraqi chemical artillery shells in ammunition dumps, but there was no evidence that CW had been used.

Iraqi use of the Scud missiles brought a resurgence of public attention to the problem of ballistic missile proliferation and the Group of Seven's 1987 **Missile Technology Control Regime (MTCR)** agreement. In February 1990 the Soviet Union had indicated that it would abide by MTCR export guidelines [*F.A.S. Public Interest Report* 44, no. 2 (3-4/91):3]. Proposals for conventional arms control in the Middle East after the war reflected the realization of major arms suppliers that they had just fought a war against an adversary they themselves had armed in the preceding decade.

On May 29, in a speech at the Air Force Academy, President George Bush proposed that the world's five major arms suppliers—China, France, Great Britain, the United States, and the Soviet Union—establish guidelines to constrain arms transfers to the Middle East. The plan called for the five nations to curb the sale of the most destabilizing conventional weapons to states in the region. Bush proposed a freeze on the purchase, production, and testing of surface-to-surface ballistic missiles and a verifiable ban on the production and acquisition of nuclear weapons materials. He urged all states in the region to sign a global ban on chemical weapons and to abide by the 1972 biological weapons convention [*The New York Times*, 5/30/91]. A few days after the Bush speech, France called for global controls on weapons production and transfers [*The New York Times*, 6/4/91]. Talks were held in Paris, July 8–9, and agreement was reached to reconvene in September.

But negotiating arms export limits did not mean that weapons sales to the region would be ended. U.S. Secretary of Defense Dick Cheney, on a trip to the Middle East, said that the United States "cannot fall into the trap" of saying that "arms control means we don't provide any arms to the Middle East." The United States announced its intention to give ten used F-15 fighters to Israel, to continue funding Israel's Arrow antiballistic missile system, to sell helicopters to the United Arab Emirates and Bahrain, and to consider selling tanks and other armored vehicles to those two Arab states [*The New York Times*, 6/5/91].

As a result of the end of the Cold War, discussions in the 1990–91 General Assembly and Conference on Disarmament continued the recent trend toward focusing on substantive issues and reducing the time and effort devoted to purely symbolic matters. General Assembly **First Committee** members urged continued reduction and consolidation of agenda items to be carried over to future sessions of the Committee and the Conference. They expressed impatience with the pace of progress toward a CW treaty and with the obstruction of a CTB agreement. They greeted progress in CFE and START negotiations enthusiastically and encouraged continuation of both processes. They were more optimistic than in previous years in their official outlooks on multilateral arms control and disarmament efforts, mirroring the general improvement in U.N. morale since the end of the Cold War. Renewed progress in the CW negotiations, movement on U.S.–Soviet strategic arms talks, and the likelihood of multilateral discussions on conventional arms transfer limitations were positive signs in mid-1991. Optimism was tempered by the apparent stalemate on CTB and continued arms sales, especially to states in the Middle East.

1. Nuclear Arms Control and Disarmament

Essential agreement on a bilateral U.S.–Soviet **Strategic Arms Reduction Treaty (START)** had been reached by the time of the 45th Session. The draft treaty limits the United States and Soviet Union to 6,000 warheads each, but the counting rules are such, especially for bomber-based weapons, that the actual numbers of deployed warheads will be higher.

Under the draft treaty, no more than 4,900 warheads may be deployed on submarine-launched ballistic missiles (SLBMs) and land-based intercontinental ballistic missiles (ICBMs). The remaining 1,100 warheads covered by the treaty may be deployed on heavy bombers as bombs, air-launched cruise missiles (ALCMs), or short-range attack missiles (SRAMs). The total number of delivery vehicles for the 6,000 warheads is limited to 1,600. Either side can shift warheads under the limits from ballistic missiles to bombers, but not the other way around.

Submarine-launched cruise missiles (SLCMs) with ranges exceeding 600 kilometers will be limited to 880 for each side under a separate agreement. The Soviets will be limited to 500 medium-range Backfire bombers, and the Soviets have agreed not to modify the bombers to enable in-flight refueling. Neither the SLCMs nor the Backfires will count under the START 6,000 warhead or 1,600 delivery vehicle limit.

It was estimated in April 1991 that the agreement would reduce the total numbers of strategic nuclear warheads from 12,081 to 10,395 for the United States and from 10,841 to 8,040 for the Soviet Union. Soviet land- and submarine-based ballistic missile warheads would be reduced by approximately 48 percent, from about 9,396 to 4,900, while U.S. missile warheads would decline by about 35 percent, from 7,506 to 4,879. U.S. air-launched cruise missiles (ALCMs) would likely increase from about 1,600 to 1,860, while Soviet ALCMs could expand from 480 to

1,300 [*Arms Control Today* 21, no. 3 (4/91): 30–31]. Under the START agreement, the Soviet Union will reduce its deployment of "heavy" ICBMs from 308 to 154, thus significantly reducing the total "throw weight" of its strategic nuclear forces. Mobile land-based ICBMs will be permitted under the agreement, limited to 1,100 warheads for each side.

Although the agreement was largely complete, in the early part of 1991 momentum toward its final signature decreased. An early conclusion to the treaty was delayed by the Gulf war, U.S.–Soviet disagreement on CFE interpretations [ibid., no. 2 (3/91):25], U.S. worries about Soviet internal politics, and differences within the U.S. administration over treaty details [*The New York Times*, 6/7/91]. In the spring, momentum recovered and it appeared that the treaty would be signed at a Moscow summit in the summer. Three substantive issues were still under negotiation in June: test telemetry, "downloading," and the definition of new types of missiles.

The **telemetry** question hinged on what, if any, exemptions there would be from the agreement to broadcast openly test data from ballistic missiles during flight testing. The **"downloading"** issue had to do with how many warheads would be counted as typical of a multiple warhead system after the number of warheads was reduced from an earlier figure. If numbers were revised downward, then the two sides could redeploy the same number of warheads on more missiles and then "break out" by adding warheads quickly above treaty limits. The **"new types" issue** concerned how big a change would constitute an (unlimited) new type of missile system. The United States wanted a "new type" definition that would allow minor changes to an existing system. It was concerned that an existing system (in which there were already many missiles) could be slightly modified, redefined, and then rapidly deployed with a large number of warheads [*Arms Control Today* 21, no. 2 (3/91): 25-28].

The 45th Session welcomed "positive developments" in U.S.–Soviet bilateral nuclear disarmament efforts and called upon them to sign a START agreement and to "intensify" efforts to reach agreements in other areas, particularly a comprehensive nuclear test ban and an agreement to ensure that outer space is kept free of all weapons [A/Res/45/59B]. It can be expected that note will be taken at the 46th Session of the further progress of START negotiations, and the two states will be urged to pursue further bilateral arms reductions and confidence-building measures (CBMs) in a **START II** process.

2. European Security

Questions of European security have essentially disappeared from the U.N. agenda. The 45th Session took place while the final divisions of

Europe were disappearing, and it can be expected that by the 46th Session further progress will have been made to end the armed confrontation that for so long dominated European relations.

At the **November NATO-WTO summit meeting in Paris,** agreement was reached on the CFE treaty that had been in the works for the previous one and a half years. The treaty creates numerical limits for deployments of five types of weapons in Europe from the Atlantic to the Urals by all 22 WTO and NATO countries, and establishes a verification and information exchange regime for the area. The two sides are each limited to 20,000 tanks, 30,000 armored combat vehicles, 20,000 artillery pieces, 6,800 combat aircraft, and 2,000 attack helicopters. No single country can have more than about one-third of the total of such arms, which is essentially a limitation on the size of Soviet forces in Europe.

Under CFE treaty Article VII, NATO and the former members of the WTO will allocate deployments among themselves and then announce how many of the weapons will be deployed in each country. These will become binding limitations on deployments until general notification of a reallocation is made. Regional sub-limits prevent destabilizing force concentrations. Even with the breakup of the WTO, its former members will still negotiate among themselves to establish individual limits. The CFE treaty does not include personnel limits, a topic that absorbed considerable attention during the spring and summer of 1990 [see *Issues Before the 45th General Assembly,* pp. 72–74]. Personnel limits, aerial inspection measures, and "stabilizing measures" (such as limits on military exercises, call-ups of reserves, and transfers of troops within Europe) are to be addressed in negotiations called **CFE IA** after full agreement is reached on CFE I.

On May 28 the German Defense Minister Gerhard Stoltenberg and British Defense Minister Tom King, with the agreement of U.S. Defense Secretary Dick Cheney, announced that NATO would radically **reduce and restructure its forces** in the decade beginning in late 1994. The cuts would turn NATO into a smaller, more mobile standing force with additional units in reserve. The resulting force would have four main components: a brigade-sized (15,000-person) mobile unit for rapid reaction to a crisis; approximately four divisions capable of responding in five to seven days; seven defense corps each of 50,000 to 70,000 troops to operate in Central Europe; and another force of active and reserve troops, probably American, that could reinforce the existing units in case of imminent war. The U.S. force level in Europe would be reduced by at least 50 percent from its current 320,000 [*The New York Times,* 5/21/91, 6/9/91].

Discussions on **Confidence- and Security-Building Measures**

(CSBMs) among the 34 **Conference on Security and Cooperation in Europe (CSCE)** members also continued. Current plans are to complete both CFE IA and CSBM agreements by the time the March 1992 CSCE review meeting opens. A follow-up **CFE II** is to begin thereafter, expanded to include the 34 members of the CSCE.

Under the November 21 Charter of Paris, following the 1992 CSCE meetings the CSBM and CFE negotiations will be merged into the 34-nation CSCE process [*Arms Control Today* 21, no. 1 (1-2/91): 12-16]. The November summit reached agreement that heads of state would meet every two years for CSCE consultations and that their foreign ministers would meet annually. A small secretariat is to be established in Prague, an election observation office will be established in Warsaw to oversee democratic elections in member states, and a conflict prevention center is to be established in Vienna [*The Christian Science Monitor*, 11/21/90].

While ratification of the CFE treaty appeared imminent in the winter of 1990–91, progress slowed as the United States and its European allies shifted their attention to the Gulf crisis and questioned Soviet transfer of ground forces from the CFE-counted army land forces into naval units [*The New York Times*, 2/15/91]. Eastern European states remained concerned about Soviet armed intervention in the Baltic states, and U.S. members of Congress were reluctant to press ahead with CFE while it appeared that Soviet politics might be shifting toward greater repression. Negotiations continued in mid-March, but the two sides apparently made little progress toward final agreement on interpretations of CFE. The United States indicated its belief that without agreement, further progress on the START negotiations would be difficult [*Arms Control Today* 21, no. 3 (4/91): 20]. In June the United States and the Soviet Union announced that they had reached agreement on CFE and were proceeding to resolve their differences over START. A summit conference appeared probable for later in the summer [*The New York Times*, 6/4/91].

Efforts to negotiate limits on **short-range nuclear forces (SNF),** following Soviet proposals of summer 1990, slowed as the CFE talks accelerated. NATO countries agreed in July to take up the SNF issue once CFE was signed, but because of the welter of other issues—final CFE discussions, START, Middle East arms control, and the Gulf war—attention was diverted from SNF. For U.S. decision-makers, the massive reductions planned under the CFE treaty reduced the urgency of agreement on an SNF, and some apparently felt that reductions would take place more rapidly if they did so de facto rather than under a perhaps slowly forthcoming negotiated framework [*Arms Control Today* 21, no. 1 (1-2/91): 17–21].

By the time of the 46th Session further progress in CFE IA is quite likely, and the START treaty may have been signed. At the 45th Session laudatory messages and calls for further progress were the main references to the European security situation, and this can be expected again at the 46th Session.

3. Chemical and Biological Weapons

In addressing the 45th General Assembly, President George Bush again called for the completion of an international ban on the production, possession, and use of chemical weapons, citing tensions in the Gulf as reason to focus on the issue again [*Bulletin of the Atomic Scientists* 46, no. 10 (12/90): 8]. The United States and Soviet Union had made considerable progress over the previous summer, agreeing bilaterally to cease production of CW agents, on the size of their respective stockpiles, and on the desirability of large-scale reductions [see *Issues Before the 45th General Assembly*, pp. 75–76]. However, progress in the CD over the draft treaty slowed in the winter due to concerns about chemical weapons in the Middle East and about U.S. and Soviet determination to delay full destruction of their chemical weapon stockpiles until the control regime was in place and accepted by all states with CW capabilities. The pace of the negotiations picked up again in the spring.

In the October 1990 meetings of the CD and at the April 1991 session of the CD's **Ad Hoc Committee on Chemical Weapons,** the United States proposed a treaty provision under which countries with chemical arsenals could retain up to 500 tons of nerve gas (2 percent of the current U.S. level) for eight years if a "special conference" of treaty members decided that not enough countries were participating in the convention to warrant complete stockpile elimination. For the United States, "sufficient" treaty participation apparently would mean the adherence of all countries with chemical weapons capabilities. The United States justified its stand by asserting that it was intended to encourage adherence to the treaty. The Soviets accepted the U.S. position. Critics of the superpowers' position called for a commitment to destruction of all chemical weapon stocks, as had been negotiated before the October proposals. Critics further noted that an exception that permitted a two-tier system, like that of the NPT, would permit other chemical weapons states, such as Iraq and Libya, to retain CW stockpiles [*Bulletin of the Atomic Scientists* 46, no. 10 (12/90): 48–49].

At the 45th General Assembly the superpowers' position was criticized by advocates of the existing CW treaty draft text. For example, the Mexican representative to the First Committee argued that the proposals were "aimed at placing conditions on and postponing a decision on the total elimination of chemical weapons, and would give greater rights to States that possess them. If these proposals were accepted there could emerge a sort of juridical limbo with regard to the scope and implementation of the multilateral convention" [A/C.1/45/PV.7: 17]. Meanwhile, at least in the United States, efforts were under way to tighten export controls over CW technologies [*The New York Times*, 3/6/91].

On May 12, President Bush announced that the United States was "forswearing" the use of chemical weapons "for any reason" and that it would destroy all CW stockpiles once a treaty was signed [ibid., 5/14/91]. The U.S. timetable called for completion of the CW treaty near the end of 1991, with Senate ratification being sought in spring 1992 [*Arms Control Today* 21, no. 4 (5/91): 4].

The 45th Session adopted without vote **three resolutions** dealing with chemical and biological weapons. First, it called upon states to observe the 1925 Geneva **Prohibition of the Use in War of Asphyxiating, Poisonous or other Gases and Bacteriological Methods of Warfare,** welcomed U.S. and Soviet agreement to cease producing chemical weapons and to begin their destruction, urged the CD to reestablish its Ad Hoc Committee on Chemical Weapons, urged states to provide information on their CW stockpiles and capabilities to "promote confidence and openness in order to contribute to an early agreement on, and universal adherence to" a CW convention, and included the issue of CW and BW on the agenda of the 46th Session [A/Res/45/57A].

Second, it noted that the second preparatory committee meeting for the **Third Review Conference of the Parties to the Convention on the Prohibition of the Development, Production and Stockpiling of Bacteriological (biological) and Toxin Weapons and on Their Destruction** would be held in April 1991. It recalled that the Secretary-General had been asked by the 44th Session to circulate among parties to the Convention a report on implementation of confidence-building measures relating to the Convention, and it called for universal accession to and ratification of the Convention by states that had not yet done so [A/Res/45/57B]. The April 8–12 preparatory meeting set the review conference for September 9–27, 1991. The Conference will consider "the impact of scientific and technological developments relevant to the Convention," the relevance to it of progress on the CW treaty, and whether further measures are needed to improve the Convention [U.N. press release DC/2358, 4/19/91].

Third, the 45th Session condemned violations of the **1925 Geneva**

Protocol on CW and BW, called upon states to observe it, endorsed the establishment of a group of experts to investigate reports of the use of such weapons, and underlined the continuing importance of Security Council Resolution 620 of 1988, which calls for effective measures in the event of the use of such weapons in violation of international law [A/Res/45/47C].

The Bacteriological Weapons Convention Review Conference and the 46th Session's consideration of CW and BW issues will be strongly affected by the progress, or lack thereof, in the 1991 discussions of the CD's Ad Hoc Committee on Chemical Weapons. If, as it appeared would be the case in mid-1991, significant progress is being made and a CW treaty is imminent, the 46th Session should reflect renewed optimism over the prospects for multilateral arms control measures.

4. Nuclear Nonproliferation and Nuclear Weapon–Free Zones

The **Fourth Review Conference of the Parties to the Treaty on the Non-Proliferation of Nuclear Weapons (NPT)** was held just prior to the 45th Session, from August 20 to September 15, 1990. The conference was considered particularly important because in 1995 the 25-year-old NPT will come up for termination or extension, as required by NPT Article X. Despite large areas of agreement, the confence of 84 signatory governments ended without adopting a final document. Diasgreement over the **Comprehensive Test Ban (CTB)** disrupted emerging consensus.

In the end, the United States and Mexico could not agree on references to the importance, role, and necessity of negotiating a CTB treaty. The Mexican–U.S. disagreement was over language on which other participating states were apparently willing to compromise [*Bulletin of the Atomic Scientists* 46, no. 10 (12/90): 39–44]. The Conference president, Oswaldo de Rivero Barreto of Peru, sought a compromise by which divergent views would be summarized in the final text, but Mexico refused to accept the proposed text [U.N. press release DC/2326, 9/17/90: 2].

Despite the lack of consensus, some major strides were made at the Review Conference. For the first time, nuclear technology supplier states agreed to require a commitment from recipients not to acquire nuclear weapons and to accept **International Atomic Energy Agency (IAEA)** safeguards on all their peaceful nuclear activities—so-called full-scope safeguards—as a condition for the transfer of nuclear supplies to non-nuclear weapon states. France and China, not having signed the NPT, would not have been bound by such an agreement, but pressure from the other suppliers might have moved them toward full-scope safeguard commitments [*Bulletin of the Atomic Scientists* 46, no. 10 (12/90): 41].

The draft declaration called on the IAEA to study the possibility of inspecting suspicious nuclear facilities in NPT member states not declared to the Agency under its safeguards agreements. If carried out, this would be the first step toward broadening IAEA inspection activities to include a form of "challenge" inspection and on-site observation of undeclared facilities, activities that the IAEA is authorized to take under its Statute, but never implemented [ibid.].

The conference agreed to consider further a Nigerian proposal for multilateral security assurances to non-nuclear states in the event that they were threatened with, or attacked by, nuclear forces. The draft document urged states that had not yet reached safeguards agreements with the IAEA under the NPT to do so, adding that security assurances from the nuclear weapon states would aid in this process. These declarations emerged from a discussion of North Korea's failure to complete its safeguards agreement with the IAEA and to submit technical information about its nuclear facilities to the agency in a timely fashion (thus possibly being in violation of the treaty) despite having signed the NPT [*Bulletin of the Atomic Scientists* 46, no. 10 (12/90): 43; U.N. press release DC/2326, 9/17/90: 4]. Similarly, the 45th Session passed a resolution endorsing CD negotiations toward binding security assurances, and placed the issue on the agenda for the 46th Session [A/Res/45/774].

The draft final document of the NPT review also endorsed the further establishment of **Nuclear Weapon–Free Zones (NWFZs)**, commending operation of the 1968 **Treaty for the Prohibition of Nuclear Weapons in Latin America (Tlatelolco Treaty)**, and taking approving note of the 1986 **South Pacific Nuclear Zone Treaty (Treaty of Rarotonga)**. It endorsed the idea of a Middle East Nuclear Free Zone, declared that development of nuclear weapons by the Republic of South Africa would undermine the NPT, called on South Africa to sign the NPT and accept safeguards on all its nuclear facilities, and took note of efforts of the **Association of South-East Asian Nations (ASEAN)** to establish an NWFZ. The conference reviewed treaty provisions on the peaceful uses of nuclear energy, agreeing on a statement declaring attacks against safeguarded nuclear facilities as matters warranting U.N. Security Council action, and agreeing too that the unsafeguarded programs of non-NPT parties, particularly Israel and South Africa, constituted threats to the peaceful uses of nuclear energy. It urged states that had not done so to sign and ratify the NPT and complete safeguards agreements with the IAEA. There are now **141 states parties to the NPT**, the most recent adherents being **Mozambique** and **Albania**. France's announcement that it would sign the NPT left China as the only treaty holdout among the original five nuclear weapon states [*The New York Times*, 6/4/91].

On June 9, 1991, North Korea informed the IAEA that it would sign safeguards agreements required under the NPT. Although North Korea signed the treaty in 1985, it did not complete safeguards agreements with the agency within the required 18-month time period. Until June 9 it had been demanding that the United States remove its nuclear weapons and troops from South Korea as a condition for completing the agreement. During the year, North Korea was heavily criticized for activities at its Yongbyon nuclear complex, which observers claimed had nuclear weapons applications. The United States, the Soviet Union, and Japan were pressuring North Korea to complete its safeguards arrangements [ibid., 6/9/91].

Pakistan's Prime Minister Nawaz Sharif proposed on June 6, 1991, that the United States, the Soviet Union, and China bring India and Pakistan together to discuss regional denuclearization [ibid., 6/7/91]. U.S. assistance to Pakistan was suspended in the fall of 1990 upon the failure of the U.S. administration to certify to Congress that it was not developing nuclear weapons. On June 7 a representative of India's External Affairs Ministry rejected the Pakistani proposal for regional negotiations, calling instead for a "nuclear-free world" [ibid., 6/8/91].

U.N. Security Council **Resolution 687** required **Iraq** to report on the location and condition of its CW, biological weapons (BW), and nuclear facilities, materials, and stockpiles in order for a permanent cease-fire to come into force. In a series of letters in April, Iraq reported to the IAEA and to the United Nations that 24 nuclear installations were destroyed, and that it retained more than 25 pounds of highly enriched uranium fuel from France, 66 additional pounds of enriched uranium from the Soviet Union, 6 tons of depleted uranium, and 1.8 tons of low enriched uranium [ibid., 5/1/91, 5/17/91].

IAEA inspections of Iraq's nuclear facilities began in mid-May. A defecting Iraqi nuclear scientist's revelations led to challenges of the government's descriptions of its nuclear inventory and to repeated inspections. On July 8, Iraq admitted it had produced highly enriched uranium in clandestine nuclear facilities. It thus became the first NPT member explicitly to have violated the treaty. Observers estimated that Iraq might have produced 55 pounds, enough for a weapon [ibid., 7/9/91.]

Having received a report from the Secretary-General on conditions for the **Establishment of a Nuclear Weapon–Free Zone in the Middle East** [A/45/435, Annex], the 45th Session urged that steps be taken toward establishment of an NWFZ; called upon those Middle Eastern states that had not done so to submit to IAEA safeguards; invited them to support the NWFZ idea; called upon states in the region not to develop, produce, test, or acquire nuclear weapons or permit them to be stationed on their territories; invited the nuclear weapon states and all others to help establish the NWFZ; and requested that the Secretary-General submit to the 46th Session a report on the implementation of the resolution, including it in the agenda [A/Res/45/52].

The 45th Session passed a resolution reiterating earlier condemnations of Israel's refusal to renounce nuclear weapons and its military cooperation with South Africa. It expressed concern regarding Israel's continuing production, development, and acquisiton of nuclear weapons and testing of their delivery systems, called upon it to place its nuclear facilities under IAEA safeguards and not to attack others' facilities, called on other states not to cooperate with Israel in military or nuclear areas, requested the Secretary-General to report to the 46th Session on Israeli nuclear developments, and included the item "Israeli Nuclear Armament" on the agenda [A/Res/45/63]. Also on the agenda for the 46th Session is an item deferred from the 45th, dealing with "Armed Israeli aggression against the Iraqi nuclear installations and its grave consequences for the established international system concerning the peaceful uses of nuclear energy, the nonproliferation of nuclear weapons, and international peace and security" [A/Res/45/430].

On September 24 at the 45th Session, Brazilian President Fernando Collor de Mello called on all Latin American and Caribbean states to ban all nuclear explosives. Collor revealed a long-standing, secret Brazilian nuclear weapons program, which he had placed under a new director opposed to weapons development. On November 28, he and Argentine President Carlos Saul Menem signed a declaration that the two will jointly negotiate full-scope safeguards agreements with the IAEA and move to bring into force the Tlatelolco Treaty for their two countries [*Arms Control Today* 20, no. 10 (12/90): 14–15; *IAEA Bulletin* 32, no. 4 (4/90): 45–46]. The 45th Session again deplored France's failure to ratify its signature of Protocol I of the treaty, under which it would bind itself not to emplace nuclear weapons in, or transfer them through, the treaty area, and placed the issue on the agenda for the 46th Session [A/Res/45/48].

At the IAEA General Conference in September 1990, South African Foreign Minister Roelof "Pik" Botha reiterated his country's willingness to accede to the NPT "in the context of an equal commitment by other states in the southern African region." Although none of South Africa's neighbors are anywhere near a nuclear capability, several of them have not signed the NPT. Reports indicate that there is disagreement within the South African government over what, if any, conditions should be fulfilled for South Africa to agree to sign. One possibility is that South Africa will seek lifting of the boycott on its export of uranium as a condition for its accession. Meanwhile, Botha promised to negotiate with the IAEA on the possible form of safeguards eventually to be implemented on his country's extensive nuclear facilities [*Bulletin of the Atomic Scientists* 47, no. 1 (1–2/91): 27–28]. The General Conference again passed a resolution condemning Israel's refusal to place its nuclear program under IAEA safeguards [GC(XXXIV)/Res/526]. Over the objections of mostly Western European and North American states, it resolved that the 1991 General Conference would consider and take a decision on previous recommendations by the IAEA Board of Governors to suspend South Africa from "the exercise of the privileges and rights of membership of the Agency" [ibid.].

The 45th General Assembly called upon all states to abide by the **Declaration on the Denuclearization of Africa** adopted by the **Organization of African Unity (OAU)** in 1964. It condemned South Africa's pursuit and development of a nuclear capability and the cooperation extended to it by other states, especially Israel. It called for safeguards on all of South Africa's nuclear facilities and for monitoring of its nuclear development, asked the Secretary-General to assist the OAU in convening a meeting of experts in Addis Ababa in 1991 to consider preparing a convention or treaty on the denuclearization of Africa, called for termination of all forms of nuclear and military collaboration with South Africa, and requested that the Secretary-General report to the 46th Session about South Africa's "evolution in the nuclear field," placing the issue on the agenda of the 46th Session [A/Res/45/56 A, B]. South Africa's July signing of the NPT should alter the tone and substance of future discussions of its nuclear program and policies. It may now resume its former place on the IAEA's Board of Governors as the African state most advanced in the development of nuclear technology.

On October 1, 1990, the United States suspended approximately $700 million in aid to Pakistan when the U.S. executive branch failed to certify to Congress that Pakistan was not developing nuclear weapons. In November, Prime Minister Nawaz Sharif stated that he would accelerate Pakistan's nuclear power program, asserting that Pakistan was opposed to the destructive use of atomic power and was pursuing a peaceful program [*The New York Times*, 11/8/90]. The 45th Session called for **Establishment of a Nuclear Weapon–Free Zone in South Asia,** placing the issue on the agenda for the 46th Session [A/Res/45/53], with only Bhutan, India, and Mauritius voting negatively. The 45th Session also adopted a resolution again endorsing **Implementation of the Declaration of the Indian Ocean as a Zone of Peace,** calling for preparations for a Conference on the Declaration to be held in Colombo, Sri Lanka, in 1992, and asking the Ad Hoc Committee on the Declaration to report to the 46th Session on implementation of the Declaration. The resolution passed by a vote of 128–4–17, with France, Japan, the United Kingdom, and the United States opposed [A/Res/45/77].

Once again endorsing the idea that one way to limit incentives for nuclear proliferation would be to increase the security of non-nuclear weapon states, the 45th Session passed a resolution on Conclusion of effective international arrangements to assure non-nuclear-weapon States against the use or threat of use of nuclear weapons. The resolution particularly urged that negotiations in the CD on this topic continue, noting that no objections in principle to the concept had emerged in ongoing negotiations. It called for the item to be discussed again at the 46th Session [A/Res/45/54].

5. Nuclear Testing

Over the summer of 1990 the United States and the Soviet Union agreed on verification procedures for the 1974 **Threshold Test-Ban Treaty (TTBT)** and the 1976 **Peaceful Nuclear Explosions Treaty (PNET).** On September 25 the U.S. Senate gave its consent to the ratification of the two treaties. On October 9 the Supreme Soviet approved them. Under the TTBT, the two countries limited underground nuclear weapons tests to a yield of 150 kilotons. The PNET established the same ceiling for all nuclear explosions. Attached to the U.S. Senate ratification were contradictory declarations that both endorsed a U.S. commitment to negotiate a CTB and called for continued weapons testing. The Soviet ratification appealed for a total test ban.

Initiated in 1985 by six nonaligned states—Indonesia, Mexico, Peru, Sri Lanka, Venezuela, and Yugoslavia—the six-year effort by non-nuclear weapon states seeking to press forward with a CTB forced the **PTBT** depositary states—the United States, the United Kingdom, and the Soviet Union—to convene an **Amendment Conference on the Treaty Banning Nuclear Weapon Tests in the Atmosphere, in Outer Space and under Water,** January 7–18, 1991, in New York [see *Issues Before the 44th General Assembly:* 66–67; *Issues/45:* 77–78; *Arms Control Today* 20, no. 9 (11/90); *Bulletin of the Atomic Scientists* 47, no. 3 (4/91): 10]. Having managed to postpone the meeting until after the NPT review, the United States and the United Kingdom made it clear at the

January meeting that they were opposed to a CTB at that time, although they accepted the concept as a long-range objective.

The United States objected to the amendment process on both substantive and procedural grounds. Substantively, it argued that since international security and stability depended on nuclear deterrence, continued testing was essential in order to detect possible weaknesses in weapons safety, effectiveness, and survivability. A testing halt would, without preventing production of nuclear weapons, create uncertainty about the safety and credibility of the weapons stockpile. Procedurally, the United States argued that it was inappropriate to use the amendment process to convert the PTBT (the purpose of which, it argued, was not to ban nuclear tests but primarily to prevent radioactive pollution from such explosions) into a CTB, which would be a wholly new treaty. It therefore announced its refusal to take part in or to finance any continuation of the conference beyond the January meeting, and indicated that it would veto any amendment to the PTBT that came to a vote in the conference. The United States proposed instead that a CTB should be pursued in the CD, through the Ad Hoc Committee established for the purpose [U.S. Mission to the U.N., Press Release USUN 01-(91), 1/10/91: 8].

The United States and the United Kingdom announced that they would reject any amendment to the PTBT, so the other participants called instead for a vote on continuation of the negotiations—which would not require unanimity to pass. The proposal to continue negotiations passed by a vote of 74 to 2 with 19 abstentions. It was the first time an amendment procedure had been invoked under any disarmament treaty and the first time the non-nuclear states had proposed detailed verification and sanctions provisions for a nuclear limitation treaty. The conference called upon its president, Foreign Minister Ali Alatas of Indonesia, to undertake consultations to achieve "progress on those issues" and to reconvene the conference "at an appropriate time" [*Bulletin of the Atomic Scientists* 47, no. 3 (4/91): 10–11; *Arms Control Today* 21, no. 2 (3/91): 14–17].

The 45th General Assembly, while urging states to negotiate toward a CTB at the Amendment Conference, called on all states to stop nuclear testing, urged the CD to reestablish its Ad Hoc Committee on a Nuclear Test Ban, reaffirmed its conviction that "a treaty to achieve that prohibition of all nuclear-test explosions by all states in all environments for all time is a matter of fundamental importance," urged the CD to encourage worldwide technical measures to develop verification methods, called upon the CD to report to the 46th Session, and placed three items dealing with the CTB on the agenda [A/Res/45/49–51].

6. Special Sessions on Disarmament and General and Complete Disarmament

At the 46th Session, as at the 45th, a series of agenda items will be considered that brings before the General Assembly the resolutions of the General Assembly Special Sessions on Disarmament (SSODs), reiterates past resolutions under the rubric of General and Complete Disarmament (GCD), and serves as a way for the General Assembly to urge continued progress in ongoing negotiations outside of its own forums.

Multilateral arms control measures appear at present to be making substantive progress in the CD, in conferences reviewing particular treaties, such as the NPT, and as a consequence of regional negotiations, such as the CFE/CSCE process. The resolutions flowing from the omnibus multilateral approach of the Special Sessions have become essentially pro forma reminders by the General Assembly of issues still requiring action, and exhortations for progress in other forums.

Under the rubric of matters implementing the decisions and resolutions of the **first SSOD** (Tenth Special Session), the 46th Session will receive reports from the Disarmament Commission and Conference on Disarmament [A/Res/45/62 B, D] and from the Advisory Board on Disarmament Matters [A/Res/38/183O], as well as reports on the status of multilateral disarmament agreements [A/Res/36/92H]; on the activities of the United Nations Institute for Disarmament Research [A/Res/39/148H]; on the economic and social consequences of the armaments race and its extremely harmful effects on world peace and security [A/Res/43/78J]; on the progress of the Comprehensive Programme of Disarmament [A/Res/44/119/A; 45/62E]; on the cessation of the nuclear arms race and nuclear disarmament [A/Res/45/62C]; and on the prevention of nuclear war [A/Res/45/62C].

From the **second SSOD** (Twelfth Special Session), the 46th Session will consider reports of the Secretary-General on regional disarmament [A/Res/44/117B]; on the U.N. disarmament fellowship, training, and advisory services program [A/Res/45/59A]; on the World Disarmament Campaign [A/Res/45/59C]; on the nuclear arms freeze [A/Res/45/59D]; on U.N. regional centers for peace and disarmament in Africa and in Asia, from the Pacific and U.N. regional center for peace; and on disarmament and development in Latin America and the Caribbean [A/Res/45/59E].

Under resolutions addressing GCD, the 46th Session will deal with notification of nuclear tests [A/Res/42/38C]; international arms transfers [A/Res/43/75I and decision 45/415]; implementation of General Assembly resolutions in the field of disarmament [A/Res/44/116G]; conversion of military resources to civilian purposes [A/Res/44/116J]; the relationship between disarmament and development [A/Res/45/58A]; prohibition of the development, production, stockpiling, and use of radiological weapons [A/Res/45/58F]; conventional disarmament [A/Res/45/58G]; prohibition of attacks on nuclear facilities [A/Res/45/58J]; prohibition of the dumping of radioactive wastes [A/Res/45/58K]; prohibition of the production of fissionable material for weapons purposes [A/Res/45/58L]; charting potential uses of resources allocated to military activities for civilian endeavors to protect the environment [A/Res/45/58N]; regional disarmament [A/Res/45/58P]; naval armaments and disarmament [decision 45/416]; and conventional disarmament on a regional scale [decision 45/418].

7. Other Issues

The 46th Session will consider multilateral agreements to create "transparency" of and reductions in military budgets [A/Res/44/114A, B]; compliance with arms limitation and disarmament agreements [A/Res/44/122]; and education and information for disarmament [A/Res/44/123]. Questions regarding arms control and international cooperation in outer space will also be considered [A/Res/45/55A; A/Res/45/72]. The 46th Session will review the operation of the **Convention on Prohibitions or Restrictions on the Use of Certain Conventional Weapons which May Be Deemed to Be Excessively Injurious or to Have Indiscriminate Effects** [A/Res/45/64], consider security and cooperation in the Mediterranean region [A/Res/45/79], review the implementation of the **Declaration on the Strengthening of International Security** [A/Res/45/80], and consider measures for the protection and security of small states [A/Res/44/51].

III
Economics and Development

1. The World Economy: Restrospect and Prospect

Nineteen ninety began by posing two questions of vital interest—(1) Would the strong rates of economic growth enjoyed since 1983 be sustained? and (2) What might reduce or reverse them?—and ended by offering decisive but not necessarily reassuring answers. Moreover, it left for its successor, 1991, a number of even more momentous questions: Would the Persian Gulf crisis, which began with Iraq's invasion of Kuwait on August 2, erupt into war? How long would a war last? Would a war result in serious damage to Middle Eastern oil fields and refineries? Would the crisis lead to a global recession? Would a long or deep recession turn into a depression? Would the world's trading system unravel?

Answers to the year's initial questions were provided on the one hand by the dramatic rise in the price of oil—from about $15 per barrel in July to about $33 in the aftermath of the invasion of Kuwait—and on the other hand by the somewhat delayed but nevertheless chilling effects of tightened macroeconomic (especially monetary) policies in the major industrial countries. Other contributing factors were adverse economic developments in Eastern Europe and the Soviet Union; economic stabilization measures in Latin America; and non-oil-related Gulf crisis developments, including the flight of foreign workers from Iraq and Kuwait, which created refugee crises in several countries in the region and the loss of those workers' remittances to their home countries. Together, these factors produced a world economic output growth rate of 2.0 percent, down from 3.25 percent in 1989 and 4.1 percent in 1988 [International Monetary Fund (IMF), *World Economic Outlook* (hereafter *WEO*), 5/91, p. 1]. Significantly, per capita world output declined for the first time since 1982 [United Nations, "The World Economy at the End of 1990: Short Term Prospects and Emerging Issues," E/1991/INF/1, 1/91, p. 1].

Attention naturally and appropriately focused on the international economic impact of the Gulf crisis, which dominated the second half of

93

the year in every respect. However, economic activity during the first half of 1990 was shaped principally by restrictive macroeconomic policies first adopted in mid-1988 by the major industrial countries (especially Germany, Japan, Canada, and the United States) in response to inflationary pressures. This helps explain, among other things, why both Canada and the United States slipped into recession before the Gulf crisis erupted [*The New York Times*, 4/27/91, p. 1].

The effect of the Middle East crisis was to tilt the wavering world economy toward recession. The conflict's principal economic result was a "spike," i.e., a sharp but temporary increase in the price of oil, which "left no country untouched" [E/1991/INF, p. 1]. The oil price shock, like its predecessors in 1973–74 and 1979–80, was expected to have negative price and income effects, or, in other words, to be both inflationary and recessionary. Moreover, it was generally expected that most countries would opt to give priority to fighting the inflationary effects of the oil price increase, a strategy that would reinforce recessionary tendencies. In short, slower growth seemed a certainty, which it proved to be.

In 1991 the rate of world output was expected to decline still further to 1.2 percent as negative influences that appeared during 1990 continued to operate and, in some instances, worsened. Specifically, it was anticipated that disruptions resulting from the Persian Gulf crisis, recessions in North America and the United Kingdom, a continuation of restrictive monetary policies in the industrial countries, and continued economic disarray in Eastern Europe, not to mention near-collapse in the Soviet Union, would contribute to a continuation of overall worldwide decline.

Many analysts attribute the decline to the restrictive monetary policies being followed in the major industrial countries. As mentioned above, these policies were initiated in response to steadily increasing average consumer price inflation in those countries between 1986 and 1989. The threat of an increase of unknown duration in oil prices during the second half of 1990 reinforced policy-makers' determination to restrain price levels. As oil markets calmed in late 1990 and early 1991, a looming question was whether the macroeconomic policy–induced recessions of 1990–91 would swiftly and decisively weaken underlying inflationary tendencies—and thereby permit a resumption of noninflationary expansion—or instead fail to dampen those tendencies, prompting policy-makers to 'stay the (restrictive) course' [Organization for Economic Cooperation and Development (hereafter OECD), *Economic Outlook*, 12/90, p. vii]. A clear indication came in late April 1991, when the other members of the Group of Seven (G-7) finance ministers rejected a U.S. plea for coordinated reductions in interest rates made by Treasury Secretary Nicholas Brady and strongly backed by President George Bush [*The Wall Street Journal*, 4/29/91, p. 2]. Thus, despite rising unemployment, especially in North America and the United Kingdom, **inflation** continued to be the primary target of the largest industrial countries as a group. In the United States, however, and to some degree in Canada and the United Kingdom, a consensus was emerging that the risk of global recession had overtaken the risk of global inflation and, therefore, that the stance of policy should shift from restrictive to expansionary [ibid., p. 1], at least in the short run. There were warnings, however, including some from the U.S. Federal Reserve, that premature and/or excessive easing of U.S. policies could lead to a surge of inflation alongside a U.S. recovery expected to begin in late 1991.

The Industrial Countries

There were two principal developments among the industrial countries in 1990. One was a **continuation of the slowdown in growth** that first appeared in 1989. Among the 24 OECD countries, growth averaged 2.8 percent in 1990, compared to 3.4 percent in 1989 and 4.4 percent in 1988 [*Economic Outlook*, p. viii]. The second development was a **growing disparity between two sets of industrial countries**—Japan and Germany on the one hand and, on the other, the United States, Canada, and the United Kingdom. Japanese growth actually increased in 1990, to 5.6 percent from 4.7 percent in 1989, and German growth (not including eastern Germany) rose to 4.5 percent from 3.8 percent. In contrast, U.S. output fell sharply in 1990, to 1 percent from 2.5 percent in 1989. (See Table III–1.) Canadian output fell to 1.1 percent from 3.3 percent, and British output fell to 1.6 percent from 2.2 percent.

Such clear evidence that the major industrial countries were at significantly different stages of the business cycle implied differences in macroeconomic policies and, in turn, more difficulty in coordinating economic policies. This difficulty revealed itself at the previously de-scribed meeting of G–7 finance ministers. The deep discord among the participants could not be masked by a statement of general agreement issued when the meeting adjourned [*The Wall Street Journal*, 4/29/91, p. A2].

Considering the fact that since early 1989 industrial countries' economic policies generally, and their monetary policies specifically, have mainly targeted inflation, it is important to ask whether any improvement was evident in this regard in 1990. Among the seven largest industrial countries consumer prices continued to rise, as they have since 1986 when the annual rate of increase was only 2.0 percent. However,

Table III–1
World Output, 1986–90

	1986	1987	1988	1989	1990
Output (percentage annual change)					
World	3.1	3.4	4.5	3.3	2.1
Advanced industrial countries	2.7	3.3	4.5	3.3	2.5
United States	2.7	3.4	4.5	2.5	1.0
Japan	2.6	4.3	6.2	4.7	5.6
West Germany	2.2	1.5	3.7	3.8	4.5
Developing countries	4.0	3.7	4.5	3.1	0.6
Africa	1.7	1.3	2.9	3.3	1.9
Asia	6.9	8.1	9.0	5.5	5.3
Middle East	−0.7	0.1	4.7	3.2	−1.5
Latin America	4.7	2.4	0.2	1.5	−1.0

Source: IMF, *World Economic Outlook*, 5/91, Table A1.

the rate of acceleration of price increases clearly slowed in 1990. Consumer prices rose 4.7 percent from 4.2 percent in 1989 and 3.1 percent in 1988 [WEO, 5/91, p. 140]. Among the G–7, the United Kingdom recorded the highest rate of consumer price inflation in 1990, 9.5 percent, up from 7.8 percent in 1989 and 4.9 percent a year earlier. Italy's rate was nearly unchanged at 6.5 percent. In the United States, consumer prices rose 5.3 percent in 1990, compared to 4.8 percent in 1989 and 4.1 percent in 1988; and Canada's rate fell slightly from 5.0 percent in 1989 to 4.8 percent, after having come in at 4 percent in 1988.

Japan and Germany tend to have a much lower tolerance of inflation and, therefore, a much lower threshold for activating anti-inflationary policies. (It is worth noting in this regard that while U.S., Canadian, British, and French inflation averaged between 6 and 9 percent per year between 1978 and 1987, both Japanese and German rates averaged about 3 percent per year during the same period.) Japan's inflation rate reached 3.1 percent in 1990, up from 2.3 percent in 1989 and, more important, from 0.1 percent in 1987. West Germany's experience was comparable. At 2.7 percent, German inflation in 1990 was virtually unchanged from its 1989 rate. However, the 1989 rate was significantly higher than the 1987 rate of 0.2 percent. Thus it was not surprising that the industrial countries, which had entered 1990 with anti-inflationary priorities, responded to the post–August 2, 1990, oil price shock by tightening those policies even further.

Interestingly, however, because of a slowing of labor force growth, the effects of nearly two years of restrictive macroeconomic policies were not immediately evident in OECD labor market indicators for 1990. Although the **unemployment rate** rose slightly in the United States and Canada, the average OECD unemployment rate actually fell slightly, to 6.2 percent from 6.4 percent. Japanese and German unemployment rates declined. Similarly, the number of unemployed workers in OECD countries fell 0.3 percent to 24.5 million. However, evidence of contraction was apparent elsewhere, namely, in the change in the rate of growth of employment in OECD countries, which fell from 1.8 percent in 1989 to 1.3 percent in 1990 [*Economic Outlook,* p. 20.]. Among the larger industrial countries, employment growth rates fell sharply between 1989 and 1990: in the United Kingdom from 3.1 percent to 1.1 percent, and in the United States and Canada from 2 percent to about 1 percent.

Despite the oil price shock in the second half of the year, 1990 witnessed continued progress in reducing large **current account imbalances** among the three major industrial countries—the United States, a deficit country, on the one hand, and Japan and Germany, both surplus countries, on the other. The U.S. current account deficit peaked in 1987 at $162.3 billion or 3.6 percent of gross national product. Since then, the deficit has narrowed steadily, reaching $99 billion or 1.8 percent of GNP in 1990. Japan's current account surplus peaked at $87 billion, also in 1987. (See Table III–2.) As a percent of GNP, Japan's surplus was greatest in 1986 at 4.4 percent. By 1990 the surplus has shrunk to $36 billion and only 1.2 percent of GNP. Germany's surplus rose to $55.4 billion or 4.6 percent of GNP in 1989, then narrowed in 1990 to about $45 billion or 3.0 percent of GNP as the two Germanies merged [*WEO,* 5/91; also *Economic Outlook,* 12/90].

In welcome contrast to the troubling events of the mid-1980s, these favorable current account developments have allowed the major industrial countries, on the whole, to focus on domestic rather than external economic policy objectives. However, because each country's circumstances differ, such objectives vary, and disagreements among the major industrial countries about appropriate macroeconomic policies now promise to become more frequent and perhaps more heated.

The improvement in current account imbalances among the major industrial countries was facilitated by the coordinated **realignment of exchange rates** beginning in late 1985. The decline of the U.S. dollar against the Japanese yen and German mark helped restore the competitiveness of U.S. products internationally and thereby improved the U.S. current account balance. After partial recovery in 1987–89, the dollar's decline continued during 1990 until it established record lows against the mark, yen, and Special Drawing Right (SDR). For different reasons, this

Table III–2
Payments Balances on Current Account, 1986–90

	1986	1987	1988	1989	1990
Payments balances on current account (billions of dollars)					
Advanced industrial countries	−25.1	−54.8	−52.4	−82.4	−110.7
United States	−145.4	−162.3	−128.9	−110.0	−99.3
Japan	85.8	87.0	79.6	57.2	35.7
West Germany/ Germany	39.7	45.8	50.4	55.4	44.5
Other	−5.3	−25.2	−53.6	−85.0	−91.7
Developing countries	−41.8	1.7	−14.0	−15.9	−29.0
Africa	−10.3	−5.1	−10.3	−8.9	−4.0
Asia	4.2	20.5	8.8	−1.9	−3.7
Middle East	−17.2	−4.2	−8.4	0.3	13.8
Latin America	−16.7	−10.4	−10.8	−8.9	−12.0

Source: IMF, *World Economic Outlook*, 10/90 and 5/91, Table A30.

continued decline troubled policy-makers of the United States and its major trading partners. The former feared the weak dollar's inflationary effects, while the latter feared its trade effects. However, there seemed to be broad agreement, at least for the time being, that improvement in the U.S. current account deficit warranted incurring both types of risk.

Looking ahead, the OECD expects its 24 mainly industrial member countries to record an average growth rate of only 1 percent in 1991, down from 2.8 percent in 1990. After 1991, however, more healthy growth rates are anticipated, beginning with a 3 percent increase in 1992 [*The Wall Street Journal*, 5/20/91, p. A15]. The IMF expects output among the seven largest industrial countries to expand at a rate of only 1.3 percent in 1991, down from 2.5 percent in 1990. However, the group's growth rate is expected to rise to 2.8 percent in 1992 [WEO, 5/91, p. 131].

Despite their relative optimism regarding 1992, both the OECD and the IMF believe that the situation in early 1991 requires that their forecasts be qualified. Much depends, they say, on the course of the U.S. recession, which began by mid-year 1990 and had been forecast by some analysts to end at mid-year 1991. In short, the recession was supposed to be short and shallow. If for any reason, however, it should become either a long or a deep recession, or both, most of the rest of the world, especially other industrial countries, would also probably be unable to grow as fast as expected in 1992. Among the most often cited factors that could extend or deepen the U.S. recession are a lack of business or consumer confidence in the United States, renewed U.S. concern about inflation, and an unexpected increase in oil prices. In early 1991, U.S. officials added to this list the restrictive policies of Japan and Germany, which would tend to dampen foreign demand for U.S. exports at a time critical to U.S. recovery.

It is not surprising, then, that the attention of the industrial countries in early 1991 seemed to focus on U.S. economic prospects. In April the IMF predicted that U.S. output would grow at a rate of only 0.2 percent in 1991, compared to 1 percent in 1990 and 2.5 percent in 1989. However, ceteris paribus, U.S. growth would rebound in 1992 to a more respectable 2.7 percent. (The OECD was somewhat less pessimistic about 1991— forecasting about 1 percent growth—and less optimistic about 1992— forecasting about 2 percent growth.) There seems little doubt that Japan's growth rate in 1991 will be significantly below its 1990 rate of 5.5 percent. The OECD predicts Japanese output of 3.7 and 3.8 percent in 1991 and 1992, respectively. The German growth outlook is perhaps the most interesting because of the ongoing integration of the West and East German economies, which began on July 1, 1990. Despite the virtual collapse of the economy of what was once East Germany, and consequent extremely high rates of unemployment in that region, the economic unification process is expected to be fundamentally inflationary. This is in part because of the nature of the monetary unification process, which was very generous toward holders of East German marks, and also because the massive reconstruction of the economy in eastern Germany may cost approximately 1 trillion marks during the next decade.

There was in early spring 1991 a general expectation that the central banks of both Japan and Germany would maintain their restrictive anti-inflation stances and that this would, again, probably limit the degree to which Japanese and German demand for U.S. exports could contribute to a U.S. recovery. It was this realization that prompted U.S. policy-makers to ask Japan and Germany to relax those policies in April 1991, and it was their counterparts' fear of inflation that prompted them to refuse the request. Thus, the situation was one in which, on the one hand, U.S. policy-makers feared that a prolonged U.S. recession, combined with restrictive policies in Japan and Germany, could produce a global recession by 1992 and, on the other hand, Japanese and German policy-makers believed that a premature relaxation of macroeconomic policies could abort the current effort to wring inflation out of the world economy and force not only an early resumption but also an intensification of painful anti-inflationary measures.

By July 1991 certain elements of this scenario had begun to change. On July 1, two weeks before the annual meeting of the Group of 7 heads of state, the Bank of Japan lowered its discount rate by one-half of a percentage point. Some observers attributed the shift to a slowdown in Japanese construction, industrial production, and capital spending, as well as to a reduction in inflationary pressures [*The New York Times*, 7/2/91]. In Germany, however, where inflationary tendencies remained strong, the Bundesbank came under pressure to raise, not lower, interest rates [ibid., 6/28/91].

The Developing Countries

The developing countries, on the whole, could not escape the combined effects of contraction in the developed world and the Gulf crisis. Not surprisingly, therefore, they recorded lower growth in 1990 (0.6 percent) than in 1989 (3.1 percent) [ibid.]. However, there were great differences of experience, both individually and regionally, among developing countries. (See Table III–1.) Asian developing countries, for example, grew at a very respectable rate of 5.3 percent, essentially unchanged from 1989 but noticeably lower nonetheless than rates recorded during the 1983–88 period. The four newly industrializing economies (NIEs) of Asia— Singapore, Hong Kong, South Korea, and Taiwan—did even better than the region as a whole, recording a growth rate of 6.8 percent in 1990, following 6.9 percent growth in 1989. Not unlike the developed countries, most of the more advanced Asian economies have had to respond to inflationary pressures rooted in the late 1980s' boom period by tightening monetary policy. Singapore, Taiwan, Indonesia, and Thailand adopted a more restrictive stance, as did China in 1989. A notable exception was South Korea, where monetary policy was not tightened and increased domestic consumption and booming construction generated a 1990 growth rate of 8.5 percent, despite an export slowdown associated with the U.S. recession. In addition, China's success in reducing inflation in 1989 permitted a relaxation of monetary policy in 1990. China recorded 4 percent growth in both 1989 and 1990.

At the other end of the developing-country spectrum (excluding Eastern Europe and the Soviet Union, which are discussed below) were the developing countries of the Western Hemisphere. While individual countries' experiences varied, the region as a whole fared poorly in 1990, recording a growth rate of − 1.0 percent, compared to + 1.5 percent in 1989, a 1981–86 average of 1 percent per year, and a 1972–78 average of about 5 percent [ibid.] Among the factors contributing to the poor performance of such countries as Argentina, Brazil, and Peru were either serious domestic disequilibrium unaddressed by adjustment measures or restrictive anti-inflationary adjustment policies, as well as the U.S. recession, the continuing external debt crisis, and, for oil-importing countries, the Gulf crisis–related increase in oil prices.

Some countries fared better than others, however. Mexico, for example, enjoyed windfall income of at least $3 billion as a result of the oil price increase [*The New York Times*, 2/12/91, p. D6]. Mexico was also one of several countries (e.g., Chile, Colombia, Uruguay, and Bolivia) that had both undertaken successful stabilization policies in earlier years and, more recently, consolidated their positions by adopting moderate fiscal and monetary policies.

Africa, including North Africa, recorded slower growth in 1990 (1.9 percent) than in 1989 (3.3 percent). Even before the Gulf crisis hurt oil-importing countries in Africa, prices of primary commodities, which contribute significantly to output, revenue, and export income, had declined noticeably. In addition, the Gulf war created a refugee crisis of immense proportions in some countries. The latter had especially negative economic implications for Egypt. In addition, wars, civil disorder, and famine hindered or obstructed economic activity in a number of African countries. In sub-Saharan Africa, growth declined to 1.5 percent in 1990 from 2.3 percent in 1989, further worsening the situation in one of the most desperate regions of the world. (See the discussion of efforts to aid the least developed countries below.)

The Gulf crisis had immediate and major consequences for the developing countries of the Middle East. Iraq's invasion and occupation of Kuwait resulted in a U.N. embargo against exports, principally oil, from Kuwait and Iraq, thus depriving the affected area of revenues from the sale of a combined total of about 4.3 million barrels of oil per day. Simultaneously, massive numbers of foreign workers, primarily from the Middle East, North Africa, and Southwest Asia, began to flee or be expelled from Kuwait and Iraq, further disrupting production in the area. This created massive refugee problems for such countries as Jordan, Pakistan, and Sri Lanka and deprived the workers' home countries of substantial wage remittances. Jordan was hit especially hard; and its lost production, along with that of Kuwait and Iraq, more than offset the growth of other countries in the region, especially oil exporters. The IMF and the World Bank, as well as the United States, the European Community, and Japan, provided aid and/or debt relief to the most seriously affected. Overall, Middle Eastern growth fell sharply in 1990 to − 1.5 percent from 3.2 percent in 1989 and 4.7 percent in 1988 [*WEO*, 10/90, p. 6].

On the whole, developing countries made important progress in containing inflation in 1989 and 1990. Argentina and Brazil achieved significant reductions in 1990, and other countries, such as Bolivia, Mexico, Uganda, and Vietnam, which had begun the process earlier, consolidated their gains.

As a group, developing countries' external balances deteriorated during 1990. Non-oil-exporting countries were especially affected. Their combined current account deficits swelled from about $10 billion in 1989 to about $38 billion in 1990 [*WEO,* 5/91, p. 162]. In contrast, oil-exporting developing countries enjoyed a significant improvement, swinging from a current account deficit of $6 billion in 1989 to a surplus of about $8.5 billion in 1990.

While some analyses were pessimistic about developing countries' prospects for 1991 [see, for example, E1991/INF/1], the OECD's forecast was neutral [see *Economic Outlook*] and the IMF's was, on balance, optimistic [*WEO,* 10/90]. The IMF expects growth to rebound to more than 2 percent in 1991, with all geographic areas, except the Middle East, participating in the recovery. Asian developing countries, led by the Asian NIEs, are expected to maintain strong growth at a rate of 5 percent. Western Hemisphere developing countries, according to the IMF, should swing from negative growth in 1990 to a positive growth rate of 1 percent in 1991. The Fund expects both African (at 2 percent) and even European (at 1.5 percent) developing countries to show improvement over 1990. The IMF attributed the projected decline in Middle East growth in 1991 (− 3.3 percent) to the costs of the Gulf war and the continuing loss of export earnings from workers' remittances and tourism receipts [*WEO,* 5/91, p. 17].

With the end of the Gulf war in late February 1991 came the prospect of stable, and perhaps even temporarily very low (e.g., $10 per barrel), oil prices. However, in March 1991 the Organization of Petroleum Exporting Countries (OPEC) successfully restored production restrictions and the price stabilized at about $20 per barrel, compared to an average of more than $30 per barrel during the crisis and the alarming predictions that prices would average from $50 to $100 per barrel if war broke out. The situation at mid-March 1991 tended to confirm the more optimistic expectation of many mainstream analysts that the **overall effects of the crisis-related increase in oil prices** would be smaller and more temporary than in 1973–74 and 1979–80.

Development Assistance

In 1989 net official development finance to developing countries (ODF), which excludes IMF transactions, increased in nominal terms by 4.5

percent, to $69 billion from $66 billion in 1988. In inflation-adjusted terms at constant exchange rates it increased by about 5 percent [OECD, *Development Cooperation*, 12/90, p. 122]. Official Development Assistance (ODA), which accounts for about one-half of ODF, rose slightly in nominal terms to about $53 billion from about $51.5 billion in 1988. Japan ($8.95 billion) surpassed the United States ($7.66 billion) as the largest donor in absolute (as opposed to percentage of GNP) terms—though perhaps only temporarily due to the unusual factors that influenced the U.S. total. Japan (0.32 percent) also provided more than twice as much ODA as the United States (0.15 percent) as a percentage of GNP. Norway (1.04 percent) and Sweden (0.97 percent) continued to lead all donor nations according to the share-of-GNP criterion.

The Fourth Development Decade

As anticipated in *Issues Before the 44th General Assembly of the United Nations* (hereafter *Issues/44*) [United Nations Association, 1989, p. 80], the U.N. General Assembly met in late April 1990 to lay the groundwork for discussions about a fourth "development decade." However, in contrast to the contentious atmosphere that prevailed in 1988, there was a "high degree of consensus" on fundamental goals and strategies [OECD, *Development Co-operation*, 12/90, p. 26]. Meeting in a **Special Session Devoted to International Co-operation,** the General Assembly adopted a declaration stating that an opportunity exists to restore a long-term approach to development and to move beyond short-term adjustment. The Declaration stated further that a primary objective of development must be to "respond to the [health, nutritional, housing, population, and social] needs of all members of society." It also emphasized the responsibility of the developing countries themselves and looked forward to continued work on the issue later in the year.

The Least Developed Countries

Nine years after the First U.N. Conference on the Least Developed Countries, the second such conference was held in Paris in September 1990 [see "Development and International Economic Co-operation: Review and Appraisal of the Substantial New Programme for the 1980s for the Least Developed Countries," A/45/695, 11/90]. One hundred fifty governments participated in the conference, which was held to "draw world attention to and bring into focus the problems of the [41] weakest and poorest members of the international community," 28 of which are in Africa. The conference was planned when it became clear that despite increases in development assistance and trade preferences granted by developed countries, economic conditions in the least developed countries had continued to decline during the 1980s. The conference adopted a Programme of Action, which included four options by which donors would promise more development aid to the least developed countries. The conference also approved a strategy for addressing those countries' external indebtedness. All creditors were urged to cancel or provide equivalent relief for bilateral concessional debt. Creditor governments were also urged to apply less stringent "Toronto terms" (see Section 3 below regarding the external debt crisis) to nonconcessional bilateral debt. Multilateral institutions were asked to give serious attention to debt-relief measures for these countries. The new Programme departed significantly from the previous one by stressing the importance of private-sector initiatives. It also emphasized democratic participation, respect for human rights, population policy, and the potential role of women and nongovernmental organizations in promoting development. Given the contentiousness of some of the issues, some observers and participants had expected the conference to end in failure. That it ended in success instead was gratifying to all participants, especially the organizers, not least of all the Secretary-General of the Conference and of the U.N. Conference on Trade and Development (UNCTAD), Kenneth K. S. Dadzie.

Economies in Transition: Eastern Europe and the Soviet Union

Nineteen ninety was the first full year of the "new," or post–Cold War, Europe. The anticommunist, prodemocracy revolutions of 1989 had swiftly displaced the old Stalinist regimes in several Eastern and Central European countries. Western observers, amazed and generally delighted by the speed and extent of political change in the former Eastern-bloc countries, eagerly awaited indications of the ramifications for economic organization in those countries. They perceived, as the IMF noted, that a broad consensus seemed to be emerging in favor of market-oriented economic systems. However, significant divergence about the pace of reform and the sequencing of reform measures arose both between and within many of the countries [WEO, 10/90, p. 22]. These two issues were especially controversial in the Soviet Union, and political polarization with respect to them contributed to an image and reality of a country that was disintegrating both politically and economically. Moreover, along with labor restiveness and open ethnic conflict, the heated public and private debates over the course of economic reform contributed to a

3 to 5 percentage point decline in Soviet economic output in 1990 [*Economic Outlook*, p. 31]. The Soviet experience was replicated to some degree in certain other Eastern European countries, including **Romania and Bulgaria.** Like the Soviet Union, both suffered from the combined effects of the collapse of central planning mechanisms and the delayed introduction of market-based methods of economic organization. Romania's economy, for example, was estimated to have contracted by 15 to 20 percent.

However, while some Eastern European countries hesitated, others took major steps toward economic transformation. Though these measures tended to be extremely painful in the short term, they were expected to make those countries that were among the first to adopt serious reform measures also among the first to reap the anticipated benefits of a market-based economy. **Poland** is perhaps the most often mentioned country in this regard. Even though it experienced a sharp decline in output in 1990, estimated in the 15–20 percent range [ibid.], Poland was able to eliminate hyperinflation and begin establishing a firm base for future growth [*WEO*, 10/90, p. 23].

Czechoslovakia and Hungary fell somewhere between the two types of experiences just described. Czechoslovakia, by opting to postpone major economic reform, avoided a major reduction in output (a decline of only 1 percent in 1990 was recorded) but also virtually guaranteed that its eventual transition to a market economy would be even more painful and costly than it might otherwise have been. Hungary's experience was similar: Output declined only 1 to 3 percent in 1990. Yet Hungary's approach differed from that of both Czechoslovakia, which chose deliberate procrastination, and Poland, which "went cold turkey." Hungary, according to one analysis, has simply "drifted" toward a course of reform [*The Economist*, 4/28/90, p. 21].

The external accounts of Eastern European countries, excluding the Soviet Union, improved temporarily in 1990, mainly because domestic economic weakness reduced demand for imports. However, it was generally anticipated that these balances would worsen significantly in 1991 for at least two reasons: the phasing out or collapse of the Council for Mutual Economic Assistance's (CMEA) preferential trade arrangements and the related necessity to buy from and sell to Western markets; and the new necessity to conduct trade with the Soviet Union at world market prices, both because of new general Soviet policies in this regard and, more specifically, because of the termination of Soviet oil price subsidies. The OECD forecast a deterioration of approximately $10 billion in these countries' overall trade balance [*Economic Outlook*, p. 31]. Separately, the Soviet Union's external imbalance was expected to worsen in 1991. Despite benefits from higher oil prices both globally and in the former Eastern bloc, Soviet oil production was declining rapidly [*The New York Times*, 9/27/90], while non-oil exports were stagnating and imports were increasing rapidly to compensate for lost or inefficient Soviet production.

Clearly, both the Soviet Union and the former Soviet-bloc countries continue to need significant if not massive outside assistance to complete successfully their transitions to market-based economies, assuming that they are committed to following through on such transitions. **Poland** has almost certainly been the most visible beneficiary of Western economic support so far. In early 1991 the Polish government reached an unprecedented agreement with the Paris Club of creditor governments that would in effect cancel half of Poland's debt to those governments. Under the agreement, these governments also retained the option to offer Poland further debt concessions. The United States chose to exercise its option in this regard when the new Polish president, longtime political activist and the embodiment of Polish resistance to communist rule, Lech Walesa, paid a state visit to Washington, D.C. [*The Financial Times*, 3/16/91, p. 2]. The **Soviet Union** also found favor in the West in 1990, although political strife and economic disarray in that country worked to undermine Western interest in intervening economically. In late 1990 both the European Community and the United States responded positively to Soviet President Mikhail Gorbachev's appeals for food aid. The European Community pledged to send about $250 million in direct aid and to offer $750 million in credits to allow the Soviet government to buy food [*The Boston Globe*, 12/15/90, p. 2]. President Bush authorized between $500 million and $1 billion in federally guaranteed loans for the purchase of food supplies from the United States [*The New York Times*, 12/13/90, p. 1]. In early 1991, however, Western attitudes toward the Soviet Union began to change for the worse in response to the Soviets' use of military force against the secessionist Baltic republics. This military response was especially troubling because it appeared to reflect a sudden swing toward authoritarianism by Gorbachev, who had previously portrayed himself as a moderate reformer [*The New York Times*, 2/6/91, p. A8]. The resignation in January 1991 of Soviet Foreign Minister Eduard Shevardnadze, a popular and trusted figure in the West, reinforced Western leaders' fears. At the time of his resignation, Shevardnadze warned of an impending return to dictatorship either by Gorbachev or his would-be successors. Thereafter, a palpable coolness characterized Western relations with Gorbachev's government. Perhaps the most indicative demonstration of Western displeasure was Japan's flat rejection of Gorbachev's appeal for investment and aid during a long-planned and heavily publicized state visit to Tokyo [*The New York Times*, 4/18/91, p. A1].

By June 1991 relations between the Soviet Union and the advanced Western democracies had improved significantly. In response to Soviet overtures and economic and political reforms, the Group of Seven agreed to offer the Soviet Union associate membership in the International Monetary Fund and to confer with Gorbachev immediately after the mid-July 1991 meeting of G-7 in London.

Western interest in the economic and political transformation of the former Eastern-bloc countries remained high even as relations with the Soviet Union fell and rose. In late 1990 and early 1991 many in both the East and West looked forward to the contributions to Eastern European renewal that they hoped would flow from the newly created **European Bank for Reconstruction and Development.** Capitalized initially at $13 billion, a relatively low level, the London-based bank, under the leadership of France's former economic advisor Jacques Attali, was established to invest in private or privatized ventures in formerly socialist economies, help improve the infrastructure in those countries, and provide management training for people running privatized companies [*The Wall Street Journal*, 11/26/90, p. A5C]. Its inaugural loan was made to a privatized bank, which planned to relend the money [ibid., 6/26/91].

2. The External Debt Crisis

By 1988 the collapse was obvious not only of the Baker plan of 1985 but indeed of the entire approach to the management of the developing countries' external debt crisis, which had exploded onto the world economic scene in 1982 [*Issues/44*, p. 83]. Most of the largest debtors were worse off than in either 1985 or 1982. Most were no closer to restoring external creditworthiness, and commercial lenders were no closer to resuming voluntary lending. In June 1988, at a meeting of the G-7 countries in Toronto, Canada, a new range of debt-relief options covering official debt was formulated. Initially limited to African countries but later extended to certain others, the so-called **Toronto terms** urged creditor governments to forgive one-third of the debt service due and reschedule the rest, extend the maturity date on loans, or reduce interest rates to below-market levels [United Nations, "Debt: A Crisis for Development," DPI/NGO/SB/90/13, 4/90]. Then, in early 1989, U.S. Treasury Secretary Nicholas Brady proposed yet another approach to commercial debt. The **Brady plan** broke new ground by calling for debt reduction. In return for guarantees from the IMF and the World Bank, commercial banks were asked to provide voluntary reductions of troubled debts through reductions in principal or interest payments [*Issues/44*, p. 85]. Within about a year, however, the Brady plan was perceived by some observers as underfunded and as neither making the desired cuts at the desired pace nor attracting the desired amount of new money to the countries in need [United Nations, "Statement by the Secretary-General's Personal Representative on Debt," EC/2692, 7/9/90].

In December 1989 the 44th General Assembly, asserting that existing policy approaches to the developing countries' external debt crisis were inadequate and that the crisis had become "a political problem" [DPI/NGO/SB/90/13], adopted Resolution 205, which "spelled out a number of measures that would be required . . . to ensure that recent initiatives on debt . . . have an effective and comprehensive impact on the reactivation of economic growth and sustained development in the developing countries" [United Nations, "External Debt Crisis and Development: The Recent Evolution of the International Debt Strategy; Report by the Secretary-General," A/45/656, 10/23/90]. Simultaneously, the Secretary-General, to support the enlargement of international agreement on policy approaches to debt problems, appointed a **Personal Representative on Debt,** the Honorable Bettino Craxi, former prime minister of Italy.

Craxi reported that the developing countries' foreign debt had soared to about $1,200 billion in 1990 from about $600 billion in 1980 [A/45/380, 7/90]. (In a separate report, the World Bank estimated 1990 external indebtedness at about $1,340 billion. See Table III–3.) Moreover, Craxi said, scheduled annual debt service payments had climbed to about $175 billion from $90 billion a decade earlier, despite the Baker plan, the Toronto terms, and the Brady plan. After 1983, he stated, the next flow of financial resources was reversed from annual net transfers to the developing from the developed countries to annual net transfers from the developing to the developed countries. In 1990 the amount of that transfer was said to be about $10 billion. Thus, Craxi called for priority to be given to "correcting this anomaly and resuming transfers in the opposite direction." To this end, he proposed a 15-point plan that called for, among other things:

- Strengthening the Brady plan through larger resources;
- Further alleviating the burden through debt rescheduling and reductions of interest rates;
- Debt service forgiveness for the poorest countries;
- Reaffirmation of the objective of 0.7 percent of GNP for official development aid allocated by industrialized countries.

In October 1990 the Secretary-General reported, among other things, that the Gulf crisis would probably have a major impact on a number of debtor countries, though he hoped that the impact would be relatively short lived and largely offset by additional external finance [A/45/656].

Finally, in December 1990 the World Bank warned that "the debt crisis is not over," despite certain positive developments, including increased financial flows to developing countries [World Bank, *World Debt Tables, 1990–91,* 12/90, p. 3]. According to the Bank, the Gulf crisis was expected to benefit indebted oil-exporting countries, at least temporarily, and hurt indebted oil importers. Ultimately, however, 1990 witnessed the first increase (6 percent in dollar terms) in developing countries' debt in two years. However, the debt-export ratio was expected to continue to decline from its 1987 peak of 232 percent of exports. Still, the Bank feared that, in the absence of new net private lending, the pattern of limited external finance and dependence on foreign official flows and foreign direct investments would prevail even as the debt crisis eased, as a result of debt relief and restructuring programs and the strong export performance of some countries. The Bank concluded that developing countries would

Table III–3
Developing Countries' External Debt, 1986–90

	1986	1987	1988	1989	1990
Total external debt (billions of dollars)					
Latin America and Caribbean	410	445	427	422	428
East Asia and Pacific	185	205	206	206	224
Sub-Saharan Africa	114	139	141	147	161
North Africa and Middle East	107	120	122	124	133
All developing countries	1,127	1,268	1,265	1,261	1,341
Long-term debt	867	980	960	959	1,015
Official sources	357	433	437	454	521
Private sources	511	547	523	505	494
Short-term debt	118	128	142	156	169
Debt-export ratio		232	201	187	
Debt-service ratio		28	27	22	

Note: The debt-service ratio is the product of the debt-export ratio and the average rate of debt service (interest plus amortization divided by the debt stock).

Source: World Bank, *World Debt Tables, 1990–91.*

need to rely on their own savings, multilateral institutions would remain an important link between international capital markets and developing countries, and developing countries would have to work to protect their creditworthiness [ibid.].

3. Trade and the Trading System

Trade Volume and Value

The volume of world exports rose 5 percent in 1990, slower than 1989's 7 percent growth and 1988's 8.5 percent but significantly faster than the growth rate of the world economy as a whole in 1990 (2.1 percent). According to the **General Agreement on Tariffs and Trade (GATT)**, this suggests that the world's economies are becoming increasingly reliant on trade and, therefore, more interdependent [GATT, *Annual Survey of International Trade*, 4/91; GATT, *International Trade, 1989–90; The Wall Street Journal*, 4/26/91, p. A19; *The Economist*, 4/27/91, p. 110].

The value of world exports reached $3.5 trillion, an increase of $405 billion or about 13 percent over 1989. Germany ($421 billion or 12.1 percent of the total) overtook the United States ($394 billion or 11.4 percent of the total) as the world's largest exporting nation. (See Table III–4.) However, the dollar's 16.5 percent depreciation against the German mark skewed the results as measured in dollars. Japan finished in third place with exports valued at about $287 billion or 8.2 percent of the total. France, with exports of about $220 billion or 6.2 percent of the total, overtook the United Kingdom, which posted exports of about $185 billion or 5.3 percent of total exports. The growth rate of all the Western European nations' trade, taken together, exceeded the world average. Among the 25 leading exporting nations, Austria, at 28 percent, enjoyed the most rapid growth in 1990. Three Asian newly industrializing economies (NIEs)—Hong Kong, South Korea, and Taiwan—accounted for more than 6 percent of the world total. Among the worst performances were those of the Soviet Union and Brazil, both of which registered absolute declines. One of the most significant developments, mentioned earlier, was the continued narrowing of the U.S. trade deficit and the Japanese and German trade surpluses.

Regarding the near-term future, it is generally expected that the volume of world exports will increase at about the same rate in 1991 as in 1990 (5 percent). Shaping this projected outcome will be the generally recessionary environment, which will almost certainly be sustained at

Table III–4
Merchandise Exports, 1990 Value;
Share of World Total

Country	Value ($ billions)	Share (percent)
TOTAL	3500	100.0
Germany	421	12.1
United States	394	11.4
Japan	287	8.2
France	217	6.2
Britain	186	5.3
Italy	172	4.9
Holland	137	3.9
Canada	133	3.8
Belgium/Luxembourg	119	3.4
Soviet Union	105	3.0
Hong Kong	84	2.4
Taiwan	67	1.9
South Korea	67	1.9

Source: *The Economist*, 4/27/91.

least through mid-1991 if not into early 1992, and German reunification, which is expected to result in a significant diversion of exports from the former West Germany to the five new *länder* which comprised the former East Germany. The United States and Germany are expected to secure nearly equal shares of about 13 percent of the world market for non-oil exports. Japan's share, which peaked just above 11.5 percent in 1986, is expected to level off at the 9 percent level recorded in 1990. The four Asian NIEs will likely gain about an 8.5 percent share in 1991, down from 9 percent in 1989 but still very impressive, especially considering that their 1980 share was about 5 percent. Canada's share is projected to decline to less than 4 percent after having peaked at nearly 5.5 percent in 1984 [*WEO*, 10/90, p. 27].

Terms of Trade

Despite the strong positive effects of higher oil prices, the developing countries, including oil exporters, enjoyed virtually no improvement in their terms of trade in 1990. (See Table III–5.) While oil exporters enjoyed an 11 percent gain, non-oil exporters suffered a 2.9 percent decline; and while oil prices rose more than 28 percent on average during the year, the prices of non-oil primary commodities—the principal exports of non-oil-exporting countries—declined by about 8 percent [*WEO*, 5/91, p. 151]. Sharp declines in the prices of tropical beverages, such as coffee, cocoa, and tea, contributed significantly to the overall decline. Recession in major developed markets and supply increases among producing countries were the principal market forces at work. The IMF noted that between 1980 and 1990 non-oil commodity prices fell by about 40 percent relative to the export prices of the industrial countries' manufactured goods. A further decline of 2.5 percent was anticipated in 1991, while manufactured goods' prices were expected to rise again (by 8.3 percent) after having climbed 9.6 percent in 1990 [ibid.].

The International Trading System

Developments in 1990 raised serious doubts about the future of the nearly 45-year-old GATT-centered international trading system. In mid-December 1990 the **Uruguay Round** of multilateral trade negotiations appeared to have collapsed. The reasons for this failure may be found in part in events that occurred during the preceding 20 months. In April 1989 the GATT's Trade Negotiating Committee had broken impasses on four issues that had threatened since mid-1988 to scuttle the negotiations—agricultural trade reform, textiles and clothing, industrial safeguards, and intellectual property rights [*Issues/44*, p. 94]. Then, in July 1989, a schedule had been established that called for completion of the Round in early December 1990. In July 1990 the Trade Negotiating Committee expressed disappointment "at the degree to which the negotiations had fallen behind and the apparent lack of political will to resolve the basic difficulties." The Committee, therefore, called for "substantive bargaining to begin without delay" [*WEO*, 10/90, p. 94].

Table III–5
Developing Countries' Terms of Trade, 1986–90

	1986	1987	1988	1989	1990
	(annual changes in percent)				
All regions	−16.4	1.8	−3.4	1.9	0.2
Africa	−25.4	0.5	−4.4	−1.6	−1.8
Asia	−3.6	1.7	0.3	1.7	−1.0
Middle East	−44.5	8.5	−19.0	10.8	8.6
Latin America	−10.3	−2.0	−2.2	0.2	−1.5
Fuel exports	−46.7	9.4	−18.4	10.7	11.0
Nonfuel exports	0.8	−0.9	1.7	0.1	−2.9
Manufactures from developed countries	17.7	11.9	6.1	−0.4	7.9

Source: IMF, *World Economic Outlook*, 10/90 and 5/91, Table A28.

Final negotiating positions were to have been set by October 15, 1990, so that final bargaining could commence. By that date, however, the principal actors' positions—especially those of the European Community (whose agricultural policies had been targeted by the others), the United States, and the Cairns Group of agricultural exporting nations— remained essentially unchanged. The United States and the Cairns Group threatened to quit the negotiations entirely. Shortly afterward, the European Community offered a new proposal—a 30 percent reduction in overall farm subsidies over ten years from peak 1986 levels. The proposal was promptly and emphatically rejected by the Community's major trading partners, which calculated that the effective reduction would be closer to 15 percent by 1996. The United States and the Cairns Group were demanding overall reductions in subsidization on the order of 75 percent (including 90 percent cuts in export subsidies) over a ten-year period beginning in 1991. The Europeans' offer proved to be unacceptable even as a basis for negotiations. Moreover, while the Europeans stalled on agriculture, the United States separately began to retreat on freer trade in services, something the United States had been promoting aggressively since the early 1980s. Ultimately, however, it was because of the European agricultural policies that negotiations collapsed temporarily on December 7, 1990, threatening not only gains made in a number of other areas but also the future of the trading system itself. U.S. officials angrily declared that it was up to the Europeans to resurrect the negotiations, if indeed they were ever to resume [*The New York Times*, 12/10/90, p. D5]. Widespread speculation about the future of the international trading system began immediately. Some observers hoped and called for a prompt resumption of negotiations, while others, such as *The Wall Street Journal*, proclaimed "GATT Riddance" [12/12/90, p. A16]. Still others, noting U.S. agreements or proposed agreements with Canada, Mexico, and a number of other Western Hemisphere countries, feared a breakup of the international trading order into regional blocs, followed perhaps by trade wars [*The New York Times*, 12/10/90, p. D5].

However, beginning in mid-January 1991 there was tentative movement toward a resurrection of the Round. GATT's Secretary-General, Arthur Dunkel, took the lead [ibid., 1/16/91, p. D2] and was followed first by the European Community, then by business groups from throughout the world that adopted a resolution at a conference in Washington, D.C. [ibid., 1/27/91, p. 6], and finally by the U.S. government. In mid-February 1991, Dunkel announced that arrangements had been completed for a **resumption of the Round** [ibid., 2/16/91, p. 37]. However, at least one major obstacle remained: U.S. **"fast-track"** negotiating authority, which limited Congress's opportunity to modify any proposed agreement, was about to expire and would have to be renewed by a Congress that was by now disenchanted with GATT and overtly hostile to a U.S.–Mexican free trade agreement (expected to subsume the existing U.S.–Canada free trade agreement), which President Bush strongly favored but would have to be negotiated under the same fast-track extension. By late April 1991 prospects for a resumption of negotiations were improving as the Bush administration brought its domestic political assets to bear against fast-track opponents in Congress. In late May 1991 congressional approval was secured. The multilateral negotiations resumed and the OECD countries committed themselves to completing them by the end of the calendar year.

4. Transnational Corporations and the Global Economy

The United Nations has new issues and themes for developing the global economy in the 1990s. There is an effort to harmonize the needs of commerce and investment with development issues within countries, and to reconcile both with the need for international security and environmental safety. Direct investment, privatization, and entrepreneurship are seen as the new ingredients of successful development. A stable set of common international standards of trade, environmental safety, and accounting practices is the recipe for a flourishing commerce.

Such issues and themes derive from real changes in world economic power: The Soviet-influenced economies are in near collapse, the newly industrialized countries are prospering, and the least developed countries are losing ground. Direct investment and increased trade are the most available avenues for developing countries hoping to escape the cycle of debt and impoverishment. The competition for foreign aid has been eliminated by the fading of the Cold War, and the Eastern nations that were once a source of development aid are now at the head of the receiving line.

In a report reciting the lessons of the 1980s and looking toward the decade ahead, the U.N. Conference on Trade and Development (UNCTAD) focused on the divergence of Asia's newly industrialized countries from the path taken by the economies of Africa and Latin America. The conclusions can be summed up as follows:

• Transnational corporations (TNCs) can bring large infusions of capital and assist in the development of technological infrastructure.

- Protectionism can lead to entrenched "infancy," but subsidizing infant industries and making capital available is probably healthy.
- Successful economies can be built around imported technology.
- Entrepreneurship and free enterprise can facilitate growth.

Only a few years ago the U.N. organizations concerned with development were defensive and suspicious of multinational investment; they now openly seek ways to facilitate it. This is certainly attributable, at least in part, to a remarkable maturing of competency and confidence by **the U.N. Centre for Transnational Corporations (CTC)**. The stage is now being set for true global investment and multinational business for large, medium, and small enterprises, North and South.

Transnational Corporations and Foreign Direct Investment

For much of the last decade and a half, acting under the guidance of the U.N. Economic and Social Council's (ECOSOC) Commission on Transnational Corporations (TNCs), the CTC emphasized the marginal, if not negative, impact of foreign direct investment (FDI) on employment generation, manufacturing exports, and balance of payments and exchange rates, and advocated a wide range of national controls on the activities of TNCs in developing countries.

The CTC was instrumental in encouraging **national regulations on TNC operations in developing countries** that ranged from liberal competitive rules tempered by entry and supervisory controls in Southeast and East Asia, to a combination of free-operating environment and strict financial controls in Latin America, to a myriad of entry, participation, operating, financial, and terminal controls in South Asia. The motivations behind the imposition of such controls by developing countries generally related to dissatisfaction with the development impact of TNCs as well as to fear that TNC intercompany fund movements might threaten national policies affecting exchange rates, balance of payments, domestic credit availability, and viability of local firms. Such subjective perceptions were often reinforced by objective U.N. studies of the impact of TNCs on developing countries. For example, studies by UNCTAD and CTC showed that, on the whole, TNC FDI tended to have marginal effects on manufacturing exports and negative direct effects on the balance of payments of several developing countries ["Transnational Corporations: Direct Effects on Balance of Payments," E/C.10/84, 4/6/85].

As TNCs used increasingly sophisticated management techniques in developing countries, the CTC also saw the need to provide **advisory services** to these countries to strengthen government supervision over TNC activities with the aim of ensuring an equitable distribution of benefits between the TNCs and the host country. The CTC likewise took on the task of helping these countries develop their negotiating skills as well as their foreign investment policies, laws and regulations, contractual arrangements, and national information systems relating to TNCs.

Since the fundamental objectives of TNCs (maximization of global profits) and host developing countries (maximization of national gains) are essentially contradictory, the outcome of their negotiations is determined in large part by the bargaining leverage of each. The CTC has played a valuable role in strengthening the bargaining capacity of developing countries by highlighting policy options available to them, including various forms of intervention. More recently, the CTC has identified a number of new areas where national controls can be strengthened—among them, intermediary services provided by transnational banks, technical service agreements, and transfer pricing.

Historically, **wholly owned foreign affiliates** have been the TNC's preferred form of FDI, but host developing countries began to insist on **equity-sharing** arrangements as well as on such **nonequity financing methods** as licensing, management contracts, and turnkey arrangements, and today joint ventures and nonequity forms of participation are the predominant ways of doing business in these countries. Over many years the CTC was an active advocate of equity-sharing and an active promoter of short-term contractual relationships and turnkey projects.

Recently, however, the CTC's hostility toward FDI has given way to recognition of FDI's benefits for the national economies of developing countries. The catalysts for this attitudinal change were many:

1. Since the 1980s, many developing countries have been liberalizing their national laws and regulations regarding the role of the private sector in development. These changes were a response to harsh economic realities in countries that had seen the **failure of central planning** to solve the basic problems of chronic unemployment, acute balance of payments deficits, and severe foreign exchange shortages.

2. The realization that, under the impetus of "**Reaganomics**" and **deregulation** in industrialized countries, there was increasing competition in international markets for foreign investment, and developing countries could be bypassed by TNCs in this new competitive environment.

3. The **dismantling of the socialist regimes of Eastern Europe and the Soviet Union,** the transition of these economies from centrally planned to market economies, and the demand for U.N. technical assistance in all areas relating to private enterprise and FDI.

4. The emergence on the global scene of **multinational corporations based in the newly industrializing countries** themselves (as well as some based in socialist countries)—dubbed "Non-Conventional TNCs" by the CTC.

In response to these fundamental changes, a major recent CTC initiative has been to sponsor seminars and workshops on negotiating joint-venture agreements; on establishing stock exchanges, offshore banking centers, and free enterprise zones; and on improving accounting standards for the private sector.

An ongoing CTC initiative has been the development of guidelines for the behavior of TNCs—a difficult task, as indicated by the international community's experience to date. The instruments that exist, such as those issued by the Organization for Economic Cooperation and Development (OECD), tend to be issue-specific and concrete—dealing, for example, with the protection of foreign property. The U.N. effort, entitled **"The International Code of Conduct for Transnational Corporations,"** is the only truly global attempt to formulate a code of conduct for transnationals. Prolonged negotiations have succeeded in producing a draft text on which there is agreement to about 80 percent of the provisions. If and when adopted, the code would set standards for both the conduct of TNCs in host countries and the treatment of TNCs by host countries. The guidelines have already raised global awareness of appropriate behavior and appear to be changing the behavior of some corporations.

The CTC has also played a role in developing regional guidelines for the behavior of TNCs, and its advisory services have helped governments to "unbundle" the package of services offered by TNCs. (Since unbundling can be an expensive proposition at the purely national level, the U.N. efforts here have strengthened the collective bargaining position of several developing countries vis-à-vis the TNCs.) Further, the CTC has been helping to strengthen national efforts at monitoring both rapidly changing technologies and dynamic corporate responses to them, and helping to upgrade the managerial skills involved in tracking ever-changing products and process technologies and obtaining the required intra-firm product or skill transfers.

As hostility toward TNCs continues to give way to a more open policy aimed at attracting FDI, the CTC will have to undertake further research on the implications for developing countries of the 1992 integrated market program of the European Community, as well as on the impact of the recent changes in Eastern Europe and the Soviet Union on FDI flows to developing countries [Commission on Transnational Corporations, Report on the Sixteenth Session, E/C.10/1990/19].

Increasingly, the focus of CTC's future analytical work will be on maximizing the intangible benefits of FDI and on resolving outstanding issues in such areas as the environment, intellectual property rights, trade-related investment measures, small and medium-sized enterprises, and on promoting greater collaboration among developing-country firms to enhance regional cooperation among developing countries.

Privatization and Entrepreneurship

Beyond assisting developing countries in monitoring and controlling the dealings of TNCs, the CTC is now actively working with transnational corporations and their international business associations to create standards that help developing countries exploit what the TNCs are ready to offer. In addition, it has been directing developing countries to pay more attention to a variety of benefits the multinational presence offers somewhat less directly. The 45th General Assembly's Special Session on Development and International Economic Cooperation reviewed some of these. "Foreign direct investment," noted one report, "can make an important contribution . . . as a means of providing access to modern environmentally sound technologies, skills and markets." And further: "Entrepreneurship should be encouraged at all levels and in all sectors in the setting up of industries" [A/45/849/Add. 1].

The global shift in attitude toward **entrepreneurship** goes hand in hand with the global trend toward **"privatization"** of enterprises that were formerly the preserve of government. Whether through the sale of state-run industries in Eastern Europe or the auctioning of entire telecommunications systems in Latin America, the prevailing belief today is that governments can afford to relinquish ownership to private businesses or even multinational corporations [see, for example, "Privatization Takes Hold in Eastern Europe," in the CTC quarterly newsletter, *Transnational*, 12/90]. The selling of assets is seen as a logical way to attract capital, pay off debts, promote entrepreneurship, and make the most efficient use of commercial technology.

Outside Europe and the United States, where privatization and deregulation began accelerating over a decade ago, this reversal in world view has been remarkable for its suddenness and momentum. From a few debt-for-equity swaps under what amounted to extreme duress a couple of years ago, the financing of privatization has moved into the global market. International accounting standards are needed to accommodate this phenomenon, and the CTC has begun studying ways to develop such standards [E/C.10/AC.3/1991/1.3/Add. 5]. Business enterprises will also be seeking guarantees that deals they have struck with governments will be judged by global standards rather than local law, e.g., conforming to the arbitration standards set forth in the U.N.–sanctioned "New York Convention," already ratified by 82 countries (rather than to any of the regional conventions adopted by developing countries, such as the InterAmerican Convention ratified by 12).

Environmental Issues

Throughout the last two decades the United Nations has sought better means to ensure that the TNCs employing **chemical, nuclear, and other technologies** do not abuse the environment or engage in practices that endanger host country **health and safety.** The underlying assumption was that multinational businesses will attempt to get away with substandard practices if not closely monitored. One of the United Nation's responses has been to promote responsibility on the part of multinational companies themselves to disclose all risks and refrain from industrial practices that are below home-country standards.

The effort to **monitor and regulate TNC behavior** continues, with continued improvement in information-gathering about the products and practices of the largest corporations. Considerable effort is being expended on preparations for the 1992 World Conference on Environment and Development. The CTC has made compelling arguments for keeping the focus on those corporations that, by sheer volume, dominate world production in petrochemicals, forest products, and other industries of environmental concern.

Here too, however, the trend is toward cooperation. Many of the multinational companies targeted as potential violators are adopting higher standards and policing themselves, and the CTC has cited favorably the efforts of such mammoths as General Motors, ICI, and DuPont in this regard. (The lead article in one issue of CTC's quarterly newsletter, *Transnational,* went so far as to proclaim: "Environmental Concerns Set Global Regulatory Trend: Companies Responsive, Some Announcing Plans to Go Beyond Current International Measures.") A considerable number of the leading TNCs have now announced that environmental health and safety are part of what a quality-conscious, risk-sensitive business must take into consideration if it is to remain profitable in the long term. Many of the largest have instituted **global environmental audits** as a routine part of doing business.

The United Nations now faces the reality that member nations themselves, both knowingly and unknowingly, are endangering the environment—and that many have strong economic incentives to permit environmentally unsound practices, whether by indigenous enterprises or foreign businesses. Development itself creates the conditions for international ecological disasters, contributing to global warming, acid rain, nuclear fallout, deforestation, and chemical discharges. As developing countries struggle between feeding today's population and preserving the environment for future generations, there are difficult choices to be made. The state-controlled economies of Eastern Europe and the developing world have shown themselves to be just as capable of miscalculation and willful abuse as are multinational corporations.

The issues were easier to address when TNCs were viewed as the prime culprits. To address the same practices now is to raise additional, **complex questions of sovereignty.** How does the United Nations respond when developing countries insist on retaining the right to make their own cost-benefit calculations in assessing environmental risks? Should Côte d'Ivoire be allowed to provide landfill for multinational toxic wastes? Does Brazil have the right to exploit its gold fields while leaching mercury into the rivers? Should the 10,000-year-old forests of Tierra del Fuego be harvested—and how carefully? These are the types of questions the United Nations is beginning to address.

And what is to be done in the case of the country that attempts to attract direct investment in manufacturing by relaxing environmental standards, having decided that the need for local jobs is more pressing than environmental protection? The largest multinationals are bound, in theory, by a U.N. code of conduct that forbids them to shop around for easier regulations, and it is they who are being assigned responsibility for ensuring that the .technology supplied is appropriate and within the ability of the host country to control. The loopholes are potentially endless, and accountability and enforcement are still in their infancy.

In the case of domestic industries, the temptation has been to ignore unsafe practices when the local plant lacks the capital for purchasing the technology for lower emissions or detoxifying wastes, allowing it to survive. Today, however, there is greater likelihood of an international outcry. And the very multinational entities that have been the target of reform efforts are now calling for the enforcement of standards on pragmatic grounds: They do not want to have to compete with companies that are able to avoid the costs associated with ensuring environmental safety.

Environmental safety is also becoming a **trade issue.** The costs of remediating air, water, and ground pollution are increasingly factored in as a cost of business. The CTC is taking a lead role in setting the stage for international accountability for environmental damage, and justifiably claims it "has served as a catalyst for a number of national institutes" that are setting national standards [E/C.10/AC.3/1991/5]. Developed nations are beginning to bar imported goods produced in ways that do not conform to good environmental practice. In the United States and Western Europe, domestic manufacturers and labor alike contend that imported products are cheaper and compete unfairly because they contain a hidden environmental subsidy. Those seeking access to developed-country markets, for their part, tend to view environmental regulations as nontariff barriers to trade—a "protectionist ruse." Among the items barred have been crops containing safe levels of pesticides whose use has been banned in the United States, and manufactured products from countries in which worker safety is substandard or air pollution controls are lacking.

With time has come much clearer recognition that nations and corporations often **share the blame for pollution** and must cooperate in environmental regulation and in the clean up. Activities in the wake of the Chernobyl accident and ongoing efforts regarding the ozone layer provide examples of such international cooperation. The wartime polluting of the Persian Gulf and the setting of oil-well fires, as well as continuing revelations of pollution by state-run industry in the Eastern bloc, have widened the focus of concern and increased awareness of the need for cooperation from many quarters. CTC data and counseling have helped to raise this awareness.

One area in which the United Nations has been expected to achieve success without directly confronting sovereignty issues is in the **ban on drift-net fishing.** But here, as in the case of international whaling conventions, it has met resistance from nations that perceive such activities as vital to their economies. No sooner had the 44th General Assembly passed Resolution 225 on drift-net fishing than violators shifted to flags of convenience. The Secretary-General advised the 45th Session that "complete implementation . . . requires further measures in the form of national legislation governing activities of the flag State's vessels on the high seas" [A/45/663].

The U.N. system's decade-long efforts—on ozone protection and acid rain and in the aftermath of Bhopal and Chernobyl—have laid the groundwork for additional guidelines for the international community as well as TNCs as they confront an ever-wider array of environment-related issues.

Technology Transfer

Developing countries have for years tried to bargain access to their markets for access to the newest technology, whether molecular genetics, materials sciences, or advanced electronics. Now it is generally recognized that a transfer of the basic technologies of business—automation, communications, and computers—offers more immediate benefits. What is more, as these technologies and business skills come together, developing countries are able to acquire specific new technologies on far more favorable terms and enter the competition for global markets. The success of the economies of South Korea, Taiwan, Thailand, and Singapore provides a powerful example to developed and developing countries alike. These countries' early welcoming of direct investment has made them highly competitive technology exporters in just a few years. Nonetheless, their economic booms appear to have come at some social and ecological cost.

Newly recognized in discussions at the CTC and at the U.N. Industrial Development Organization (UNIDO)—the specialized agency that serves as intermediary between developing and developed countries in the cause of industrialization—is the responsibility of the technology supplier to provide **appropriate technology** to fit a strategy of sustainable development. This implies that it is the technology supplier's responsibility to ensure that the host country is able to provide environmental safeguards, that the technology will fit the growth capabilities of the country, and that the country will not put the technology to ill purpose (e.g., the making of weapons of mass destruction). There is a clear message that the technology supplier may have continuing liability even after the technology has been sold. Litigation over Bhopal continues to break ground in this area. In the case of weapons technology, the focusing of attention on the suppliers of nerve gas capability to Iraq has embarrassed home countries (e.g., Germany), some of which are attempting to prosecute exporters and pass new legislation.

The enforced embargo and the dismantling of Iraqi weapons technology, now under way, are potent examples of what U.N. resolutions can accomplish when there is force behind them. However, what the Security Council could accomplish in times of stress will not be easy to sustain in the months ahead. The permanent members of the Security

Council are the leaders of the weapons trade and home base for the most technologically volatile industries. The corporations and state enterprises continue to sell weapons at a time when the appetite of other sovereign nations for these weapons has been whetted by the demonstration of their effectiveness in the Middle East. Here, as with the environmental issues discussed above, the interests of the owners of technology, of sovereign nations, and of the world community need to be harmonized.

Until now, embargoes on technology and weapons have been effective only when focused on a single country. Yet companies and countries readily circumvent the rules, as was the case during the early years of the international sanctions against South Africa.

South Africa and Transnational Corporations

Today, 30 years after the United Nations first called for economic sanctions against South Africa, both time and internal developments have diminished the attention given to such issues as trade embargoes and the monitoring of disinvestment. Recently, the Organization of African Unity reasserted the need to continue sanctions against South Africa, and although some of the OECD countries have shown signs of relaxing sanctions, the worldwide network of civic and religious groups, cooperating enterprises, and local and municipal governments remains alert to the prospect of achieving the aim of such constraints: the **dismantling of apartheid.**

It is perhaps too soon to herald this victory, but the very fact of putting the **sanctions** into place and monitoring progress is remarkable enough. No issue has been more effective in shaping an international alliance to bring economic pressure on one country as well as on the nations and enterprises that circumvent the U.N. sanctions against it.

Documentation of the complexity—and limitations—of the financial pressure applied on South Africa is contained in the Secretary-General's report to the 45th General Assembly, "Policies of Apartheid of the Government of South Africa" [A/45/539]. The monitoring of government trade credits, bank lending, strategies of disinvestment, and import restrictions appears to have achieved a real reduction in South Africa's Gross Domestic Product of at least 20 percent, and the country's economic outlook, in the absence of trade and credit markets, became decidedly worse.

This impact has taken decades to achieve, due to a very slow learning curve that accelerated dramatically over the past few years. At first, each strengthening of the sanctions was matched by the actions of TNCs and

South Africa to evade them. This led to further rounds of monitoring and economic pressure, which had the additional effect of raising international awareness of the complexity of global business and financial transfers. The result has been both greater competence in and appreciation of the need for international accounting standards for transnational business.

International Accounting Standards

Few activities of the United Nations are likely to have a more enduring and substantial impact on international economics than are those in the little-known area of accounting standards, the bailiwick of the CTC's **Intergovernmental Working Group of Experts on International Standards of Accounting.** In a few short years this group has moved from trying to tabulate the accounting practices of developed and developing countries to setting the ground rules for keeping score in an increasingly globalized economy.

This committee of umpires is assuring that the rules will be essentially the same for both the home team and the visiting team on any playing field in the world. They have enlisted the cooperation of international securities associations, global accounting firms, associations of financial executives, and tax and trade authorities from both the developed and the developing countries. Their forums are becoming the focal point for discussions of the tradeoffs of environmental impacts, the economics of ownership for public and private enterprise, the international transfer of wealth through subsidiaries, joint ventures, trading partnerships, and other issues that affect the free flow of wealth across national borders. This knowledge is essential for the success of a global economy, and the United Nations has begun to play a lead and catalytic role in developing it.

The findings and recommendations of these studies can be deceptively simple. According to one, "Accounting by joint venture entities should follow the generally accepted principles of the country where the joint venture operates; however, internationally acceptable accounting standards should be used as the benchmark" [E/C.10/AC.3/1991/4]. This report provides the terms for one of the fastest growing and most effective ways for multinational corporations to work within developing countries, gradually transferring technology and establishing transactions on a partnership basis. Without such ground rules, developing nations will not readily permit TNCs to operate freely, investors will be reluctant to supply funds, and opportunities for sustainable development are liable to dissolve in a morass of legal and accounting disputes. Among the other particular issues addressed in the accounting standards arena are securities and publicly traded companies, environmental accounting, investment and disinvestment, and privatization.

The guidelines that emerge must catch up with the leaders of the global economy. The truly transnational corporations, including the global accounting firms, securities traders, and banks, already know how to keep score. They are accumulating wealth and power outside any one set of laws, even as they are providing much of the needed infrastructure of the global economy. If the United Nations is to help all its members become players, then its powers—to monitor, recommend, and educate—are urgently needed in this arena.

IV
Global Resource Management

1. Food and Agriculture

Contrary to many predictions, the 45th General Assembly saw little action on food and agriculture. It was instead preoccupied by the deteriorating situation in the Persian Gulf and by the pressing need to deal with the conflict precipitated by Iraq's invasion of Kuwait. While specific attention was paid to situations in particular regions, such as the Horn of Africa, Bangladesh, and the Kurdish areas of Iraq, Iran, and Turkey, the general world situation with regard to food and agriculture received little attention in the broader arena of debate.

The **World Food Council (WFC)**, the United Nations' highest policy body in this area, held its 16th session in Bangkok May 21–24, 1990 [Suppl. No. 19: A/45/19]. After reviewing individual government policies, as well as the findings of its four regional consultations (in Bangkok, Paris, Cairo, and San José, Costa Rica), the Council, in a spirit of optimism, expressed the hope "that the 1990s provide an historic opportunity to reverse the trend of growing hunger and jointly build a more equitable, just, peaceful world which will be a better home to live in for all people" [ibid., p. 4]. This optimism was dashed shortly after the meeting by the events of August 1990 in the Gulf.

Acknowledging that in the previous decade the number of hungry people had increased to more than 550 million (the most conservative figure offered by any international agency), the Council nevertheless saw possibilities for amelioration in the progress it observed in the GATT negotiations, the adoption of the Food Aid Sahel Charter by the CILSS (Comité Internationale pour la Lutte Contre la Secheresse du Sahel), and the generally increased interest among governments in dealing with the issues of hunger and malnutrition.

The Council agreed on four goals for the 1990s: "the elimination of starvation and death caused by famine; a substantial reduction of malnutrition and mortality among young children; a tangible reduction in chronic hunger; and the elimination of major nutritional-deficiency diseases" [ibid., p. 15]. Documents prepared for the 17th session of the WFC, scheduled for Helsingør, Denmark, June 5–8, 1991, suggest that very little progress has been achieved toward any of those goals.

The Bangkok WFC meeting emphasized that the debate on food and agriculture has in recent years moved beyond that sector and into the context of the global economic structure. This shift reflects the growing perception that food and agriculture are central factors in development and that hunger is, at root, a symptom, symbol, and signal of underdevelopment. It also reflects the growing emphasis on environmental problems and their impact on both the conceptual framework and the practices of the development community. It is expected that these questions will be central to the agenda of the June 1992 U.N. Conference on Environment and Development (UNCED) in Rio de Janeiro, Brazil. Indeed, the WFC declared that "there is now greater concern to make the improvement of the human condition a central objective of development" [ibid., p. 2].

The Council, repeating the basic conclusion of the 1974 World Food Conference that more food must be grown where the hungry people are, said: "Within the food-strategy framework, greater efforts will be needed to increase the productivity and incomes of small farmers and encourage them to adopt environmentally sustainable production practices; to promote rural and urban employment-generation policies and programmes; to implement more effective targeted food-subsidy and nutrition programmes; to promote measures in support of women, which take into consideration their needs and full contribution to the development process; to strengthen and build domestic institutions, with appropriate emphasis on private-sector and 'grass-roots institutions' " [ibid., p. 18].

Anticipating the World Bank's *World Development Report 1990*, the Council called for "integrating food-security and poverty-alleviation objectives into economic adjustment programmes to ensure not only that the food-security levels of low-income groups are protected during adjustment, but also that adjustment leads to long-term, sustainable reductions of hunger and malnutrition" [ibid., p. 19].

Elsewhere in the U.N. system, the **Food and Agriculture Organization's (FAO) Committee on World Food Security,** meeting in Rome, March 11–15, 1991, noted that because of a record world production of staple foods, supply had exceeded utilization for the first time in five years and that cereal stocks were expected to rise for the first time in several years [CFS:91/2]. This increase in global cereal stocks was expected to result in a decline in some cereal prices—a fact confirmed by producers in many exporting countries. To some extent the increase in stocks also reflected a decline in world trade in those commodities and consequently a lowered per capita food consumption in some low-income, food-deficit countries, mainly in sub-Saharan Africa. These observations further underscore the holistic character of the global economy; reduced consumption results from the economic and financial difficulties (i.e., external debt) afflicting several developing countries and from the general global recession.

Thus the slight overall improvement in food security in 1990 continues to mask chronic and deepening regional problems, particularly in sub-Saharan Africa. Although unwise development policies and hostile climatic conditions are generally cited as the predominant causes of hunger in Africa, it is equally clear that military conflicts in the Horn of Africa—Sudan, Ethiopia, and Somalia—as well as in Liberia, Mozambique, and Angola, have been major contributors. Hope has been expressed that the recent peaceful settlement in Angola will begin to alleviate the situation, which is likely to be exacerbated by expected crop failures in four major war-devastated provinces. In any case, all these countries remain in need of food aid to tide them over until the hoped-for period of development arrives. Meanwhile, the impact of the Persian Gulf war and the disaster in Bangladesh have strained the resources of aid-giving agencies, even when commodities are available.

Ironically, record world food production did not result in record food aid, the major operational response to hunger by the development community. On the contrary, the Committee on World Food Security projected that food aid would decline from 11.5 million tons in 1989–90 to 9.9 million in 1990–91, despite the record harvest—although budgetary allocations by major donors were expected to maintain their previous level [ibid.]. At the same time, the U.N./FAO's World Food Programme was undergoing a fundamental review of its governance and rationale by a subcommittee of the Committee on Food Aid Policies and Programmes, for which it was commended by the General Assembly [A/Res/45/218].

That review involved a new look at the question of how to make **food aid** contribute more effectively to **food security.** This question has often been addressed by the Committee on World Food Security and other groups and individuals interested in stimulating development through the provision of commodities rather than funds or technical assistance. Food aid has been provided as humanitarian assistance, as development assistance, and as assistance in emergency situations. The humanitarian motivation for food aid often springs from the guilty feeling that the unmarketable surpluses in some countries should be used to reduce endemic or intermittent starvation in others.

This matter has not been debated in the General Assembly in a long time, but the new emphasis on development, both bilateral and multilateral, and the growing conviction among food-aid donors that the development uses of that aid are of increasing importance and that improvement of ways in which food aid can add to food security, both directly and in conjunction with development programs, have led to greater attention to this kind of aid. Food aid is clearly an additional resource transfer and a part of official development assistance (ODA); yet it has been used or withheld for political purposes by many donors, and it has been frequently criticized as dependency-creating and a disincentive to domestic food production in recipient countries. For these reasons the General Assembly welcomed the new focus [CFS 91/3, passim].

Discussion in the General Assembly and elsewhere on these and related issues continues to take place against the background of worsening development problems. In the food area alone, the FAO expresses little optimism about future crop prospects in southern Africa and North America and expects no more than good or fair harvests in other regions. Cereal prospects in Asia are normal, but the situation in Latin America is uncertain. On a global basis, a supply adequate for this year's food needs appears likely, but the situation continues to deteriorate in Africa, where a variety of weather-threatened crops are grown on different production timetables. As a result, one can point to subregional differences in central, western, eastern, and southern Africa.

Joining the FAO in the concern for agricultural development are the **U.N. Development Programme (UNDP)**, whose first "Human Development Report," published in July 1990, broke new ground in dealing with hunger and poverty issues; the **International Fund for Agricultural Development (IFAD)**, which continues to concentrate on the smallest farmers and pays particular attention to low-input agriculture and to the role of women; and the **U.N. Children's Fund (UNICEF)**, whose annual report on the state of the world's children provides graphic and compelling information on the extent of hunger and malnutrition among the most vulnerable victims of underdevelopment. All three of these U.N. agencies conduct and support activities that contribute to food security.

The **General Assembly's** primary involvement in food and agricultural issues includes the reports it receives from the operating agencies and the policy analyses and proposals of the World Food Council—often via the U.N. Economic and Social Council (ECOSOC). Certain ad hoc U.N. events, like the **World Summit on Children,** which convened more than 60 heads of state at the end of September 1990, and the upcoming Conference on Environment and Development, focus indirectly on these issues and generally raise public awareness, at least when they receive media coverage.

Sectoral emphases, such as food and agriculture, are increasingly dealt with in the context of broader debates on subjects like the environment, development, trade, and finance. It becomes increasingly clear that the interdependence of these topics and the problems of dealing with them rule out treating them as separate matters. The GATT negotiations, the environmental debate, the urgent problems of more than 15 million refugees in various parts of the developing world, the handling of external debt, the war in the Persian Gulf, the development models of the World Bank and other aid donors—all these have much more bearing on food and agriculture than almost any specific debate in the General Assembly. Indeed, there have been few such debates on this sector.

The problem of world food security, which is what the sectoral emphasis on food and agriculture was originally about, is now understood to be a pervasive matter and is touched on in all major debates. The documents prepared for the upcoming 17th session of the World Food Council—documents that will establish the policy debate framework that will be reported to the 46th General Assembly via ECOSOC—bear out this judgment in considerable and convincing detail.

The first such document, "Food Security Implications of the Changes in the Political and Economic Environment," begins with a segment entitled "Overall Economic Outlook and Prospects for Poverty Alleviation in the 1990s" [WFC/1991/3]. The document deals with the impact of the political changes in Eastern Europe and the economic integration of Western Europe (Europe 1992) on the battle against world hunger. It concludes that external support for Eastern Europe and the Soviet Union will change agricultural and other trade patterns, as well as foreign aid allocations, most likely with negative effects for the food-deficit developing countries.

With respect to the GATT negotiations, it notes that the difficulty of reaching agreement in the agricultural sector imposes serious costs on the world's poor people. The document also points out the serious economic losses sustained by Turkey, Jordan, Egypt, and, of course, Iraq. It concludes that "the current and prospective global economic environment is not conducive to meeting these challenges and points to the need for special efforts by the council to maintain the political momentum for fighting hunger and malnutrition as a central objective of the International Development Strategy for the 1990s, adopted by all members of the United Nations" [ibid., p. 45].

A second document, "Focusing Development Assistance on Hunger- and Poverty-Alleviation" [SFC/1991/5], summarizes earlier efforts to direct aid toward poverty alleviation and concludes that "the international community is giving clear signals of its intention to give increasing attention to problems of poverty, hunger, and malnutrition." At the same time, the document notes that "the continuing growth in the number of hungry people testifies that neither domestic policies nor external development assistance . . . have been effective in addressing hunger and poverty problems" [ibid., p. 5].

Most aid, the document says, does not reach the poor, partly because that has not been its main purpose; rather, politics, commerce, and strategy have played the most decisive roles in foreign aid allocations by most countries. The document continues to advocate enhanced policy dialogue among the donors, but acknowledges that the increasingly critical nature of financial problems has made structural adjustment the dominant element in that dialogue and rendered the urgently needed emphasis on poverty-focused activities much more difficult to achieve.

In its discussion of the food security implications of the GATT negotiations, the WFC secretariat's brief report, "The Consequences for Food Security of the Multilateral Trade Negotiations in the Uruguay Round" [WFC/1991/4], stresses the importance of a successful outcome, especially of the efforts to liberalize agricultural trade, but acknowledges that the food security considerations that have constituted the agenda of the Council since its formation in 1975 have not been accorded the attention that their urgency warrants. The main area of debate has been between the somewhat limited proposal by the donors to initiate negotiations for a new Food Aid Convention and the broader measures for differential treatment proposed by the food-deficit developing countries.

In April 1991 the World Food Council, fulfilling a mandate from its 1990 Bangkok meeting, convened a consultation in Cairo to discuss more fully the results of the regional meetings that had preceded the Bangkok session. The information made available to the consultation was far from upbeat ["Meeting the Developing Countries' Food Production Challenges of the 1990s and Beyond," WFC/1991/6].

Although the Council had called for a renewal of the Green Revolution as the central focus of the thrust toward food security and against hunger, the consultation was inclined to circumscribe that endorsement, recognizing that the benefits of the Green Revolution in South Asia and elsewhere had not been equitably shared and that the circumstances of sub-Saharan Africa, for example, raised questions about its direct adaptability. "In particular," the study noted, "there has been much controversy about the Green Revolution's socio-economic benefits in terms of sustainable food security for all people and the alleviation of poverty. The general conclusion is that neither the Green Revolution nor the slow spread of other agricultural technology has done much to reduce hunger or poverty" [ibid., p. 35].

The report described the year 2000 outlook for Africa as "alarming," citing studies by the World Bank and the International Food Policy Research Institute. Similar concern was expressed about Central America and the Caribbean region. In both instances the fragility of the resource base appeared to be a major factor on the supply side, and on the demand side the political and social institutional infrastructure was a major impediment to equitable distribution. Because specific policy changes would have exceeded the mandate of the consultation, the major recommendation was to strengthen, upgrade, and expand the research and technology capacities of countries at risk.

It seems almost too obvious to point out that all four of these preparatory documents have much more to do with food security than with food production (that is, with food rather than agriculture, or with the demand rather than the supply side of the famous equation). This reflects the inexorable shift of emphasis, beginning with the 1974 World Food Conference, from production to distribution. As long as population continues to increase more rapidly than food production, especially in the food-deficit areas, consideration must be given, of course, to increasing supply; and the supply-side elements of land, water, energy, research, technology, and climate must receive major attention.

At the same time, it has to be acknowledged, as every official and responsible report and study does, that enough food is produced every year to provide every human being on earth an adequate (not just a minimal) diet. However, each person must have access to it, and, for all practical purposes and in normal circumstances, access is a function of income. Therefore hunger (i.e., lack of food security) is a function of poverty. Poverty itself results from underdevelopment—or inadequate sharing of the benefits of development. This shifts the debate to the demand side—away from the "easier" problems of technology, research, and farming practices to the more intractable ones of distributive justice. Who will benefit when the majority of potential beneficiaries have no part in the decision about the sharing?

Considerations such as these lead to discussions about:

a. Why concessional aid is declining as a proportion of resource transfers and is being allocated less and less in terms of genuine need and authentic development;

b.. How the developing countries' growing external debt burden (up 6 percent in 1990, to $1.341 trillion, according to the World Bank's 1990 *World Debt Tables*) is to be handled without condemning the debtors to unending stagnation;

c. How unofficial financial transfers, mainly via private investment, are to be increased without at the same time increasing dependence and worker exploitation in the host developing countries;

d. How the deteriorating terms of trade for those developing countries that mainly export primary commodities are to be reversed, so that they can earn the foreign exchange without which development, in the current global economic order, is almost impossible;

e. How the development sought by all, in both quality of life and quantity of GNP, is to be achieved in a participatory, equitable, and sustainable fashion.

2. Population

The world's population, now at 5.4 billion, will most likely reach 10 billion by the year 2050, according to revised projections published by the U.N. Population Fund (UNFPA) in its 1991 *State of World Population* issued in May. Earlier U.N. projections estimated that global population would stabilize at 10.2 billion by the year 2085, but under the new scenario, world population is expected to grow into the 22nd century and to stabilize at a level of more than 11.6 billion [UNFPA, Report of the Executive Director, *State of World Population 1991*, p. 3].

The U.N. medium projection of a 10 billion population level in the year 2050 is dependent on the number of developing-country couples using contraception increasing from 381 million to 567 million by the year 2000 [ibid., p. 6]. World population could stabilize at just over 9 billion within the next century if universal access to and widespread use of family planning were achieved in this decade. However, if family planning programs and contraceptive use expand more slowly and birth rates fall more gradually, world population could exceed 14 billion before stabilizing [Population Crisis Committee, *1990 Report on Progress Towards Population Stabilization*].

The U.N. medium projection is contingent on 59 percent of developing country couples practicing family planning by the year 2000, up from 51 percent in 1990 [UNFPA, *State of World Population*, p. 6]. However, a stable world population will not be achieved until about 75 percent of couples in the world use contraceptives and a two-child family average is reached, as is the case in most developed countries today.

The average number of children born to a woman in her reproductive years is declining in all major regions of the world. Population Council researchers estimate that world population would be 412 million people larger today in the absence of organized family planning programs ["The Demographic Impact of Family Planning Programs," *Studies in Family Planning*, 11–12/90]. Even in areas where fertility is high and contraceptive use low, such as South Asia and Africa, women are having fewer children now than in the early 1960s. In South Asia, fertility is expected to decline to 4 children per woman by the late 1990s and then to 2.2 children in 2020–25, based on the new U.N. medium projections. In Africa, fertility is projected to decline to 3 children per woman by 2020–25, down from 6.2 today [UNFPA, *State of World Population*, p. 7].

The countries facing the greatest increases in population are those least able to afford universal access to family planning. The expansion of family planning necessary to achieve these declines in fertility cannot take place without help from the international community. Self-reliance is the goal of population activities, but it will remain beyond the reach of the least developed countries, including most of sub-Saharan Africa, during the 1990s.

One key to breaking the cycle of poverty is to enable couples to plan the size of their families. Continuing population pressures have made efforts to alleviate poverty more difficult, and some countries are falling further behind. As the number of people increases, per capita incomes are declining in many parts of the world. In some countries in Latin America and most of sub-Saharan Africa, the 1980s were a lost decade, with declining real per capita income and living standards [World Bank, *World Development Report 1990*, p. 2]. In 1985 more than one billion people, or almost a third of the developing world, were living on less than $370 a year [ibid., p. 28]. The number of people with a per capita income below $300 is projected to increase rather than decrease by the year 2000.

One billion people will be added to the world's population over the next 10 years under the U.N. medium projection. Ninety-five percent of this projected growth will occur in developing countries. South Asia, which includes India, Bangladesh, Pakistan, and Iran, will have the largest numerical increase, from 1.2 billion today to 1.5 billion people by the end of the century. Africa will experience the greatest percentage increase—38 percent—from 650 million today to 900 million by the year 2000. In Latin America and the Caribbean, the population will reach 540 million by the century's end, an increase of 100 million [UNFPA, *State of World Population*, p. 3].

On the other end of the spectrum, East Asia, which includes China and Japan, is growing very slowly. Japan is already below replacement-level fertility, an average family size of less than two children. China, Korea, and Thailand are close to replacement level. The countries of North America and Europe, with few exceptions, have growth rates of less than one percent, and the average family has less than two children. Most of these nations appear to be on their way to population stabilization; but in some, immigration remains an important source of growth.

By the year 2000, UNFPA estimates that a total of 567 million of the 980 million couples in developing countries will practice family planning, an increase of 186 million couples. The average annual cost of providing comprehensive family planning services is $16 per couple. About 140 million of the anticipated additional users of family planning will be in Asia, with the remaining 46 million divided among Africa, Latin America and the Caribbean, and the Arab states [ibid., p. 6].

The cost of providing these services will require at least a doubling of expenditures over the course of the 1990s. Developing countries now pay about two-thirds or $3.5 billion of the $4 to $4.5 billion annual cost of family planning programs [ibid., p. 34]. Total international assistance, including World Bank contributions, adds another $760 million a year [UNFPA, *Global Population Assistance Report 1982–1989*, p. 20]. Ten countries provide about 95 percent of all international population assistance. The United States is the largest single contributor and gives more than $300 million annually. Japan has become the second largest donor, contributing more than 10 percent. Other significant contributors are Canada, Denmark, Finland, Germany, the Netherlands, Norway, Sweden, and the United Kingdom. Of these ten countries, only the United States makes no contribution to UNFPA.

Half of the $9 billion minimum needed for family planning services by the year 2000 should come from the developing countries themselves. Bilateral and multilateral donors and nongovernmental organizations are to provide the remaining $4.5 billion, including substantial increases from the World Bank. The General Assembly has endorsed the mobilization of these financial resources for international population assistance, as outlined by the Amsterdam Declaration, and reaffirmed the importance of the role of population policies in development [A/Res/45/199]. A similar official endorsement for greater family planning funding is contained in a policy statement, *Development Cooperation in the 1990s,* adopted by the Development Assistance Committee of the OECD. UNFPA hopes to increase its own expenditures on family planning to $500 million by 1994 and to $1 billion by the year 2000 [*Population,* 3/91].

The message that family planning promotes human welfare and development is becoming broadly accepted by families and governments around the world. According to UNFPA, 144 countries provide either direct or indirect support to family planning programs. Only four of the world's 170 governments intentionally restrict access to family planning services [U.N., *World Population Policies,* 1990]. Prominent among the four is Iraq, where Saddam Hussein's pronatalist policies led to the highest population growth rate in the world prior to the Gulf war [Population Reference Bureau, *1990 World Population Data Sheet*]. Developing-country governments increasingly believe that rapid population growth aggravates many of their social and economic problems. Environmental degradation, food shortages, migration, rapid urbanization, deteriorating social services, and political instability are all exacerbated by ever-increasing numbers of people in the world's poorest countries.

Family planning itself has a positive impact on the health of women and children. According to the World Health Organization (WHO), half a million women die each year as a result of pregnancy and childbirth. Of these deaths, 99 percent occur in developing countries and most of them are preventable. It is estimated that between 25 and 40 percent of maternal deaths could be prevented if women could simply choose to avoid unintended and poorly timed pregnancies. Spacing the births of children at least two years apart could save the lives of almost 2 million infants and children each year. If women also waited until age 20 before having their first child, the number of lives saved would increase to 3 million, preventing one out of five infant and child deaths [Shanti Conly, *Family Planning and Child Survival* (Population Crisis Committee, 1990), pp. 13–14].

In many parts of the world, mounting population pressure on arable land, fuelwood supplies, fresh water, and other renewable natural resources has caused rapid deterioration in local ecological systems, further impoverishing the poor families who depend on the renewability of natural resources for their own survival. In just 20 years the world will need to feed a population 40 percent larger than today's. Some experts estimate that around two-thirds of recent tropical deforestation can be related to population growth, largely through its impact on the demand for more agricultural land for food production [Paul Harrison, "Too Much Life on Earth?" *New Scientist*, 5/19/90]. Even in the Amazon region, where misguided government policies are responsible for much deforestation, population pressures and poverty have driven millions of landless settlers into virgin rain forests, where most practice small-scale but unsustainable slash-and-burn cultivation.

Population growth also drives up demand for fuel, and for 2 billion people in the developing world this still means firewood. In parts of Africa, fuelwood consumption is at least four times the rate of tree regrowth. Some African women now spend as much as half their waking hours collecting scarce supplies of firewood, fodder, and fresh water [Robin Clark, "The Disappearing Forests," *UNEP Environment Brief* (3) 1988, p. 5].

A doubling of world population also has implications for global warming. Population size, together with economic activity, affects greenhouse gas emissions, but "reducing population growth alone may not reduce emission of greenhouse gases because it may also stimulate growth in per capita income" [National Academy of Sciences, *Policy Implications of Greenhouse Warming*, 1991, p. 81]. Changes in the pattern of energy use may reduce the impact of population growth and the resulting increase in economic activity.

Lack of access to safe water supplies is also exacerbated by demographic trends. At the Global Consultation on Safe Water and Sanitation for the 1990s in New Delhi, delegates learned that by the year 2000 there could be a total of three-quarters of a billion people, principally in Africa and Asia, without an adequate water supply and more than double that number without sanitation [*The New York Times*, 9/11/90].

The environmental impact of continued population growth in the developed world—most important, in the United States and the Soviet Union—cannot be ignored. Natural population increase in the United States adds 2 million people to the world's population every year, a small amount compared to India and China, which add over 18 and 15 million respectively [PRB, *1991 World Population Data Sheet*]. However, because the average American puts much greater demands on the world's natural resources, U.S. population growth makes a significant contribution to global environmental problems. As Paul and Anne Ehrlich have pointed out:

> Statistics on per capita commercial energy use are a reasonable index of the responsibility for damage to the environment and the consumption of resources by an average citizen of a nation. By that measure, a baby born in the United States represents twice the disaster for Earth

as one born in Sweden or the USSR, three times one born in Italy, 13 times one born in Brazil, 35 times one in India, 140 times one in Bangladesh or Kenya, and 280 times one in Chad, Rwanda, Haiti, or Nepal ["Too Many Rich Folks," *Populi* 16, no. 3, 9/89, p. 25].

It is becoming clear in this last decade of the 20th century that human populations are, with current technology and patterns of consumption, already threatening the earth's ability to support life. The U.N. Conference on Environment and Development in 1992 presents the world's peoples with a unique and timely opportunity. By means of the proposed **Earth Charter** and **Agenda 21**—the former a set of principles guiding the conduct of nations regarding sustainable development, the latter specific actions to implement these principles—the countries of the North and South, East and West could strike a new global bargain based on a true sense of common destiny and shared responsibility for the planet. However, any new global bargain to preserve the earth and the life it sustains must begin with an understanding of the widespread poverty, the mounting pressures of human numbers, and the degradation of natural resources as three problems so closely intertwined that one of them cannot be solved without progress on the others.

While a new global bargain must include a greater cooperative effort to stabilize world population, clearly it must also include a demonstrated commitment on the part of the industrialized countries to reduce their profligate use of natural resources and to increase support for the development and worldwide dissemination of appropriate technologies for natural resource conservation and environmentally sustainable agricultural and industrial development. All parties must agree to share in the responsibility to reverse worldwide the loss of forest, the degradation of soil, the contamination of air and water, and the disappearance of plant and animal species [InterAction Statement of Principles on Sustainable Development, 11/90].

All of these efforts will require substantial new investments, but population stabilization requires the smallest. Compared to the cost of reforestation, adaptation to energy-efficient technologies, or sewage treatment plants, for example, the price tag for universal availability of family planning is very small. For about $5 billion a year now and about $10 billion a year by the year 2000, every couple of childbearing age could gain access to safe and effective fertility control by the end of this decade. Population would stabilize short of another doubling over the next 60 years. If this is not accomplished, the costs in human suffering and in irreversible environmental damage will be incalculable.

According to UNCED organizers, preparations for UNCED include discussion of population growth as one of several crosscutting development issues [*Earth Summit News*, 3/91]. Some are looking to the conference to produce a worldwide commitment to achieving early population stabilization and universal access to family planning by the year 2000. The prospects for the conference taking such action are encouraging. Several of the conference documents, prepared by the UNCED secretariat and presented at the preparatory committee meeting in Geneva in March 1991, include fair, balanced, and thoughtful discussions of population-environmental linkages in the context of crosscutting themes [A/Conf. 151/PC/15 and 16]. Strong statements on population and environmental issues were made at the March meeting by the delegations of Finland, Canada, the Netherlands, the United Kingdom, and the United States, with support from Australia, Senegal, and Jamaica [Philander Claxton, "Report to NGOs on Second Preparatory Committee on UNCED"]. With additional encouragement from governments, the secretariat may be prepared to expand coverage of population issues.

Although the original General Assembly resolution mandating the conference did not include any reference to population matters, in December 1990 the Assembly specifically emphasized the importance of "addressing the relationship between demographic pressures and unsustainable consumption patterns and environmental degradation during the preparatory process of the United Nations Conference on Environment and Development" [A/Res/45/216]. Despite the passage of this resolution, some continue to make the argument that UNCED is not authorized to consider population issues. However, the conference may certainly do so if member governments wish to raise the topic.

Unanimity among governments does not exist, of course, on the importance of discussing population as a crosscutting issue at the conference. Although committed to national population policies and family planning programs at home, many developing countries want to be sure that the conference adequately recognizes the share of responsibility for global environmental problems borne by the industrialized world and its wasteful consumption patterns. These nations fear that discussions of population problems could be used to shift the blame unfairly. Developing countries are concerned that the conference preparations have given too little weight to development issues and to the need for debt relief, technology transfer, and increased aid flows, if they are expected to address environmental problems. In addition, some point to the international conference on population in 1994 as the appropriate forum for discussion of population issues. Therefore, a strong outcome on population is unlikely at UNCED unless developed countries press for it and unless they respond appropriately to the concerns of developing countries.

Despite the mounting evidence that world population will probably at least double and could almost triple to 14 billion by 2100 without a large infusion of resources, political controversies in the United States still threaten to undermine the global consensus on the need for expanded family planning and population programs.

Ignoring calls for better international cooperation, the United States no longer contributes to UNFPA, an institution it was instrumental in establishing over 20 years ago, because of UNFPA's program in China. In 1985 the **U.S. Agency for International Development (AID)** withheld $10 million of an earmarked $46 million for UNFPA, claiming the organization was involved in comanaging China's population program and that the Chinese program relied on coercive abortion and involuntary sterilization to implement its one child per couple policy. In the five years since, the administration has not changed its view of UNFPA and has withheld all funding of the agency, despite repeated attempts by Congress to reinitiate funding.

As the basis for its decisions to withhold funds, AID has cited what has come to be known as the Kemp-Inouye amendment, originally part of the supplemental foreign aid appropriation in 1985. The amendment prohibits U.S. funding of any organization that "supports or participates in the management of a program of coercive abortion or involuntary sterilization." AID has established conditions under which U.S. contributions could be resumed: China must prevent coercion by punishing abuses or UNFPA must "radically change its assistance to the China program . . . such as by supplying only contraceptives" [AID administrator M. Peter McPherson to Senator Mark Hatfield, 9/25/85].

AID has continued to maintain that the activities of neither the Chinese government nor UNFPA have changed sufficiently to warrant renewed U.S. support. UNFPA has repeatedly denied the allegation, pointing out that it does not support abortion in China or anywhere else in the world since the international community does not consider abortion to be a method of family planning. In addition, UNFPA denies the charge that it "manages" China's program. The size of UNFPA's contribution relative to the Chinese government's expenditures ($10 million versus $1 billion annually, or 1 percent of the total) and the number of UNFPA staff in Beijing compared to the employees of the State Family Planning Commission (4 versus 160,000 family planning workers, plus numerous volunteers, scattered throughout the countryside) suggest that allegations that UNFPA helps manage the Chinese program are far-fetched. Of the funds that have been allocated by UNFPA for projects in China under the five-year program that began in 1990, only 1 percent has gone to the government of China, with the remainder administered through "executing" agencies, such as WHO, UNICEF, FAO, and nongovernmental organizations [UNFPA, "Facts About UNFPA and China," 10/90].

Critics of U.S. policy have long maintained that U.S. birth control opponents have never been able to produce evidence of UNFPA complicity, a fact confirmed by a 1985 review of UNFPA's assistance to China, which concluded that UNFPA "neither funds abortions nor supports coercive family planning practices" [AID, "Review of UNFPA Program for Compliance with U.S. Law and Policy" (executive summary), 3/85]. Prior to 1989, the United States had never formally expressed any concern about the China program in the UNDP/UNFPA Governing Council, the appropriate institutional forum. The Governing Council approved five-year China programs in 1980 and 1984, and subsequent annual meetings were notable for the absence of any expressions of concern about the China program from the United States. Many critics of U.S. policy marshal such facts to support the contention that the withdrawal of U.S. funding from UNFPA was primarily a concession to a vocal domestic political constituency rather than an expression of concern about alleged human rights violations in China.

Defenders of UNFPA believe that the organization plays a positive role by strengthening voluntarism in the Chinese population program. Since 1980, UNFPA has supported modern contraceptive production to improve the typically low quality of contraceptives manufactured in China. Its funds have provided production equipment, analytical instruments, and technical assistance to 18 factories and two training institutions. The wide availability of higher quality contraceptives promotes voluntary participation in the population program by reducing the incidence of unplanned pregnancies resulting from contraceptive failures and discontinuation of use. For example, one study of the impact of Chinese women replacing primitive steel rings with modern copper-bearing IUDs, manufactured by two factories built with UNFPA support, estimates that 324,000 unplanned pregnancies, many of which would be aborted, are prevented each year [personal communication, 11/89].

UNFPA is currently in the second year of a $57 million assistance program in China for the period 1990–94, which was presented for approval to the 48-member Governing Council in June 1989. The program concentrates on three priority areas: contraceptive production and research, maternal and child health programs, and the training of demographers. Assisting in the implementation of major components of the new program will be UNICEF and WHO [DP/FPA/CP/48]. The composition of the new program eliminates some of the activities that UNFPA funded in China that the U.S. government found most objectionable, such as technical assistance in census taking and other demographic data collection and analysis. Despite these UNFPA and Chinese efforts at accommodation, the U.S. delegate to the Governing Council expressed strong opposition to the new cycle of U.N. assistance to China. Acceding to the demands of anti-abortion legislators and pressure groups, the Bush administration stated that the United States "strongly oppose[s] the program as currently formulated and dissociate [sic] ourselves unequivocally from any interpretation of this body's consensus that suggests we approve the family planning program in the People's Republic of China" [AID press release, 6/7/89]. No other country rose to criticize the new program. Four nations—Australia, Bangladesh, Romania, and the Federal Republic of Germany—spoke in its favor, and the program was approved by consensus.

In response to the Bush administration's refusal to restore U.S. support to UNFPA, family planning supporters in the U.S. Congress have unsuccessfully attempted to pass legislation to force AID to fund UNFPA. An amendment to the fiscal year 1990 foreign aid appropriation bill, sponsored by Senator Barbara Mikulski (D–Md.), earmarked $15 million for UNFPA and stipulated that UNFPA was to maintain the U.S. funds in a segregated account, none of which could be used in China. The Mikulski amendment was adopted by both houses of Congress as a reasonable compromise to break the impasse over UNFPA funding. It was sent to President Bush as part of a $14 billion foreign aid appropriation bill. Rather than sign the bill with the Mikulski amendment, President Bush vetoed the legislation, refusing to fund UNFPA's program, which he described in his veto message as "inconsistent with American values" and contrary to the "human rights character of our foreign policy around the world" [*Congressional Quarterly*, 11/25/90, p. 3266]. During 1990, Congress failed to adopt legislation restoring the U.S. contribution to UNFPA.

In June 1991, UNFPA supporters in the House of Representatives attached amendments to both the foreign aid authorization and appropriations bills earmarking a $20 million contribution to UNFPA in fiscal year 1992. Anti-abortion forces attempted to remove the amendment to the authorization bill but failed on a vote of 234 to 188. Action by the Senate was pending at press time. However, even if congressional initiatives to refund UNFPA are successfully attached to foreign aid bills in

1991, vetoes by President Bush are expected, barring a major shift in the political risk-benefit calculation at the White House. Such a shift may be more of a possibility than previously thought because the issue of refunding UNFPA has become enmeshed in a much larger foreign policy debate between the President and Congress over renewal of most favored nation trade status for China.

Despite the absence of U.S. participation, contributions from other donor governments in 1990 pushed UNFPA income over the $200 million level for the first time. Donor assistance grew from $125 million in 1980 to $210 million in 1990. However, adjusted for inflation and for declines in the value of the U.S. dollar, contributions were worth about 60 percent less. As a result of the lack of resources, $300 million worth of developing-country projects cannot be funded [*Population*, 3/91].

Another example of the contentious abortion issue's intrusion into the work of the United Nations is the **threat to the U.S. contribution to WHO** because of its involvement in the development and alleged promotion of RU-486, the so-called French abortion pill. John Bolton, Assistant Secretary of State for International Organization Affairs, wrote to WHO Director-General Hiroshi Nakajima requesting information on WHO's abortion research activities [letter from Bolton to Nakajima, 3/14/91]. The inquiry was made on behalf of members of Congress and organizations opposed to abortion, perhaps foreshadowing legislative initiatives to cut off or reduce U.S. funding for the agency. The U.S. inquiries come at a time when member states are urging WHO to pay greater attention to high population growth rates in light of advances in basic health and accompanying reductions in death rates [*Population*, 4/91].

WHO has denied that its RU-486 research has in any way violated the conditions under which it receives funding from the United States. WHO serves only as the executing agency for the Special Programme of Research, Development, and Research Training in Human Reproduction, which has conducted research on RU-486. The Special Programme receives voluntary contributions from a number of bilateral donors (not including the United States) and the World Bank, WHO, UNFPA, and UNDP. Compared to WHO's total annual budget of $654 million, expenditures for research on RU-486 were minuscule—a mere 1.7 percent of the Special Programme's $20.7 million budget in 1989 [*The New York Times*, 4/7/91]. WHO has previously stated that "safe and effective medical methods of early termination of pregnancy have the potential for less adverse effects than surgical abortion." Therefore, the organization believes that scientific research on RU-486 is appropriate and necessary and has noted that "it is up to Member States to formulate their own policies on abortion" [WHO Statement on RU-486, 3/89]. The recipients of the **U.N. Population Award** for 1991 are Dr. Julia Henderson, who served as Secretary-General of the International Planned Parenthood Federation from 1971 to 1978 after a distinguished career at the United Nations; and the Centro de Estudios de Poblacion y Paternidad Responsable of Ecuador, a demographic research institution [*Population*, 3/91].

3. Environment

Safeguarding the future of the planet from environmental degradation has emerged as one of the most urgent priorities on the international agenda in the 1990s. New and startling scientific data about the rapid pace with which **chlorofluorocarbons (CFCs) and halons** are destroying Earth's ozone layer moved 93 nations to strengthen the **1987 Montreal Protocol on Substances that Deplete the Ozone Layer** in June 1990. The Montreal Protocol, negotiated under the auspices of the **United Nations Environment Programme (UNEP)**, called on signatories to halve CFC production by 1998 [*The New York Times*, 6/30/90]. The new agreement, calling on nations to halt CFC production by the end of the century, was nearly undermined when the United States reversed an earlier decision to support the establishment of a multilateral fund to help developing countries phase out CFCs. Under heavy fire from its European allies, the United States reversed its position again at the 11th hour. The treaty came into effect on March 7, 1991 [U.N. press release HE/735, 3/15/91].

International concern over **global warming** escalated substantially with the release of three authoritative reports by the **International Panel for Climate Change (IPCC)** in the spring of 1990. The IPCC was established by UNEP and the **World Meteorological Organization (WMO)** in November 1988 to coordinate and unify the world's scientific and policy-making communities for effective, realistic, and equitable action on climate change [*Issues Before the 43rd General Assembly of the United Nations*, p. 107]. The panel concluded that emissions of greenhouse gases (primarily carbon dioxide, but also methane, CFCs, and nitrous oxides, among others) were causing a rise in the global mean temperature and would have to be reduced by 60 percent to stabilize concentrations at today's levels [*The InterDependent* 16, no. 3, 1990]. Several attempts to reach agreement among industrialized nations on stabilizing carbon emissions have been blocked by the United States—first, at a regional conference of European and North American nations on environment and development, held in Bergen, Norway, in May 1990, and a month later when the Group of Seven industrialized nations met in Houston, Texas, for their annual summit meeting. At the **Second World Climate Conference**, held in Geneva from October 29 to November 7, 1990, 135 nations adopted a declaration calling on nations to reduce greenhouse gas emissions through national and regional actions, and to negotiate a global convention on climate change [U.N. press release ENV/DEV/26, 2/1/91]. While Japan, Canada, Australia, New Zealand, and 18 European nations pledged to cut back carbon dioxide emissions, the Soviet Union joined the United States in refusing to make similar commitments [*The New York Times*, 11/7/90].

From February 4 to 14, 1991, the United States was host to the first round of negotiations by the **International Negotiating Committee** on a framework convention on climate change, to be ready for signature in June 1992. By the end of the general debate, Committee Chairman Jean Ripert of France found several points of agreement among delegates on a global approach to climate change: The stabilization of greenhouse gas emissions should be the first step toward their reduction; measures were required to enable developing countries to become full partners in the negotiating process; and those countries would need additional financial resources and technology [U.N. press release ENV/DEV/34, 2/8/91]. *UNEP North America News* reported that "most of the 130 nations [were] confounded by U.S. reluctance" to reduce carbon emissions [Vol. 16, nos. 1 & 2].

Brazil 1992

A "landmark" decision by the 44th General Assembly to convene a **United Nations Conference on Environment and Development (UNCED)**—to be held in Rio de Janeiro, Brazil, June 1–12, 1992—has put virtually every environmental issue on the table for international negotiation in 1991–92. In a gesture symbolizing the high priority being given to the event, the 45th General Assembly urged that UNCED representation be at the level of Head of State—possibly making it the largest international summit to date.

The conference will mark the 20th anniversary of the **1972 U.N. Conference on the Human Environment** and, along with it, a change in the way nations view environmental issues. In the years since the Stockholm conference, both the developing and the developed worlds have come to see that hopes for sustained economic growth can be fulfilled only if the environment is recognized as a major factor. The 44th General Assembly made this link clear when it mandated UNCED to elaborate strategies that will promote "sustainable and environmentally-sound development in all countries" [A/Res/44/228]. These strategies are intended not only to halt but to reverse the effects of environmental degradation. "The Stockholm Conference put environment on the international agenda," writes UNCED Secretary-General Maurice Strong. "[UNCED] will move it into the center of economic policy and decision-making" [*Earth Summit News*, no. 1, 3/91].

The conference will be run from an ad hoc secretariat in Geneva with one unit in New York to act as liaison with U.N. bodies and the missions to the United Nations, and a second unit in Nairobi, Kenya, to act as liaison with UNEP, which is headquartered there. Coordinating the complex two-year planning process, drawing up the provisional agenda, and drafting all the resolutions for consideration by the conference is a preparatory committee made up of all members of the United Nations and its specialized agencies and chaired by Tommy Koh, former Permanent Representative of Singapore. At its organizational session, held in New York, March 5–16, 1990, the committee established "two open-ended working groups which would meet in conjunction with the substantive sessions of the Committee, at the same venues, and would submit progress reports to the Committee on their work" [A/Conf.151/PC/4, 6/13/90]. **Working Group I** addresses the issues of Protection of the Atmosphere by Combating Transboundary Air Pollution, Protection of the Atmosphere by Combating Climate Change, Protection and Management of Land Resources by Combating Deforestation, Protection and Management of Land Resources by Combating Desertification and Land Degradation, Conservation of Biological Diversity, and Environmentally Sound Management of Biotechnology. **Working Group II** addresses the Protection of the Oceans and of Coastal Areas, Rational Use of Marine Living Resources, Protection of the Supply and Quality of Fresh-Water Resources, Environmentally Sound Management of Toxic Chemicals, and Environmentally Sound Management of Hazardous Waste. All are to be examined from a development perspective, taking into account such matters as indigenous patterns of consumption and production, the relationship between food security and agricultural practices, and the development of human resources.

Other issues to be addressed by the preparatory committee are the Improvement of the Living and Working Environment of the Poor, Protection of Human Health Conditions and Improvement of the Quality of Life, and a variety of "cross-sectoral" issues, including the questions of Financial Resources, Technology Transfer, Legal Aspects, Institutions, and Supporting Measures [A/Conf.151.PC/5, 6/28/90].

Owing to a prolonged and heated debate among member states over the mandate of **Working Group III,** this group was not established until March 1991, during the second substantive session of the committee (PrepCom II). While most developed and some developing countries believed that Group III should deal strictly with legal and institutional matters, many developing countries supported a broader definition that would encompass the "cross-sectoral" issues of technology transfer and additional funding—the two most politically divisive issues on the UNCED agenda. In a compromise, the PrepCom gave Group III a somewhat ambiguous mandate to deal with "legal, institutional and all related matters" [A/Conf.151/PC/L.31, 3/22/91].

The Preparatory Committee, in response to a proposal by the Conference Secretary-General, is considering organizing the 1992 event around six agenda items: an **Earth Charter,** containing basic principles of conduct to promote a sustainable future; **Agenda 21,** specifying the actions to take in implementing the Charter; measures to finance those actions and to ensure developing countries the resources for promoting sustainable development; measures to ensure access to environmentally sound technologies on an equitable and affordable basis; the strengthening of existing international environmental institutions as well as the creation of new machinery that promotes the examination of environment-development issues at the highest policy-making levels of government; and conventions on climate change and biodiversity.

Formal provisions were made by the PrepComs for regional, national, and nongovernmental input. Regional meetings have been held for Africa, in Kampala, Uganda (June 1989), for Europe and North America, in Bergen, Norway (May 8–16, 1990), for the Asian region, in Bangkok (October 15–16, 1990), and for Latin America and the Caribbean, in Mexico City (March 4–7, 1991). Their final reports are to be integrated into the work of the PrepComs. Governments have been asked to submit national reports to the conference secretariat in July 1991 that assess environment and development trends and problems of the last 20 years, and that identify current policy options.

In his report to the committee's organizational session in March 1990, Conference Secretary-General Maurice Strong stressed the importance of effective nongovernmental participation throughout the process, stating that "the community of nongovernmental organizations had an extensive network and keen interest in a wide range of environmental issues" and thus could enrich the deliberations [A/Conf.151/PC/9, 6/22/90]. While many delegations viewed their participation as vital, some expressed strong concern that the PrepComs might become a free-for-all if there were no restrictions on the input of nongovernmental organizations (NGOs) [*The InterDependent* 17, no. 1, 1991]. The committee requested the secretariat to submit "at its first session suggested arrangements for involving nongovernmental organizations in the preparatory process for the Conference," and it took note of proposals from nongovernmental organizations that "regional conferences and working groups on environment and development should make use of the regional expertise of nongovernmental organizations, and that both NGOs in consultative status to ECOSOC and others with special interest in the subject matter of the Conference be invited to participate fully in it and its preparatory meetings" [A/Conf.151/PC/9, 6/22/90].

At PrepCom I in Nairobi, August 6–31, 1990, the committee gave all "relevant" nongovernmental organizations the right to make written submissions to the conference secretariat in Geneva and to address the plenary and working groups at the Nairobi session [A/Conf.151/PC/L.8, 8/14/90], but the decision came too late in the session for many NGOs to take advantage of it. The 45th General Assembly finally fixed arrangements for nongovernmental participation at the close of 1990, when it decided to apply the guidelines used at PrepCom I for future PrepComs [G/45/211, 12/21/90]. By the time PrepCom II convened in March 1991, 179 NGOs had been accredited to the meeting. Still unresolved is NGO participation in the 1992 event itself.

NGOs did not wait for a formal invitation into the process. Little more than a week after the organizational session had adjourned, 150 representatives of 115 NGOs from 40 countries met in Vancouver with UNCED Secretary-General Maurice Strong and Gro Harlem Brundtland, Chairman of the Commission on Environment and Development, to discuss NGO participation in the process and to start planning their own, **parallel "people's conference"** in Brazil. At another international meeting of NGOs, convened by the Centre for Our Common Future in Nyon, Switzerland, June 3–6, 1990, participants established an **International Facilitating Committee (IFC)** to assist organizations and networks in defining their roles vis-à-vis UNCED; to serve as an information clearing-house; to provide a forum for dialogue among the independent sectors; to promote fair and effective participation in UNCED on behalf of the independent sectors; and to assist the Brazilian NGO forum in promoting and facilitating the parallel people's conference in Brazil.

At a meeting in Cairo, November 13–14, 1990, the Steering Committee for 1992—initiated by the Kenyan-based Environmental Liaison Centre International (ELCI), and consisting of 40 NGOs from 30 countries—began preparing for a **Global NGO Conference**—sponsored by the French government—to be held in Paris, December 17–20, 1991 [*Network '92*, no. 3, 12/90]. The aim of the event is to bring together grass-roots groups (an estimated 850 participants in all) from the North and South who are working in the fields of environment and development, and "to debate and adopt guidelines for a program of action for NGOs up to and beyond 1992" [ibid., no. 6, 4/91]. The conference will also provide a platform for discussing a draft NGO document for presentation to UNCED.

An **International Round-Table on Law and Institutions Before the U.N. Conference on Environment and Development,** sponsored by the United Nations Associations of the United States, Canada, and Iowa, in cooperation with the UNCED secretariat, will convene September 22–25, 1991, to help move the international policy process forward after PrepCom III concludes in early September. Bringing together experts from government, business, environment, and development NGOs, and the media, the gathering will work to ensure that developmental considerations are fully integrated into the environmental debate at UNCED.

NGOs have their work cut out for them in attempting to ensure that governments adequately address all the issues on the UNCED plate. At PrepCom I in Nairobi, "there was endless debate on matters of procedure rather than substance," commented Curtis Bohlen, head of the U.S. delegation [*The InterDependent* 16, no. 4]. The sheer magnitude of the Nairobi agenda had much to do with the lack of progress. Delegates had five minutes to address each topic, leaving little time for a thorough examination of complicated issues. By the end of the three-week session the PrepCom had requested the Conference Secretary-General to prepare 70 reports on environmental issues for submission to the second and third PrepComs in Geneva, March 18–April 5 and August 30–September 4, 1991. Additional reports were requested on the relationship between environment and development, the relationship between economic and environmental policy, and the need to harmonize development and environmental objectives [ENV/DEV/24, 9/12/90].

Like the decisions of PrepCom I, those of PrepCom II in most cases took the form of requests to the conference secretariat for more information. Since the secretariat had not completed its comprehensive reports on oceans, seas, and coastal areas, and on hazardous wastes and toxic chemicals, the debate of Working Group II focused on new topics to be considered under these rubrics, such as "the relationship between trade and the protection of living marine resources" [*Network '92*, no. 6, 4/91]. Discussion of freshwater resources centered on the extent to which

UNCED should influence the **International Conference on Water and the Environment,** to be held in Dublin in January 1992. Forestry was the focus of Working Group I, with the U.S. delegation working hard to build momentum for a convention to be signed in 1992. Although most delegates believed there was little chance of reaching agreement on a legal instrument, the PrepCom decided to "pursue, at a minimum, a non-legally binding authoritative statement of principles."

Much of the debate on climate change and biodiversity focused on the extent to which the PrepComs should be involved with these issues, since climate and biodiversity conventions are being negotiated in separate forums. The 45th General Assembly called for a "single negotiating process" to begin in February 1991, when it established the structure of negotiations on climate [A/45/212, 12/21/90]. Negotiations on a biodiversity convention are being conducted by an ad hoc group, under the auspices of UNEP. The UNEP secretariat presented a draft of the convention at the first round of negotiations in Nairobi, held from February 25 to March 6, 1991 [U.N. press release HE/734, 3/12/91]. Developing countries would like a role for the PrepCom in both sets of deliberations to ensure that their development concerns are integrated into the conventions, but the United States and other developed countries fear that work on these conventions would be undermined or duplicated by the actions of the PrepCom. The final decision calls on the Conference Secretary-General to investigate the relationship between climate and issues on the UNCED agenda, and to report back to the next PrepCom, in August, where "related proposals for discussion" might be prepared.

A number of issues on the UNCED agenda—including ozone depletion, transboundary air pollution, desertification and drought, and human settlements—will be discussed for the first time when PrepCom III convenes from August 12 to September 4, 1991.

No progress was made at PrepCom II in addressing the most divisive North-South issues—**additional funding and technology transfer.** Developing countries held firm in their call for "new and additional" aid flows, and the United States held firm in its opposition to additional funding. Developing countries insisted on the need to transfer environmentally sound technology on a "preferential and non-commercial" basis, and the United States and other developed nations emphasized the primary role of the private sector in developing and transferring these technologies [*The InterDependent* 17, no. 3, 1991]. Bridging the gulf between North and South on these issues will be vital to achieving the goals of UNCED, since the developing countries have made it clear that they do not have the resources to effectively integrate environmental protection into their development policies. "Without effective international cooperation, the outlook for developing countries looks bleak," commented a representative of the Philippines. "How could the world's forests be preserved if the poor had to burn ancient and precious trees in order to plant food crops to still their hunger and the crying of their children?" [U.N. press release GA/EF/2468, 11/13/90].

At the PrepComs and in the General Assembly, developing countries repeatedly voiced their concern that "development" was getting short shrift in the UNCED process. To ensure that development and environment are treated equally, the conference secretariat's work program is focusing on four major sets of issues from an environmental perspective: poverty; growth patterns, consumption standards, and demographic pressures; selected international economic problems (such as debt, deterioration in terms of trade, and reverse resource flows); and policy instruments and institutions [Nita Desai, Deputy Secretary-General for UNCED, *Earth Summit News*, no. 1, 3/91].

Some very important cross-sectoral issues—including population and energy—were excluded by the 44th General Assembly when it defined the UNCED agenda in Resolution 228. Efforts are being made to integrate these issues into the process, but it remains to be seen whether the Preparatory Committee will stray from the official agenda and take significant action in these areas. A number of member states felt that UNCED should not address population since the United Nations Population Fund will be convening an **International Conference on Population and Development in 1994.** Nonetheless, the issue was addressed by the 45th General Assembly in a separate resolution that emphasized the importance of examining the relationship between demographic patterns and environmental degradation during the conference process [A/45/854, 12/21/90].

Various meetings are being held to address energy questions and related issues. On August 16–17 the U.N. Committee on the Development and Utilization of New and Renewable Sources of Energy convened a high-level meeting of experts in the field to prepare for UNCED. The UNCED secretariat had asked the committee to contribute a report on the use of renewable energy sources, to discuss a proposal to invite U.N. member states to prepare country studies on the subject, and to examine a proposal to commission a scientific review of state of the art technology in renewable sources of energy [U.N. press release EN/182, HE/714, 8/16/90]. The United Nations Solar Energy Group on Environment and Development planned to sponsor a Conference on Global Collaboration on Sustainable

Energy Development from May 25 to 28, 1991, in Snekkersten, Denmark
[U.N. press release EN/187, 4/24/91].

The Environment and Corporate Responsibility

The need to ensure that corporations take responsibility for redressing their environmental abuses was confirmed for many when the *Exxon Valdez* tanker unleashed 11 million gallons of oil into Alaska's Prince William Sound in 1989. While the world has become very concerned about maritime oil spills from tankers, a less publicized but serious case of land-based pollution by the oil industry is threatening the tropical rain-forest regions of South America. Robert F. Kennedy, Jr., cites one example:

> For almost twenty years, American oil companies, led by Texaco, have pumped oil from the Ecuadorian jungle. They have created an infrastructure that includes over 400 drill sites, hundreds of miles of roads and pipelines, and a primary pipeline that stretches 280 miles across the Andes. Ecuadorian officials estimate that ruptures to the major pipeline alone have discharged more than 16.8 million gallons of oil into the Amazon over the past eighteen years (compared to the 10.8-million-gallon Exxon Valdez spill). Discharges from secondary pipelines have never been estimated or recorded. However, the smaller tertiary flowlines discharge approximately 10,000 gallons per week of petroleum into the Amazon, and each day production pits dump an astounding 4.3 million gallons of toxic production wastes and treatment chemicals into Amazonia's rivers, streams and groundwater [*The Amicus Journal*, Spring 1991, pp. 24–25].

The high value of these petroleum resources for Ecuador's immediate economic needs (in meeting, for example, its $12 billion foreign debt obligations), as well as for a global economy highly dependent upon petroleum products, is clear. However, the resulting environmental degradation is already seriously affecting the region's quarter-million population of forest people—including eight indigenous tribes that rely on the region's natural resources—and is certain to have a long-term impact on the area's future development.

There are signs that the corporate community is at long last beginning to meet the environmental challenge. At the **Second World Industry Conference on Environmental Management (WICEM II)**, held in Rotterdam, Netherlands, April 10–12, 1991, UNEP Executive Director Mostafa K. Tolba stated:

This WICEM II meeting is clear evidence that world industry is embracing new approaches. It is increasingly committed to self-policing, to implementing proactive and anticipatory strategies. The ICC's Charter for Sustainable Development, the Global Environmental Management Initiative, and the formation of the Business Council on Sustainable Development are but three signals among many of industry's determination to safeguard the environment.

Dr. Tolba went on to emphasize five interlocking issues that should be considered key elements of the proposed world business action plan for the 1990s: compliance with existing international legal instruments; an effort by transnational corporations to work toward full disclosure of appropriate information to local governments and communities about potential risks and appropriate clean-up responsibilities; the need for innovative funding sources for meeting the increasing cost of putting in place sustainable development at the global level; compensation to the private sector for technology development and technology transfer to developing countries; and the need to weigh the cost of inaction against the cost of action.

Director-General Domingo Siazon of the U.N. Industrial Development Organization (UNIDO) warned conference participants that without more support from the North, prospects for cleaner industry in the South are bleak. Said Siazon: "Enhancing the role of environmental technology in developing countries is not merely a question of encouraging industrialized countries to increase the flow of old and new technology to developing countries. It is also a question of building up and strengthening the developing countries' capacity to develop environmentally sound technologies of their own" [UNIDO/1099, 4/11/91].

An International Conference on Ecologically Sustainable Industrial Development will be held in Copenhagen, October 14–18, 1991. Organized by UNIDO, it will address the potential for integrating the interests of industrial growth with those of a cleaner future in the Third World [UNIDO/1100, 4/11/91].

In the spring of 1991 the **U.N. Commission on Transnational Corporations** adopted a resolution by consensus on environment and development that reaffirms the need for transnational corporations (TNCs) to promote access to environmentally sound technologies in developing countries; to apply corporate worldwide environment and development policies; to practice environment and development accounting and reporting; and to maintain consistent and high environmental, health, and safety standards [E/C.10/1991/L.9]. The Commission requested the Executive Director of the U.N. Center for Transnational Corporations to prepare recommendations for the UNCED secretariat on cooperation by TNCs in protecting and enhancing the environment.

The Gulf War and the Environment

Prior to the outbreak of the Persian Gulf war in January, a group of scientists headed by Dr. Abdullah Toukan, Secretary-General of the High Council for Science and Technology of Jordan, nuclear physicist Dr. Frank Barnaby, and environmental and chemical engineer Dr. John Cox prepared a statement concerning the environmental implications of war in the Gulf. This statement, endorsed by such leading scientists as Dr. Paul Crutzen, specialist in air chemistry and Director of the Max Planck Institute, Dr. Carl Sagan, Director of Planetary Studies at Cornell University, and Joe Farman, participant in the British Antarctic Survey and discoverer of the ozone hole, was submitted to Secretary-General Javier Pérez de Cuéllar and included the following warning:

> The environmental cost of such a war is likely to outstrip all other costs, great though these will be. Burning oil fields are the most long-lasting, widespread, and severe hazard to the environment. But there are other major hazards: for example, oil pollution from damaged or sunk tankers could severely contaminate the sea and cause long-term damage to marine life, the coral reefs, and interrupt fishing, a major source of food in the region.
>
> Oil fields contain much combustible material easily ignited by direct military action or sabotage. The burning of a fair sized oil field would inject much smoke and dust into the atmosphere and there are some 750 oil wells in Kuwait alone. If a significant fraction go up in flames, it will take months or even years to extinguish them. The atmosphere will become polluted with large amounts of chemicals such as carbon dioxide, which will contribute to the Greenhouse Effect, and sulfur dioxide and nitric acids. . . . In the short period these oxides fall to the surface of the earth along with rainfall, this rainfall will have a toxic effect on whatever agricultural areas are in the region, thus further depleting scarce fertile land [Scientific statement on potential environmental damage to the Gulf: Presented to press conference in London, 1/5/91].

While the most dire prognostications for the Gulf region concerning a "nuclear winter"-type effect on the atmosphere may not have been justified, the oil spills and oil fires predicted by Dr. Toukan and his colleagues have indeed had a devastating impact upon the environment. At least 520 of Kuwait's 950 producing oil wells were still burning out of control in the spring of 1991, casting a black pall over much of Kuwait.

The Amicus Journal reported that "it may take up to two years to extinguish all the fires" [Spring 1991, p. 8]. The Saudi government's original estimate on oil spillage—up to 11 million barrels—was later revised downward: "Given the multiple sources of the spill, no one could agree on how much oil has been spilled; estimates ranged from 1 million to 4 million barrels" [ibid., p. 6]. Richard Golob, publisher of *Golob's Oil Production Bulletin*, cites data based on the size of the oil slick as evidence that up to 3.3 million barrels may have been spilled. Compounding the damage done by the Iraq-Kuwait conflict are the lasting effects of oil spills unleashed over the past decade. Oil wells damaged during the Iran-Iraq war created a spill of approximately 2 million barrels in 1983, and "some scientific estimates suggest oil exploration and traffic in the area result in average annual spills of 1 to 2 million barrels" [ibid., p. 7].

Director-General Dr. Federico Mayor Zaragoza of the U.N. Educational, Scientific and Cultural Organization (UNESCO) has called for a "pedagogy of peace" in the aftermath of the Gulf war [UNEP News Release, 1991/12]. UNCED Secretary-General Maurice Strong stated that he "was appalled that the environment should become an instrument of war in this way," and that it "demonstrates that the international community needs to pursue environmental disarmament" [*Earth Summit News*, no. 1, 3/91]. **Greenpeace International** reported that the spread of oil down the Kuwaiti and Saudi coastlines toward the smaller Gulf states threatens coastal areas, mud flats, seagrasses, and algae. "Fish, sea turtles, marine mammals, birds, and invertebrates may all become contaminated through ingestion of oiled food, or, for birds, through preening of oiled plumage [*On Impact*, Greenpeace International, 5/91]. The Gulf's fisheries have already been seriously affected: "The Saudi fishing industry is reported to have lost tens of millions of dollars," and the consumption of fish in adjacent areas, such as Bahrain, has fallen greatly despite the fact that no oil has appeared in their fishing areas. The oil spills have also threatened the Saudi Arabian desalination plants, which provide the nation with 70 to 80 percent of its drinking water [ibid.].

Initial reports predicted that the destruction of sanitation, waste water, and treatment facilities by extensive allied bombing campaigns would spread solid and chemical wastes on land and into rivers and the sea [WHO press release UN 21, 3/19/91; UNEP report, "Environmental Consequences of the Conflict Between Iraq and Kuwait," 3/8/91]. The bombing campaigns may have also caused long-term damage to the desert environment: "The ecosystems that develop under arid conditions have an easily degraded soil that supports a sparse and highly specialized biota. Such a system is readily damaged and very slow to recover" [UNEP report, 3/8/91].

Regional and international responses to the environmental crisis in the Gulf came early in the war, but even after the cease-fire "cleanup efforts [were] frustrated by a lack of equipment and water, poor communications, and unexploded land mines" [*The Amicus Journal,* Spring 1991]. During the Gulf war UNEP sent several missions to the region to obtain scientific and technical information on physical and environmental damage. The World Conservation Union (IUCN) had also sent an observer to the region, and was coordinating ecological information in conjunction with the World Wide Fund for Nature (WWF) [UNEP report, 3/8/91]. Throughout the war the environmental situation was monitored by UNEP through its **Global Environmental Monitoring System,** based in Geneva, and by the International Maritime Organization (IMO), which had established round-the-clock coordinating centers in London and Bahrain. The centers were established under the terms of the **International Convention on Oil Pollution Preparedness, Response and Coordination,** adopted by IMO member states in 1990 to facilitate international cooperation in the event of a major pollution threat [IMO/B1/91, 1/29/91; B2/91, 2/22/91].

On February 5–6, a UNEP–sponsored consultation of U.N. agencies, NGOs, and representatives of international tanker companies convened in Geneva to review the immediate and long-term consequences of the conflict on the environment. Recognizing the regional nature of the crisis, participants gave UNEP the lead in revitalizing the **Regional Organization for the Protection of the Marine Environment (ROPME)**—one of the ten regional seas programs initiated by UNEP, and consisting of all eight nations in the region. On the basis of another decision of the consultation, UNEP developed a framework for action in the region which was adopted at a second interagency consultation on March 15. The plan allocated responsibilities to a dozen U.N. agencies and other international organizations—including the IUCN and the WWF—in the four areas where action is required: oil in water, oil on land, smog in the atmosphere, and terrestrial destruction [*UNEP North America News* 6, nos. 2 & 3, 2–4/91; UNEP report, 3/8/91]. A core team of experts left for Kuwait in mid-April to carry out the initial surveys and assessments needed to guide interagency responses.

UNEP established the **Technical Cooperation Trust Fund** to finance the plan and to augment efforts by the Gulf states to strengthen ROPME. The government of Japan announced that it would contribute $1.11 million of the $2.5 million estimated by UNEP to cover the costs of the operation [UNEP news release 1991/13; *UNEP North America News,* 2–4/1991].

Chernobyl

In 1990 the fourth anniversary of the Chernobyl nuclear power plant accident was marked by the introduction of a draft resolution by the representative of the Ukraine to the Economic and Social Council [document E/1990/L.21], requesting the Secretary-General to prepare proposals for a program of international cooperation to eliminate the consequences of the disaster [ECOSOC/5232, 5/18/90]. Four years after the accident, Soviet officials admitted to "an appalling underestimation of the danger of radiation" in their original prognosis, noting that the radiation affects a "much broader region." In the years since the 1986 accident, health statistics have shown an increase in blood disease and there are reports of an increase in the incidence of freak animals and deformed plants [*Newsweek*, 5/7/90]. On the fifth anniversary of the accident, an article in the *New York Times Sunday Magazine* reported that the aftereffects of Chernobyl were truly staggering [Felicity Barringer, "Chernobyl Five Years Later: The Danger Persists," 4/14/91].

4. Law of the Sea

The 1982 U.N. Convention on the Law of the Sea (LOS) has been ratified by 45 of the 60 nations necessary to bring it into force. This makes entry into force a possibility for the near future, even though it is impossible to forecast when this event will take place. Dissatisfaction expressed by the major industrialized countries, and especially by the United States, regarding a number of the Convention's provisions on deep-seabed mining beyond national jurisdiction remains the principal obstacle to ratification. Agreement on these provisions is a necessary precondition for true universality of the Convention and for the functioning of the institutions that should be created at the moment of its entry into force: the International Seabed Authority (ISA), to be located in Jamaica, and the 21-member International Tribunal on the Law of the Sea (ITLOS), to be based in Hamburg, Germany. Unless the industrialized countries can be persuaded to become parties, there is a distinct possibility that the Convention will enter into force for a group of almost exclusively Third World states, which would encounter insurmountable difficulties when trying to give life to the above-mentioned institutions.

The need for a dialogue to foster **universal participation in the Convention** emerged at the end of the 1989 summer meeting of the Preparatory Commission for the **International Seabed Authority** and the **International Tribunal on the Law of the Sea** (Prepcom). The General Assembly's annual resolutions, adopted on November 20, 1989 [A/Res/44/26] and on December 14, 1990 [A/Res/45/145], noted with satisfaction "the expressions of willingness to explore all possibilities of addressing issues . . . in order to secure universal participation in the Convention." However, states hold different views of the purpose and scope of such dialogue. The Third World countries emphasize that they are content with the Convention as it is and indicate their willingness to explore problems other countries may have, provided that these problems are clearly identified and that the basic tenets of the Convention's deep-seabed mining provisions are not jeopardized. The industrialized states indicate that they have major problems—with the decision-making processes of the ISA, with the costs involved, and with the provisions on a review conference and those on production limits to protect land-based producers of the minerals to be extracted from the seabed. Thus, one side seems to suggest minor adjustments that can be obtained through the rules and regulations under discussion by Prepcom or through interpretative statements, while the other side thinks in terms of deeper changes requiring adoption through a binding instrument, such as a protocol that could enter into force with the Convention.

The U.N. Secretary-General responded to the widespread call for a dialogue by bringing together representative delegations on July 19, 1990, for informal consultations under his chairmanship. At the meeting there was no dissent from the opening points made by the Secretary-General, namely, that universal participation in the Convention is important, that what prevents such universal participation are certain states' difficulties with the deep-seabed mining provisions, and that it is necessary to address these problems. In order to do so, according to the Secretary-General, the parties must keep in mind the changes that have occurred since 1982. These changes were, in his opinion, the following: (a) prospects for commercial seabed mining have receded into the next century; (b) international relations in general have evolved from tension and confrontation toward cooperation; (c) the general economic climate has changed and the approaches to international economic cooperation have undergone a transformation; and (d) the work of the Prepcom has brought about a better understanding of the practical aspects of seabed mining. The first meeting was followed by a second on October 30, 1990, and a third on March 25, 1991.

What is particularly important in these meetings is the presence of the United States, which does not participate in Prepcom. During late 1989 and 1990 the United States, although not moving officially from its

negative attitude toward the LOS Convention, engaged in quiet explora-
tory talks with a number of Third World delegations. These talks elicited
sufficient interest in the need to discuss U.S. problems with the seabed
mining provisions and permitted the U.S. representatives to be present at
the meetings convened by the Secretary-General. What remains to be
seen is the effect U.S. participation in the meetings will have on the
substance of their deliberations.

Another indication of the subtly changed U.S. attitude emerged in
December 1990 when the U.S. Mission to the U.N. tried to introduce a
group of amendments to the proposed General Assembly resolution on
the Law of the Sea. Such changes, if accepted, would have permitted a
U.S. abstention, instead of the usual negative vote. The amendments,
none of which were very radical, did not go through, mainly because
they were proposed too late and at a moment when most delegations
were focusing on the Gulf crisis. The attempt was nonetheless recognized
as bona fide, and the discussions it provoked were an indication of the
importance given to the U.S. position by the Third World countries. In
explaining his negative vote on Assembly Resolution 145, U.S. Permanent
Representative Thomas Pickering reiterated the U.S. position on the LOS
Convention: "Distilled to its essence, our view is that the changed
circumstances cited by the Secretary-General in the report on his initiative [A/45/721, para. 14] suggest the need for a substantially scaled-back
institutional structure and a more market-oriented approach to the
management of the [international seabed] area and its resources—an
approach which is flexible enough to adapt to new circumstances" [A/45/
PV.68, p. 58].

The Secretary-General's initiative has made it clear that the Prepcom
is not the forum in which so-called hard-core issues, which correspond
to the main questions raised by the industrialized countries, can be
tackled successfully. The Prepcom has nonetheless been far from inactive,
especially with regard to management and supervision of the **pioneer
investors**—those enterprises exclusively authorized by the Prepcom to
conduct preparatory activities on certain areas of the deep seabed. After
long negotiations, Prepcom approved an understanding on August 30,
1990 [LOS/PCN/L.87, Annex], on the obligations incumbent on the first four
registered pioneer investors: enterprises sponsored by France, India,
Japan, and the Soviet Union. This understanding waives the $1 million
annual fixed fee that pioneer investors should have paid and foresees the
possibility of postponing the submission date of **work plans** by the
pioneer investors once the Convention enters into force. This takes into
account new circumstances that make **commercial seabed mining** a

possibility rather remote in time. The pioneer investors agree in exchange to (a) provide free training for a limited number of the future international seabed **Enterprise**'s personnel and (b) carry out the preparatory work and the first stage of a plan for the exploration of the Enterprise's first mining site, up to a cost of $3 million for each of the pioneer investors, with the exception of India. With this agreement the Prepcom shows a realistic perception of the present-day difficulties of seabed mining, while the four pioneers accept involvement in a system in which seabed mining activities conducted by an international institution are envisaged.

In 1990 an **application for registration as a pioneer investor** was submitted by China on behalf of the China Ocean Mineral Resources Research and Development Association [LOS/PCN/BUR/INF/R.9]. The Chinese application was registered by the Prepcom on March 5, 1991 [LOS/ PCN/117]. On March 13, 1991, the Prepcom received a further application for registration as a pioneer investor from Poland, on behalf of Bulgaria, Cuba, Czechoslovakia, Poland, and the Soviet Union, for the Interocean-metal Joint Organization (IOM), a consortium created by these countries in 1987. (Among the original members were Vietnam, which later withdrew, and the German Democratic Republic, whose position is described as "suspended" [LOS/PCN/118]). The IOM application will be processed, as were the previous ones, through a group of technical experts and should be accepted by the Prepcom at its 1991 summer session.

Considerable concerns were raised during Prepcom's 1991 spring session regarding China's request that its pioneer investor have the same obligations as India's and not the heavier obligations agreed upon in 1990 for the French, Japanese, and Soviet investors. In particular, the membership of the Group of 77 developing countries is concerned that, through the clauses contained in the relevant understandings providing for "similar treatment" of future applicants, the Eastern European IOM and Western "potential applicant" consortia might be entitled to claim a similar treatment, permitting them to avoid the more onerous obligations accepted by France, Japan, and the Soviet Union.

The preparation by the Prepcom of the **rules and regulations of the Authority** continued in 1991, mostly on routine items. Discussions on the Enterprise in Special Commission II and those on the problems of developing land-based producers in Special Commission I continue to show that, pending clear indications on how the hard-core issues will be solved, no flexibility is possible and that delegations tend to stick to their old positions. Special Commission III, however, has shown that some constructive give-and-take is possible on a marginal issue by agreeing on the chapter of the "mining code" concerning accommodation of activities in the area [LOS/PCN/SCN.3/1991/CRP.11].

The **Office of Ocean Affairs and the Law of the Sea (OALOS)**, administered by U.N. Under-Secretary-General Satya Nandan, has continued its activities, which go far beyond the servicing of the Prepcom. OALOS monitors trends in the implementation of the LOS Convention and provides assistance to developing countries in the preparation of ocean policies and legislation. Of particular interest is the LOS *Bulletin*, where reports of recent legislation, treaties, and state practices are published, and such publications as the new *Annual Review of Ocean Affairs*. The most important document, however, is the annual Report by the Secretary-General on the Law of the Sea [A/45/721], which reviews all developments relevant to the Law of the Sea and ocean affairs that have occurred during the year. The OALOS also prepares special reports. In 1990 it issued a report on marine scientific research [A/45/563], the first part of a report on the "Realization of benefits under the United Nations Convention on the Law of the Sea: Needs of States in regard to development and management of ocean resources" [A/45/712], as well as a report on "Large scale pelagic driftnet fishing and its impact on the living resources of the world's oceans and seas" [A/45/663].

5. Antarctica

The eighth year of debate in the General Assembly on the question of Antarctica again ended in deadlock over the traditional two-part resolution. Although the resolution was approved by majority vote, none of the parties to the **Antarctic Treaty** participated in the vote on the first part [A/Res/45/78A], summarized below, while seven supported the second, which called for exclusion of the *"apartheid* régime" of South Africa from Antarctic Treaty Consultative Meetings (ATCMs) [A/Res/45/78B]. Australia continues to speak on behalf of the parties to the Antarctic Treaty, urging that consideration of the agenda item proceed on the basis of consensus.

Other participants in the General Assembly debate have been devoting their attention to the significance of Antarctica in global research efforts, particularly in relation to climate change, and to the importance of Antarctica as a "last continental wilderness." In light of Antarctica's unique international importance, they argue, "all mankind must share responsibility in its protection and conservation. Decision making must therefore rest with the entire international community" [statement by Ambassador Razali Ismail, Permanent Representative of Malaysia to the U.N., on Agenda Item 67 of the First Committee, November 19, 1990]. In their view, the Antarctic Treaty framework should provide for **universal participation in Antarctic management decisions,** and its workings should be more transparent and accountable. The first part of the 1990 resolution expresses regret that the Antarctic Treaty Consultative Parties (ATCPs) have not heeded previous resolutions calling for the Secretary-General or his representative to be invited to their meetings, and requests that information on all aspects of Antarctica be deposited with the United Nations by the ATCPs. The General Assembly resolution takes the view that any **convention on comprehensive environmental protection** should be negotiated with the full participation of the international community and in the context of the U.N. system, and urges all members to support efforts to ban minerals activities in and around Antarctica and ensure the protection of the Antarctic environment.

Four studies are requested of the Secretary-General for the 46th General Assembly: a report on the state of the Antarctic environment and its impact on the global system; a report assessing the feasibility of establishing a United Nations–sponsored research station in Antarctica, to be produced cooperatively by the relevant U.N. programs and agencies, such as the World Meteorological Organization (WMO) and the U.N. Environmental Programme (UNEP); a report evaluating information and documents deposited with the Secretary-General, as requested; and a report on actions taken to exclude the South African regime from ATCMs.

The two reports of the Secretary-General before the 45th Assembly contained the responses by Australia, on behalf of the ATCPs, to the 1989 resolution [A/45/458, 9/6/90, and A/45/459, 9/8/90]. The former reiterated earlier responses on the question of South Africa. The latter affirmed the parties' belief that concerted international action is required to protect the Antarctic environment, as well as their commitment to continue to develop the measures necessary and make available any research results. Among the additional documents referenced were the report of the First Committee's consideration of the Antarctic agenda item [A/45/789, 9/7/90] and declarations adopted by the Ninth Conference of Heads of State or Government of Non-Aligned Countries (September 4–7, 1989) [A/44/551-S/20870, Annex], by the second meeting of States of the Zone of Peace and Co-operation of the South Atlantic (June 25–29, 1990) [A/45/474, Annex], by the Nineteenth Islamic Conference of Foreign Ministers (July 31–August 5, 1990) [A/45/421-S/21797, Annex IV, Res. 17/19-E], and by the Council of Ministers of the OAU (July 17–22, 1989) [A/44/603, Annex I].

The last year saw an alteration in the membership of the Antarctic Treaty. Two of the Non-Consultative parties (NCPs)—Ecuador and the Netherlands—attained Consultative Status (CP) on November 19, 1990, and Switzerland acceded to the treaty on November 15, 1990, as an NCP. The unification of Germany reduced the number of CPs by one, bringing the total to 26 CPs and 13 NCPs.

The **XI special ATCM** has met three times to hammer out an agreement on comprehensive environmental protection in Antarctica (November 19 to December 6, 1990, in Vina del Mar, Chile; and April 22 to 30 and June 10 to 22 in Madrid). It is expected that a **Protocol to the 1959 Antarctic Treaty** will be adopted in 1991—the 30th anniversary of the signing of the Antarctic Treaty—entering into force when ratified by all 26 CPs. Two new observers were invited to these meetings: the European Community and the nongovernmental Antarctic and Southern Ocean Coalition (ASOC).

The XVI regular ACTM meets October 14–25, 1991, in Bonn. A preparatory meeting was held in Bonn, April 22–26, 1991, at which the agenda for the fall meeting was adopted. On that agenda will be any unfinished business from the XI special ATCM, as well as the normal range of ATCM agenda items—on facilitating scientific research, on the operation of the AT system, and on tourism and various environmental matters [see Report on the XV ATCM, *Issues Before the 45th General Assembly of the United Nations;* Report on Antarctica, World Resources Institute, 11/89].

The most controversial issue before the XI special ATCM was how to deal with possible **minerals development** in Antarctica and, in particular, how to provide for lifting a prohibition on minerals activity. Although the prohibition may be lifted at any time by consensus of the CPs, after 50 years an amendment to the Protocol may be adopted at a review conference. It would enter into force once ratified by three-quarters of the CPs, to include all 26 current CPs. (The number of CPs will most likely have increased significantly after 50 years.) The parties agree that, should the prohibition be lifted, a binding legal regime—specifying the means for determining whether (and, if so, under what conditions) minerals activities could proceed—would be in place. That regime could be the 1988 Convention on the Regulation of Antarctic Mineral Resource Activities (CRAMRA) or a new regime incorporated into the amendment to the Protocol. If, three years after an amendment to the Protocol had been adopted, it was not yet in force, any state could withdraw from the Protocol. Thus, despite the presumption of a fail-safe regime to prevent Antarctica's being left open to unregulated minerals development upon termination of the prohibition, such a regime is not guaranteed.

No mineral deposits of commercial interest have yet been found in Antarctica, although there is circumstantial evidence of offshore oil. Even if major discoveries were made, the costs of extracting and marketing minerals from this remote and inhospitable area could mean that it would take decades before any venture might become economically feasible.

The draft Protocol is significant in several respects, as it addresses environmental protection in the Antarctic Treaty area (south of 60 degrees South latitude). It establishes environmental principles for the planning and conduct of all activities and provides for the establishment of a **Committee on Environmental Protection** to advise ATCMs and formulate recommendations for them in connection with the implementation of the Protocol. It is contemplated that the XVI regular ATCM in October 1991 will establish a small permanent **secretariat** to support implementation of the Antarctic Treaty, including the Protocol.

The Protocol includes four annexes, which are considered integral to it. They strengthen and give greater precision to measures previously cast in the form of Antarctic Treaty "Recommendations"—on conservation of Antarctic fauna and flora, prior assessment of environmental impacts, marine pollution control, and waste management and disposal. The obligations they contain are subject to compulsory, **binding dispute-settlement** procedures, as are obligations in the Protocol itself on environmental impact assessment, emergency response, and prohibiting minerals activities. Additional annexes may be adopted, and the XVI ACTM is likely to consider drafts relating to the designation of protected areas and to tourism. Any new annex could likewise be made subject to compulsory, binding dispute-settlement procedures. The "Protocol-with-annexes approach" also permits each annex to be amended by an accelerated procedure: Amendments adopted by consensus enter into force after one year—without subsequent ratification—unless one or more CP has objected within that period.

The Protocol stresses that scientific research in Antarctica, and preserving Antarctica as an area for the conduct of scientific research, shall be accorded priority. Its provisions reemphasize the Antarctic Treaty's call for **cooperative scientific investigation**—calling for cooperative initiatives in scientific research, location and sharing of facilities, preparing environmental impact assessments, avoiding pollution and environmental hazards, and minimizing the environmental effects of accidents.

In order to strengthen **compliance** with Antarctic measures, the

Protocol specifies their applicability to all government-sponsored activities and to private ventures for which a state party is responsible (as defined in the treaty). The Protocol's provisions would also be binding for the NCPs that accede to it. At present, NCPs are not automatically bound by Recommendations in the approval of which they do not formally take part. It is up to each individual party to ensure compliance with the Protocol and its annexes. Each must also ensure that activities for which they are responsible are modified, suspended, or canceled if they result or threaten to result in environmental impacts inconsistent with the Protocol's environmental principles. The ATCMs may supplement existing Antarctic Treaty inspection procedures by designating observers in accordance with procedures to be established in the future. Each party must also report annually on how it has given effect to the Protocol, and these reports, inspection reports, and other documents and notifications are to be made available to the public. The text also specifically requires that the ATCM consider annual reports and inspection reports—effectively calling for **active, rather than passive, review.** The parties undertake to develop rules and procedures on liability, and, pending their establishment, each party is to grant recourse within its legal system to those seeking relief for environmental damage caused by any entity subject to its jurisdiction [text of the Protocol to the Antarctic Treaty, XI ATSCM/2/30, 4/29/91]. At the 1990 meeting in Chile, a brief one-day meeting took place on the liability protocol called for in CRAMRA. Many participants urged that the question of liability be dealt with in the broader context of the Protocol [Report on Antarctica, World Resources Institute, 1/91].

The ninth annual meeting under the **Convention on the Conservation of Antarctic Marine Living Resources (CCAMLR)** took place at its headquarters in Hobart, Tasmania, Australia, October 25–November 2, 1990. Italy and Sweden joined as full Commission members, and the Netherlands acceded to the Convention. Ten new conservation measures for finfisheries were adopted, as well as one establishing a protected monitoring site. The United States formally initiated the CCAMLR inspection system during the 1989–90 season. The meeting adopted a resolution opposing any expansion of driftnet fishing in the area (where none has been reported) and endorsing the goals of General Assembly Resolution 44/225 on large-scale pelagic driftnet fishing. Efforts continue on formulating a **management policy for the krill fishery,** based on endorsement of the principles that, in the absence of essential data, very conservative catch limits are warranted, and that the development of new fisheries should not outpace the ability to give effect to CCAMLR's "ecosystem" conservation standard [Report of the Ninth Meeting of the Commission].

6. International Space Year

At the second session of the 101st Congress of the United States on January 23, 1990, the Senate and House of Representatives issued a Joint Resolution to reaffirm their support for the designation of 1992 as **International Space Year (ISY)**—a proposal generated in Congress five years earlier to commemorate the 500th anniversary of Columbus's voyage and the 35th anniversary of the International Geophysical Year. Meanwhile, the framework for international support for Congress's ISY proposal had already been established under the leadership of the United Nations. The 45th General Assembly's Resolution 46, adopted on December 8, 1989, endorsed the initiative of the international scientific community to designate 1992 as International Space Year and to promote the utilization of space science and technology to benefit all states, particularly developing ones.

The Participation of the United Nations System in International Space Year, the official record of U.N.–ISY activities, defines a three-pronged plan coordinated by the **Outer Space Affairs Division (OSAD)** of the Department of Political and Security Council Affairs. The plan calls for management of the earth's resources through space technology, long-term training for the world's scientific community, and an extensive program of public education to stimulate interest in outer space and in the specific activities of ISY. Through its own participation, the United Nations hopes to encourage member states to support ISY activities and to "undertake programs that could contribute to the understanding, management, and safeguarding of the global environment."

Workshops and training programs related to the first facet of U.N. participation, **resource management,** have been initiated with the sponsorship of member states and other relevant organizations. Plans include a 30-day training program, cosponsored by the National Aeronautics and Space Administration (NASA), in the management and utilization of remotely sensed data, to be held in Sioux Falls, South Dakota, from September 9 to October 4, 1991. The United States is also cosponsoring an international conference in Boulder, Colorado, to address the needs of developing countries that utilize remote sensing to explore their resources.

The governments of China and the Soviet Union and the European Space Agency (ESA) have likewise initiated resource management programs. And China, the Economic and Social Commission for Asia and the Pacific (ESCAP), and the U.N. Disaster Relief Organization (UNDRO) have cooperated in scheduling a regional workshop in Beijing in September 1991 to explore the use of space techniques to combat natural disasters. The Soviet Union has agreed to make available at no cost remotely sensed data acquired from a number of developing nations and then to disseminate the information to authorities in the observed areas. Similarly, the ESA initiated in 1990 a program in conjunction with the United Nations to collect data from African countries that are within the observation range of the Maspalmos and Fucino ERS-1 ground stations in Spain and Italy, respectively. The ESA will work with local authorities in Africa to coordinate data and will sponsor workshops on remote-sensing techniques in Africa in 1991 and again in 1992 [A/AC.105/445].

In an action indicative of the cooperative nature of ISY, the United Nations will extend its commitment to resource management through its affiliation with the **Space Agency Forum on International Space Year (SAFISY)**. A team of 28 space agencies and 8 affiliated organizations, SAFISY promotes the unrestricted flow of data amassed via remote sensing and the use of this data for the sustainable development of the earth's resources. With "Mission to Planet Earth" as a project theme, SAFISY has coordinated the release of the time capsule Space Arc in 1992, an animated world atlas, and the "Spaceship Earth" television series—ten short programs filmed with space-based instruments and scheduled to debut in late 1991 as a preview of ISY [*ISY News*, 11/90]. In cooperation with these activities, the U.N. Educational, Scientific and Cultural Organization (UNESCO) has sponsored and outlined a booklet on the Mission's activities.

The United Nations has endorsed and sponsored several broad-based programs within the context of the second area of participation: **the long-term education of the world's scientific community.** The most ambitious program seeks to establish **Centres for Space Science and Technology Education** in four developing regions of the world. While the Centres represent only one mandate of ISY, they are "the culmination of the efforts of ISY," according to Adigun Ade Abiodun, expert on space application at OSAD and coordinator of the project. In accordance with paragraph 9 of the 45th General Assembly's Resolution 72, which endorsed the recommendation of the U.N. Committee On the Peaceful Uses of Outer Space (COPUOS) to establish Regional Centres, OSAD published a set of working project documents to guide the effort [SAP/90/001–004].

The four regions eligible for the program are those within the operating areas of the Economic Commission for Latin America and the Caribbean, the Economic Commission for Africa, the Economic and Social Commission for Asia and the Pacific, and the Economic and Social

Commission for Western Asia. Educational programs will be established within an existing educational institution in each region and will focus on "educating the educators" of the developing world. A nine-month educational session, followed by supervision of a pilot project executed by each participant upon return to his or her home country, is intended to provide indigenous expertise in remote sensing and related technologies.

Various countries have already expressed interest in hosting the Centres, and OSAD has begun evaluation missions to potential host countries to assess their relative suitability. The working project document proposes a budget of $4 million per Centre for the initial four-year operating period to cover preliminary activities, facilities and equipment, staff, expenses of participants, and evaluation workshops. UNDP has been solicited for contributions; and in May 1991 the program coordinators began visits to European nations, regional banks, and such organizations as OPEC in search of additional funding.

Several other long-term educational initiatives will complement the establishment of these Centres. OSAD is crystalizing plans to sponsor a joint Donation Program with the International Centre for Theoretical Physics to solicit books and journals from space-faring nations, scientific associations, and publishing houses for distribution to developing countries. The joint United Nations and Economic Commission for Africa Space Congress in 1993 will unite African policy-makers with space experts to establish a feasible program for utilizing the vast resources of the region. In the framework of the U.N. Space Applications Program, an International Seminar on Communication Technology for Development, sponsored by INTERSPUTNIK on behalf of the Soviet Union, will be held near Moscow in September 1992 and will host up to 30 representatives of developing countries. The main objective of the seminar will be to familiarize participants with communication technology, paying particular attention to rural education, medicine, disaster relief, and regional/international data communication networks.

In the third facet of its participation, **public education,** the United Nations aspires to create widespread support for ISY programs and to generate interest in outer space activities, particularly among young people. This realm of activity includes a publication in support of establishing "universariums" (advanced planetariums with additional emphasis on space travel and exploration) in major cities, the development of a software package to predict satellite passes, production of special videos addressing space exploration and utilization, a telecast of a panel discussion on "Mission to Planet Earth," an international high school essay contest, and a series of exhibits at U.N. Headquarters in New York.

As the international community prepares for ISY 1992, sponsorship, consultations, and program outlines have been completed for a majority of projects in all three areas of U.N. participation. At the conclusion of its 28th session in March 1991, the Outer Space Scientific and Technical Sub-Committee surveyed the progress to date of ISY 1992, and in its report the Sub-Committee expressed concern about the lack of funding for the projects and made a special appeal to member states to sponsor ISY endeavors [A/AC.105/C.1/L.175]. The report urged particular support for the establishment of Regional Centres for Space Science and Technology Education and for efforts to help developing countries gain access to remotely sensed data. The Sub-Committee's enthusiasm for ISY is implicit in its selection of the theme for its 1992 session: "Space technology and the protection of the Earth's environment: Development of endogenous capabilities, in particular in the developing countries and in the context of International Space Year."

V
Human Rights and Social Issues

1. Human Rights

The 46th General Assembly will again address a wide array of topics when it considers human rights issues in its Third Committee on social and humanitarian affairs.

The dominant human rights issues in the 45th General Assembly, the 47th Commission on Human Rights, and the spring 1991 meeting of the Economic and Social Council (ECOSOC) were the Gulf war; the development of new thematic and country-specific mechanisms to aid in enforcing human rights; the financial resources devoted to U.N. human rights programs; and Cuban and Chinese-led initiatives—aimed at undercutting those programs—to reassert the principles of "noninterference" in internal affairs and of "nonselectivity" (read: no singling out countries for criticism) in the United Nations' human rights work. This last effort largely failed in the General Assembly and the Commission on Human Rights. Instead, the world community indicated its willingness to put teeth into some of the human rights norms and standards it has promulgated over the years. Major reform of the agendas of the Assembly and Commission was agreed upon, with the effect of biennializing some issues at the Assembly and allowing more discussion of egregious rights violations at Commission sessions.

The importance of the Commission on Human Rights in global human rights activity was affirmed during its six-week session in February and March 1991, as nearly a score of foreign ministers and other top officials journeyed to Geneva to address the body about human rights concerns and conditions, usually those in their own countries.

At the spring 1991 ECOSOC meeting, in fulfillment of past agreements, ten Third World countries were elected to the Commission, enlarging to 53 the membership of the world's highest political body specializing in human rights. This enlargement was widely viewed as part of the effort to undercut the development of effective human rights mechanisms—and, indeed, such often-cited human rights violators as Iran, Libya, and Sri Lanka are among those newly elected to the Commission. But the net result of elections for new seats and old does not yet appear as negative as many human rights advocates had feared.

Over a decade, the U.N. human rights program has developed an impressive array of new enforcement machinery—machinery that is not widely known but that has changed fundamentally what the United Nations can and does accomplish to aid individual victims of human rights violations. This development has been viewed with considerable dissatisfaction by countries that violate human rights and do not wish this information publicized at the United Nations or elsewhere.

The decade's new **human rights mechanisms** include:

- A variety of specialized "theme mechanisms" (a working group and several independent rapporteurs) to take effective action (often on an emergency basis) wherever individuals are encountering such severe human rights problems as disappearances, summary executions, torture, religious intolerance, and—a recent addition—arbitrary detention.
- Numerous "special rapporteurs" (or "representatives") to examine conditions in individual countries. (Afghanistan, El Salvador, Iran, and Romania remain on the list; Iran, occupied Kuwait, and Cuba were added this year.)
- An expansion of the activities of committees that monitor compliance with human rights treaties, several of which have new optional complaint mechanisms through which individuals can seek redress when human rights are violated.
- Substantial expansion of the Advisory Services program that offers "technical assistance" in human rights.
- An initiative to expand U.N. public information on human rights in a new world campaign designed to advance awareness of rights and of the U.N. machinery through which individuals can claim their rights.

This progress has come about in fits and starts over the past decade, but the result is an arsenal of enforcement weapons that can accomplish an enormous amount to diminish human rights violations worldwide—if its political backing remains strong, if an increasingly vocal backlash is kept under control, and if its resources continue to grow.

The 45th General Assembly was successful in obtaining the Fifth

Committee's agreement to devote additional human and financial resources for the Human Rights Centre, but most new resources were earmarked for the recent Convention on the Rights of the Child. Western governments argued that the United Nations cannot continue to assign new and more complex tasks to the Centre when its staff size is relatively unchanged from 25 years ago—a time when none of the special enforcement mechanisms or treaty committees were in place.

During its first 30 years or so, the U.N. human rights program concentrated primarily on **standard-setting**, and there were only a few, modest attempts to develop procedures for enforcing human rights standards. The important standard-setting work of the United Nations goes on, reaching into new areas: the rights of indigenous peoples; the treatment of detainees, minorities, human rights defenders, and migrant workers; mental health; and the phenomenon of disappearances. But today, most human rights advocates agree, the major challenge is to strengthen the implementation and enforcement of the human rights standards developed over these decades.

The 1991 session of the U.N. Commission on Human Rights may well be remembered as its most successful in years because of the launching of new machinery that will be helping to enforce human rights standards in the days to come. Among these are mechanisms for examining conditions in specific countries: New special investigators ("Special Rapporteurs") are to look at the human rights situation in Iraq and occupied Kuwait, respectively, and a similar investigator (formally a "Special Representative") is to report on Cuba, which had managed to fight off previous attempts to establish such a post through skillful diplomatic maneuvering. At the same time, a regionally balanced Working Group of experts has been authorized to study and take action in cases of arbitrary detention throughout the world—the newest of the Commission's theme mechanisms. Many observers have expressed the hope that this group will take action on behalf of political prisoners (called by some "prisoners of conscience") to assure that their detention and trial are based on international standards of due process and humane treatment, or that they are released. Because it is worldwide in its coverage, such a mechanism adds an important dimension to U.N. attempts to put an end to egregious human rights abuses.

Tarnishing the Commission's success, in the view of many human rights advocates, is the continuing tendency to water down the references to human rights abuses in resolutions that cite countries by name, and to avoid scrutiny of some of the worst offenders. This overlooks the abundant evidence provided by private international human rights organizations and even the findings of the Commission's own officially appointed special human rights investigators.

Disappearances

The 46th General Assembly will address the phenomenon of disappearances, examining the report of the **Working Group on Disappearances** issued in January 1991 [E/CN.4/1991/20]. This Working Group was the first of the United Nations' special theme mechanisms set up by the Commission on Human Rights and the first to intervene with governments, requesting information on behalf of individual victims and their families. Disappearances are cases in which an individual has been seized, often by persons in plainclothes and either in government service or protected by government agencies, and not seen or heard from again. The government denies any knowledge of these individuals or any responsibility for their whereabouts, and the practice has a chilling effect: eliminating citizens, terrorizing the population, and rendering the government unaccountable. It flouts all international guarantees of personal liberty and causes great anxiety among relatives and friends.

The 45th General Assembly expressed continuing concern about the practice of forced or involuntary disappearances [A/Res/45/165], noting the suffering of the families of the disappeared. The Working Group has been particularly concerned about reports of the intimidation of victims and witnesses who have contacted it, and in 1990 the Group instituted a new **"prompt intervention"** procedure to defend such individuals, in response to Human Rights Commission Resolution 1990/76 on cooperation with U.N. human rights bodies.

Pursuing a strictly "nonaccusatory approach" aimed at finding out what happened to the victim rather than at assigning blame for the act, the Working Group has examined disappearances around the world. During its 11 years of operation it has asked some 45 governments to explain more than 20,000 cases of disappearances. In 1990 the Group took action on 987 of 3,864 cases newly received; about half of these had occurred during 1990. (The Group had previously noted that only 7 to 8 percent of the disappearance cases it adopted had been formally clarified but that the rate rose to 25 percent when it came to the cases submitted promptly and taken up within three months of the event.) Although the number of new cases has declined slightly, the Group advises that there has been no let up in the phenomenon or in its work.

Of the 1990 caseload, the countries with the largest number of new reported disappearances were Iraq (464, all dating from previous years),

Sri Lanka (246/44 of 1990 vintage), Peru (268/233), Colombia (108/82), Iran (58/7), Guatemala (86/74), and the Philippines (54/43). Both the Assembly and the Commission encourage governments to respond to the Working Group's inquiries and, where appropriate, to **invite visits** that might clarify the fate of alleged victims. In 1991 the Group visited the Philippines—one of two such visits by a U.N. theme mechanism this year—and issued a 35-page report [E/CN.4/1991/20/Add. 1], which was criticized by the Philippines at the Commission. This had not been the case with the report of the Rapporteur on Torture, although it covered many of the same issues and, like the Working Group, had called for a civilian national police force, for witness protection programs, for prosecution of human rights abusers, and for establishing the jurisdiction of civilian courts when police are charged with crimes against civilians. However the report on disappearances provides other, broader recommendations: the disbanding of the Citizen Armed Force Geographic Units, groups of undisciplined volunteer reservists that are charged with many human rights violations; a narrowing of the greatly expanded powers of arrest; and combating the practice of "red labeling," whereby nongovernmental groups are listed as Communist Party sympathizers or agents and their members targeted for injury, abuse, or death.

The Working Group has sent special delegations to several countries at their invitation; two new invitations have come from El Salvador and Sri Lanka. Through such visits, which may also help to spur an official response to the Group's request for clarification of cases, national nongovernmental organizations (NGOs) become more aware of the Group and its procedural requirements. The Group has said it plans to follow up more effectively on the findings and recommendations of these visits.

The January 1991 report on the Group's work expresses concern that some countries have not acted on its recommendations (mentioning former visitees Peru, Guatemala, and Colombia), and expresses equal concern about the Commission's own treatment of the mission reports. It urges the Commission to pay more attention, "lest [these reports] receive only a passing reference during the session concerned and are forgotten soon afterwards, including by the Government addressed" [para. 413]. The 47th Commission went on record as deploring "the fact that . . . some Governments have not acted on the recommendations in the reports of the Working Group concerning them" or have not replied to requests for information. Although the reports of missions to particular countries were mentioned in the debate, not a single reference is made to them in the resolutions of the 47th session, reinforcing the view that they are soon forgotten.

The Working Group had endorsed a **draft declaration on disappearances** by the U.N. Subcommission on Prevention of Discrimination and Protection of Minorities that defines and outlaws the practice. The 45th General Assembly noted "with satisfaction" the fact that this draft would be available to the 47th Commission in 1991. At its 47th session the Commission agreed to establish a working group to consider the declaration during two weeks prior to its 48th session in 1992, "with a view towards its adoption" at that session [Res. 1991/41].

The Working Group on Disappearances has been the United Nations' most vocal critic of government efforts to give impunity to the perpetrators of this phenomenon. "Impunity was perhaps the single most important factor contributing to disappearances," the Group's Chairman, Ivan Tosevski of Yugoslavia, told the Commission. "Human rights violations appear to be accelerated and aggravated by the fact that . . . people who committed these violations were unpunished" [E/CN.4/1991/ SR.25]. He called for a study of this matter by the U.N. Subcommission on Prevention of Discrimination and Protection of Minorities, which several delegations endorsed but on which there was no action. The subject is addressed in the Working Group's report [paras. 406–10].

Summary and Arbitrary Executions

Since 1982 the means of combating summary and arbitrary executions have been addressed in the annual reports of S. Amos Wako of Kenya, who is **Special Rapporteur on Summary or Arbitrary Executions,** another theme mechanism established by the U.N. Commission on Human Rights. The 45th General Assembly discussed such practices and again adopted a resolution that "strongly condemns" them, "appeals urgently" for effective action to counter them, and asks the Rapporteur to respond effectively to the information he receives about them [A/Res/45/ 162]. Despite the importance of the subject and the strong language used, the 46th General Assembly will not discuss the Rapporteur's latest report directly, having decided that the topic would be considered biannually.

For more than a decade, U.N. human rights bodies have shown special concern about mass killings, whether conducted by governments or carried out by death squads operating outside the law. Thousands of cases have been reported in which, ignoring national laws that grant the accused the right to a lawyer or to an appeal, governments have imposed the death penalty on political opponents. Since establishment of this theme mechanism in 1982, the Commission, the General Assembly, and Mr. Wako have been **expanding the scope of the Rapporteur's efforts,** which have evolved from the scholarly—a concern for the number of actual deaths—to the activist—a focus on doing something about imminent deaths. The Rapporteur inquires about death penalty cases that appear to lack legal safeguards and about suspicious deaths at the hands of a government or its agents.

In his current report [E/CN.4/1991/36], Wako identifies the following practices as falling within his mandate: death threats, deaths in custody, executions following inadequate trial or judicial procedures, and extralegal executions in situations of armed conflict. A continuing key area of concern is deaths by torture, whether as a result of the abuse of force by police, military, or other government institutions; or assault by individuals and paramilitary groups acting in collusion or with the connivance of officials or by similar bodies opposing the government or outside its control.

In earlier reports the Rapporteur noted that summary and arbitrary executions occur in all regions of the world, and in the latest he cites an alarming increase in the number of deaths among those held in custody. The same report also notes an increase in summary and arbitrary executions during periods of internal conflict. The Commission responded by urging governments "to undertake all necessary measures to lower the level of violence and the needless loss of life consequent thereupon during situations of internal violence, disturbances, tensions and public emergencies" [Res. 1991/71]. A number of NGOs and scholars have argued that such abuses would diminish if the Rapporteur were to recommend a freeze or suspension of executions during such periods.

Of the 1990 report's 156 pages, 139 document the cases (with names and dates) the Rapporteur has raised with governments and the government replies, if any. The number of cases reported to him has grown dramatically, possibly because (he speculates) his mandate is now better known worldwide, yet only a fraction of these incoming cases will generate cables or letters from the Rapporteur, for reasons he does not detail.

In 1990, Wako contacted 49 governments, about twice the number contacted in 1987. In 25 cases the governments received an emergency cable (15 replied); in 45 the government received a letter requesting information (17 replied). These figures are somewhat better than in the past but poor nonetheless, reflecting the Rapporteur's continuing difficulty in enlisting official cooperation.

Some of the governments contacted by the Rapporteur are rarely discussed in U.N. human rights bodies. Among those mentioned in the 1991 report were China (killings in Tibet and other executions), Colombia (killings of political, union, peasant, and indigenous leaders and others—some by paramilitary groups), India (deaths in Jamma and Kashmir), Iraq (killings prior to and following the invasion of Kuwait), Somalia (summary killings connected with the internal conflict; reprisals taken against civilians, including women and children), Sudan (summary trials and legal proceedings as well as killings of civilians connected with the internal conflict), the United States (execution of a person under 18 and mentally retarded), the Soviet Union (killings in Lithuania and in the Armenian and Azerbaijani republics), and Yugoslavia (killings in Kosovo). Government responses vary: from promises to investigate and punish those responsible or provide information on investigations in progress to silence, denial of the event, denial of the fact that the execution in question was summary or arbitrary, and even the launching of a counteraccusation against the victim. As with the reports of the other theme mechanisms, there is little or no information from the Rapporteur about follow-up measures once a government has replied. Neither does the Rapporteur evaluate or comment upon the responses.

Focusing on prevention, the Rapporteur has recommended undertaking more **on-site visits,** especially to countries that are the subject of continuing and serious allegations. He has visited Suriname (1984, 1986, 1989), Uganda (1986), and Colombia (1989) and reports having received invitations from Peru, Sri Lanka, and Zaire. He also recommends the use of the United Nations' expanding Advisory Services program in human rights to advance compliance with human rights norms and help to halt extrajudicial executions. Repeating his call for training programs for law enforcement officers, he urges the teaching of human rights in primary and secondary schools as well.

Debate at the 46th Commission touched only cursorily on the Rapporteur's work. Because it is only one of many items considered under the **"gross violations"** rubric—it shares this category with numerous emergent crises as well as with the reports of "country rapporteurs"—the Rapporteur's findings and recommendations do not receive sustained attention, nor is there time to discuss his mandate itself. The Commission debate and resolutions offer little or no guidance on how the Rapporteur should address the questions about the scope of his work that he raises in his report. This situation may change in 1993 as the result of a revised agenda put forward for discussion by the Commission [Res. 1991/109] in which each of the theme mechanisms would be considered as a separate agenda item.

Some NGOs have suggested that the Rapporteur's work would have greater effect if he were to offer country-specific suggestions for overcoming these rights abuses, then follow up on their implementation. Greater and more sustained interaction with the governments in question, and regular, routinized follow up, would also help. To date, Commission member governments have failed to respond to the Rapporteur's request for support in establishing some form of **sanctions against governments that fail repeatedly to respond to his requests.** Commission and General Assembly encouragement of governmental "cooperation" has only limited effect. The Commission has likewise failed to take up the General Assembly's repeated call upon the Rapporteur to serve as **mediator between governments and the NGOs that are acting on behalf of victims.** The Rapporteur has declared that he will take on such a role, pursuant to the Assembly's mandate. In 1991, Wako reiterated his intention of using the new **Principles on Arbitrary and Summary Execution** to assess government responsibility for the summary or arbitrary executions alleged. This could herald a new phase of enforcement; developments will be closely monitored.

Financial constraints affect all Rapporteurs, limiting their ability to carry out their mandates in the most effective way. The staff is minimal; and investigation and follow up of the many serious cases presented annually—not to mention holdovers—would benefit from an increase of staff at the Geneva Human Rights Centre and greater interaction with the Vienna-based crime division in matters involving forensics and related specialties.

Torture

U.N. efforts to eradicate torture have been substantial, but, as the Special Rapporteur on Torture, Peter Kooijmans of the Netherlands, stressed again in his annual report to the Commission on Human Rights [E/CN.4/ 1991/17], the achievements to date have been mainly legal and institutional. The practice of torture continues.

Torture has been formally criminalized in a binding treaty, the **Convention against Torture** (1984), monitored by the **Committee against Torture (CAT)**, which meets twice a year. Its next report will be reviewed by the 46th General Assembly, but future reports will be considered biannually. The role of the Special Rapporteur on Torture, an ad hoc theme mechanism of the Human Rights Commission, is to examine the phenomenon; take action in reported torture cases on an emergency basis, whatever the country; and examine the current situation and the measures taken to prevent torture in these and other countries, visiting when invited to do so. The United Nations has also established a **Voluntary Fund for the Victims of Torture.**

The 46th General Assembly can be expected to adopt its traditional pro forma resolutions on CAT and on the torture of children in South Africa and Namibia. It has yet to address in a resolution the highly regarded work of the Special Rapporteur, although it regularly endorses the Commission's three other theme mechanisms.

Reports on compliance with the Convention—there were 56 states parties by June 15, 1991, and an additional 20-odd had signed—are reviewed by CAT in public session. Provision for such a committee, the Convention's only implementing mechanism, is a feature of U.N. human rights treaties. The Convention's Articles 21 and 22 provide the right of petition by individual citizens, but more than half the parties have not made the declaration that they will be bound by them.

CAT's meetings to date suggest that it may develop stricter enforcement procedures than have other treaty supervisory bodies. In CAT's 1990 report [A/45/44], members noted that the official government reports had not answered many of the questions about torture and the practices that facilitate it; and as a result CAT began requesting additional reports from some parties. For example, Chilean authorities (then representing the government of General Pinochet) were asked to supply complete data and statistics on recent cases of torture, on proceedings initiated against perpetrators, and on the compensation awarded to victims. Committee members also requested an additional report from the People's Republic of China. Among the outstanding concerns of CAT members were the use of evidence obtained by torture, the organization of the judiciary and its lack of independence, poor conditions of detention, limits on detainees' contacts with family, and the role of medical personnel in establishing the fact of torture [A/45/44, para. 500]. The review of Egypt's report elicited a demand for detailed records of court proceedings vis-à-vis alleged torturers.

This convention, unlike other human rights instruments, requires that **states parties pay independently for *all* expenses of the committee**—its meetings, documents, and staff. The uncertainty of cash flow, the experience of other treaty bodies with a pay-as-you-go provision, and financial problems that curtailed CAT meeting time during its first year have led CAT to ask the General Assembly to assure the committee's finances from the regular U.N. budget or make other financial arrangements, such as additional or temporary financing. The 45th General Assembly "welcomed," but did not endorse, the call for **more secure** financial arrangements for all human rights treaty bodies that had issued from a meeting of the chairs of the several committees; and the Commission's resolution "notes" rather than endorses the recommendation of regular-budget financing. Strenuous U.S. objections had led the 47th Commission to gut the provisions of a draft resolution that called on the General Assembly to finance the treaty bodies from the regular budget. Instead, each treaty body must pay something toward the cost even of the biennial chairpersons' meeting. Remarking on Washington's vigorous opposition to new, secure financial arrangements to allow the treaty bodies to function effectively, observers have drawn attention to the fact that the United States is not yet a party to the major human rights treaties. (By early 1991 the United States had made considerable progress in ratifying the Torture Convention, which now awaits enabling legislation by Congress.) The 46th General Assembly is scheduled to examine the implications of and prospects for regular-budget financing for the treaty bodies.

The **Special Rapporteur on Torture** intervenes on an emergency basis to protect the victims of torture and asks governments to clarify the detailed reports of torture that have been received. Over nearly a decade he has recommended an array of international and national measures to halt the practice of torture. In his 1991 report to the Human Rights Commission [E/CN.4/1991/17 and Add. 1], Professor Kooijmans again remarks that his report is longer than the previous year's and that a greater number of appeals were sent to governments—a fact he attributes to greater awareness of this theme mechanism and to the greater "transparency" of some societies (permitting the launching of appeals) rather than to any increase in the incidence of torture around the world.

The 1991 report describes the Rapporteur's urgent communications on some 70 cases to 31 countries in 1990, among them China, Saudi Arabia, Myanmar (Burma), Somalia, Cuba, Iraq, and Peru. Fifteen of these countries replied. The report also provides details of individual cases and situations involving torture in the 52 countries with which the Rapporteur corresponded on a nonemergency basis. Thirty-two governments had replied in some form by publication date, and several more by February 14, 1991, when he addressed the Commission. In the end, only 16 of this last group failed to respond (in their number were Peru, India, Guatemala, and Somalia). If some of the replies simply asserted that the allegations were baseless, other attempts to dismiss the allegations were more revealing. The Saudi government, for example, responding to charges that hands and arms of a number of individuals had been amputated as punishment, stated that "only the hand is amputated if the accusation is proved and following a confession" [ibid.]. Few governments, in any event, provide details of the investigations they report having inaugurated, and few undertake independent inquiries. The Rapporteur has suggested in the past that such details be provided in official replies. In 1991 he has encouraged states to invite him to examine the charges in person.

The Rapporteur on Torture has also offered a 21-page report on his ten-day October 1990 visit to the Philippines, where an insurgency continues and from which reports have been received of continuing human rights abuses by the government. His recommendations to the Aquino government concerning measures to deter torture give a sense of the preventive measures that can be taken to deter other human rights abuses, and they confirm the value of such country-specific investigations. Kooijmans recommended, for example, that the Philippine Commission on Human Rights be strengthened and given prosecution powers, enhancing its credibility as an independent body with all strata of society; that a national civilian police force be established; that armed forces, including the police, come under the jurisdiction of civilian courts once again; that detainees be visited immediately by doctors and lawyers; that witness-protection measures be strengthened; that adequate compensation be provided to torture victims, regardless of whether the perpetrator has been identified; that accused torturers be brought to trial speedily and, if found guilty, severely punished; that all interrogations of detainees be recorded and the names of all persons involved supplied; and that those in charge of detention centers where torture takes place be disciplined, regardless of whether the specific torturer can be found.

The Rapporteur noted the lack of follow-up correspondence about the recommendations prepared after earlier on-site visits to Peru, Guatemala, and Honduras, while welcoming a brief update from Zaire. He reiterated that an invitation to him for a visit is not an admission of torture; the primary purpose of these visits is consultative and preventative, not accustory or investigatory. And, he added, he welcomes a new invitation to visit Indonesia.

For all the international efforts and machinery aimed at eliminating torture, Kooijmans concludes, the ball is in the national governments' court; it is up to them to ensure that the promises made in international forums become a reality at home. To this end he recommends general measures all states can take to halt the practice of torture: conducting interrogations only at official interrogation centers, where blindfolding and hooding are forbidden and the names of interrogators are recorded; inaugurating periodic independent investigations of detention centers;

establishing national ombudsman-type authorities or human rights commissions with the power to investigate or prosecute cases of torture; and taking action against medical professionals who collaborate in torture. As before, Professor Kooijmans spoke of the need to utilize **U.N. Advisory Services** programs to educate and improve the behavior of police, law enforcement, and other officials.

Both the Rapporteur and the Commission have discussed the need for **periodic visits by independent experts to places of detention**—something proposed by Costa Rica in 1980 as a possible Optional Protocol to the Convention on Torture but shortly shelved. The new European Convention on Torture has a provision along these lines. At the 47th session of the Human Rights Commission a revised version of the Costa Rican proposal was raised by a number of governments [E/CN.4/ 1991/66], but the Commission decided to address the specific proposal as a separate agenda item at its 48th session [Res. 1991/107]. Its resolution on the report of the Rapporteur on Torture again noted the "importance of instituting" such a system of visits [1991/38].

Religious Intolerance

The 46th General Assembly and the next session of the Commission on Human Rights will consider measures to end religious intolerance, a matter now studied by another of the Commission's theme Rapporteurs, Angelo Vidal d'Almeida Ribeiro of Portugal. The **Special Rapporteur on Religious Intolerance**—established in 1985 and extended since then by consensus—addresses individual country situations in his reports, offering excerpts from his correspondence with the country's officials and their replies, if any.

Mr. Ribeiro's most recent report [E/CN.4/1991/56] provides information on correspondence with 21 governments in 1990 regarding allegations of religious discrimination or intolerance "inconsistent with the provisions of the **Declaration [on the Elimination of All Forms of Intolerance based on Religion or Belief]**," the principal instrument in this area. Fourteen governments replied—a response rate considerably higher than that of other theme rapporteurs.

Among the countries cited in the January 1991 report are China, the document's longest section (concerning the persecution of numerous Tibetan monks and nuns and the harassment of Catholic believers); Egypt (actions against Coptic Christians, including discriminatory measures affecting their property, churches, and associations; and Islamic violence against Christians); El Salvador (the killings of six priests and other actions, such as arrests, directed against the Catholic Church, clergy, and believers); Greece (the treatment of conscientious objectors and Greek Muslims); India (a single incident involving the Ananda Marga sect); Iran (discrimination against Baha'is and "forced Islamization" directed particularly at Armenian Christians. Iran's response included a noteworthy invitation to the Rapporteur to visit); Nepal (discriminatory laws and arrests of Christians); Pakistan (the demolition of Ahmadi mosques, arrests, and other harassment of Ahmadis); Saudi Arabia (actions prohibiting Shiite Muslims from practicing openly certain rites, e.g., commemoration of the death of the Prophet's grandson, and the detention of practitioners without charge or trial. The Saudi reply states, inter alia, "No one is forced to live and work in Saudi Arabia against his will. If he dislikes its laws . . . he should not choose to live in it" [ibid., p. 115]); Vietnam (the detention of Buddhist monks); and Burundi and Indonesia (reports of the banning and harassment of Jehovah's Witnesses).

Past reports have noted that infringements of religious freedom usually result in infringements of other human rights—for instance, an individual's freedom of movement and expression—as well as in extrajudicial killings in clashes with other religious groups or even with government security forces. The report does not, however, mention the communal clashes between the Muslim and Hindu communities in India, to take one example. These conflicts indicate the degree to which religious intolerance is interlinked with other rights, and they suggest the need to consider the role of non-state actors, including the religious communities themselves, in perpetuating conflict. The lack of such details in the report highlights one of the weaknesses of the rapporteurial mechanism: It can respond only to allegations from outside parties; if none is forthcoming, no inquiry is made.

In 1991 the Rapporteur reported on the initial replies to a questionnaire circulated among governments in which he inquired about national legislation concerning religious groups, treatment of believers and nonbelievers, and the protection of religious minorities; and about reciprocity for foreigners, conscientious objection, clashes between religious groups, actions against expressions of "extremist or fanatical" opinions related to religious groups, remedies, and conciliation mechanisms. Most of those that have replied to date paint a rosy picture of legal protections and indicate a lack of conflict among religious groups. Only a very few were as candid as Yugoslavia, which referred to religious pressures among its various nationally linked churches and spoke of the need to revamp constitutional and other protections to promote tolerance for other religions and respect for the rights of their followers.

Like the other theme rapporteurs, Ribeiro does not comment on such replies, nor does his annual report offer country-specific recommendations to promote religious tolerance and prevent the infringement of religious freedom. Still, he characterizes his work as an inquiry into situations "which seemed to involve a departure from the provisions of the Declaration," and he finds that such departures "have persistently occurred in most regions of the world." The "best guarantee" of respect for these rights, he concludes, is "the efficient functioning of democratic institutions and the rule of law," coupled with measures that will put an end to various established forms of inequality [para. 105].

By consensus, the 45th General Assembly largely reiterated its concern about religious intolerance, supporting efforts to continue measures aimed at implementing the Declaration [A/Res/45/136]. The Assembly, and the 47th Commission on Human Rights, again replied with caution to **proposals for drafting a new binding instrument on religion,** even as the Rapporteur continues to urge governments "to actively consider" one. And both Assembly and Commission referred in positive terms to a paper on the topic prepared by Subcommission Special Rapporteur Theo van Boven of the Netherlands, who saw any such new instrument only as an optional protocol to an existing treaty. References to the matter were relegated by the Commission to the preambular rather than the operative paragraphs of its lengthy resolution on religious intolerance [1991/48]. Underlying this reluctance to proceed with a separate convention is the concern that any new instrument will further erode the standards set forth in the Declaration on Religious Intolerance and other instruments.

The General Assembly and the 47th Commission once again emphasized the value of the role played by nongovernmental and religious organizations; urged states to provide adequate constitutional and legal guarantees of freedom of thought, conscience, religion, and belief, as well as effective remedies for overcoming intolerance or discrimination; and encouraged greater efforts at education. Anticipating the **tenth anniversary of the Declaration in December 1991,** the Commission requested the Secretary-General to disseminate the Declaration widely and in all official languages—something called for repeatedly since 1982 but yet to be accomplished—and asked states to distribute it in all national languages.

Country Situations

For many years the General Assembly publicly addressed human rights abuses in only three countries: Chile, South Africa, and Israel. In recent years it has been expanding its venue. Special Rapporteurs or Representatives were appointed by the 47th Commission on Human Rights to conduct fact-finding studies on Afghanistan, El Salvador, Iraq, and occupied Kuwait, reporting to the General Assembly. The Commission has also appointed special country experts to provide reports on conditions in Romania, Iran, and Cuba, but these will not be presented directly to the Assembly. Other countries, Albania among them, have been the subject of Commission resolutions, but no expert has been appointed to report on the human rights situation within their borders.

Some countries are considered at the Commission under the category of "**Advisory Services,**" which were established to provide the sort of technical assistance that a developing country might need to implement the standards set in various international covenants on human rights. At the 47th Commission the countries considered under this heading were Guatemala, Haiti, and Equitorial Guinea. Guatemala formerly was assigned a Special Representative, who reported to the Assembly, but was "promoted" to review under Advisory Services after it elected a civilian government in the mid-1980s.

Several other countries are considered by the Commission under the so-called **1503 confidential procedure** in which, meeting in closed session, the Commission considers complaints (lodged for the most part by NGOs and usually documenting numerous individual cases) about a gross pattern of violations by the government. These too do not come before the General Assembly. The 1991 Commission continued to examine under this category gross violations in Myanmar, Chad, Somalia, and Sudan. The situation in Zaire, which had been under scrutiny, was dropped. Zaire has now invited U.N. investigators for a visit.

During the General Assembly's general debate, delegates may mention human rights conditions anywhere in the world. Some governments—China's prominent among them—are sensitive even to this form of human rights scrutiny.

Afghanistan

The 46th General Assembly will receive another interim report from its **Special Rapporteur,** Dr. Felix Ermacora of Austria, based on his most recent visits to Afghanistan and Pakistan. In 1990, for the first time since his investigations began, he was able to travel to areas inside Afghanistan that are held by guerrilla forces. He notes that a "clear picture" of the situation in such areas can only be obtained through systematic visits, and he called attention to the absence of administrative structures in the opposition-controlled areas visited.

In 1990, two years after the withdrawal of Soviet troops, Dr. Ermacora concluded that their departure had diminished but not ended the human rights violations he had been investigating since 1984 [A/C.3/45/ SR.48]. Citing some "overall improvement" in the human rights situation, he said that he had found no sign of movement toward the pluralistic political system called for by the country's 1990 constitution, that no one had yet clarified the fate of 3,000 political prisoners, and that the agreement granting the International Committee of the Red Cross (ICRC) access to Ministry of State Security detention centers was not being honored, despite official promises to him—in short, that there was no democracy and no respect for the rule of law. His report [A/45/664] had discussed unsatisfactory detention conditions, and he expressed regret that he was unable to examine reported cases of torture, saying this would be a priority for his next report. The "principal" human rights problem, Ermacora reiterated, stems from the armed conflict itself, and a political solution to the war would be the most significant step toward improving the human rights situation. This call was widely echoed in speeches by Western delegates at the 45th General Assembly and the 47th Commission, and by the representatives of Pakistan and the Soviet Union as well. The Soviet delegate drew attention to his government's active collaboration with the Special Representative, pronouncing the report "on the whole, objective and balanced" [E/CN.4/1991/SR.53]. The Commission's resolution on the situation in Afghanistan was adopted by consensus, but the Soviet delegate remarked that, had there been a vote, he would not have participated.

Ermacora's 1990 and 1991 reports, like those preceding his visit to guerrilla-held areas, had much to say about Afghanistan's 5 million refugees, whose plight, he stated in the most recent report, "constitutes a human rights problem in itself" [E/CN.4/1991/31, para. 89ff]. He stresses the need for renewed efforts to bring the refugees back home, noting resistance by opposition parties and armed groups within Afghanistan. And he discusses various proposals and actions that would move the country toward free elections, urging the United Nations to play a role in this area.

Directing attention to government and rebel forces, the Special Rapporteur calls for the release of all political prisoners and detained soldiers; asks the opposition to clarify the fate of prisoners it holds and respond to lists drawn up by the Soviet authorities; asks that amnesty decrees be applied to foreign detainees as well, mentioning Soviet prisoners of war; and asks that the names of all political prisoners and detained soldiers be transmitted to humanitarian organizations. Noting the problem, as yet unclarified, of an estimated 18,000 "so-called Afghan orphans" reportedly "detained" in the Soviet Union [para. 47], he cites Soviet representations to him to the effect that 3,000 Afghan children are "studying and working" in the Soviet Union. He also cites reports of three instances of massive summary executions by the Afghan armed opposition forces, killing hundreds, for which there is "no justification."

During the General Assembly debate the Afghan government sought to affirm that it does permit the ICRC into the prisons and spoke of a prisoner amnesty. The Rapporteur's report, the government's delegate maintained, had paid insufficient attention to the problems in areas outside government control, to the great personal danger faced by refugees who do return, to deteriorating conditions facing women in the refugee camps, to the status of the Geneva negotiations, and to humanitarian efforts [see A/C.3/1991/SR.50]. Pakistan, host to millions of the refugees, criticized specific details of the report during the 47th Commission [E/CN.4/1991/SR. 36]. Ermacora replied point by point, affording a more coherent and fuller public discussion of the report than is usual in country situations [see E/CN.4/1991/SR.37]. A number of NGOs have been urging an in-depth Commission review and discussion of rapporteurs' reports, believing this a means of increasing the impact and significance of U.N. special human rights procedures.

Most, but not all, of Ermacora's suggestions found their way into the resolutions adopted by the Assembly and the 47th Commission. The Commission resolution [1991/78], mirroring that of the Assembly, noted with appreciation the Special Rapporteur's report (but did not, as in the past, thank him personally), welcomed the Afghan government's cooperation with the Rapporteur and with international organizations, including the High Commissioner for Refugees; and stressed the importance of a comprehensive political settlement, with provision for free elections, an end to hostilities, the return of refugees, and full enjoyment of human rights by all citizens. It also called for a ban on the use of weapons against civilians; for protection of prisoners from reprisals and from such rights violations as torture and summary execution; for investigations of all disappearances; for the submission of the names of prisoners to the ICRC; for guarantees of due process for all; and for assuring the ICRC access to *all* prisons and prisoners. It went on to encourage exchanges of prisoners, and—on behalf of Soviet prisoners of war being held by opposition forces—recommended that foreign detainees be included in amnesty agreements. "All parties" are asked to assure detainees fair treatment and to observe the humanitarian laws of war. The Commission resolution noted "with concern" the allegations of atrocities against Afghan soldiers and civilians, reiterating past resolutions, and concern too at the living conditions of the refugees. It called for cooperation in mine detection and removal, voicing a new concern for the safety of humanitarian workers in the area.

El Salvador

El Salvador's human rights situation has been under scrutiny in the General Assembly and Commission on Human Rights since 1981. The 46th General Assembly will consider a report on El Salvador by the **Special Representative of the Commission on Human Rights,** José Antonio Pastor Ridruejo of Spain.

In his report to the Commission in 1991 [E/CN.4/1991/SR.40], the Special Representative voiced concern at instances of politically motivated summary executions and disappearances and the practice of torture during extrajudicial interrogations of detainees, "although the Special Representative believes these practices are not widespread and do not represent offiical policy." He found an unsatisfactory judicial system ("although the main defects are to be seen in the area of investigation and fact-finding rather than in the trial and sentencing activities") and discussed the **killing in 1989 of six Jesuit priests, their cook, and the cook's daughter.** There were nonetheless some encouraging signs, said Mr. Pastor Ridruejo: In 1990 a number of sentences were handed down for politically motivated crimes of earlier years, and on his visit he found members of the military and security forces in prison, which "demonstrated that the alleged impunity of the armed forces was not absolute." He refers again to harsh treatment of the civilian population and to the economic and social problems that have resulted from the conflict.

The report devotes rather little attention to the **U.N.–brokered San José agreement,** but it cites with favor the fact of it. In this agreement, signed by the Salvadoran government and the Farabundo Martí National Liberation Front (FMLN) on July 26, 1990, both sides pledge to take immediate action to prevent infringements of the right to life and to physical integrity, and the freedom of the individual; to cease and desist from the practice of abductions and disappearances; to give priority to investigating cases of this kind so as to identify and punish those responsible; and to take immediate steps to ensure that no one is held in incommunicado detention or subjected to torture or other cruel, inhuman, or degrading treatment or punishment [A/44/971-S/2154, Annex].

As before, the Special Representative was critical of members of the government apparatus *and* members of the FMLN. In the most current report he "takes note of the continuing, obvious efforts by the President of the Republic and [others] . . . to improve the human rights situation." Although these efforts have led to a decrease in the number of violations, he points out, the violations continue. He also takes note of positive FMLN actions, such as the declaration of a cease-fire at the time of former President Duarte's death and the decision to suspend armed attacks against civilians.

The 45th General Assembly and 47th Commission resolutions mirror one another to a considerable extent. Both endorsed the recommendations of the Pastor Ridruejo reports, voicing concern about executions, abductions and disappearances, and the atmosphere of intimidation in which certain sectors of the population live. They likewise expressed concern about an unsatisfactory judicial system and deplored irregularities in the proceedings held in connection with the murder of the six priests as well as the lack of cooperation by sectors of the armed forces. The San José agreement received a welcome from both bodies.

Human rights organizations welcomed the agreement too, viewing it as a positive development, but some noted that it largely restates the government's binding human rights obligations under international law. In the days following the signing of the agreement, the government moved to fulfill its pledge by issuing new directives to the Salvadoran security forces that prohibit the use of torture and emphasize the need to halt disappearances. Nonetheless, the Representative stated, serious human rights violations have continued since the agreement was signed.

At the 47th Commission, a number of NGOs challenged Pastor Ridruejo's finding that torture is not widespread or a national policy; others argued that the present condition of the justice system is far worse than he had described, citing the poor record on prosecuting human rights violators and the continued activities of the death squads. Several governments discussed the lack of progress in pursuing a prosecution in the case of the six Jesuit priests; and most took up the Special Representative's repeated call for a negotiated political settlement to end the armed conflict in El Salvador.

The Soviet Union

For the very first time, the Commission took **formal action** regarding the human rights situation in the Soviet Union: A carefully balanced consensus "statement" (negotiated by and approved in Moscow), read publicly by the Commission's Chairman, expressed concern about **recent killings in Lithuania and Latvia** and asked to see the results of investigations now in progress. According to the diplomatic formula, the statement offers words of praise for the Gorbachev government's reform program in human rights.

Iran

Despite a serious challenge by Iran, the 47th Commission agreed to extend the mandate of its investigator (reappointed annually since 1984) for one additional year. However, in a controversial agreement with Iran that permitted the resolution to be adopted by consensus, the Commission stated explicitly that if there is "progress" toward improving human rights during the next year, it will dispense with the **Special Representative;** and it drops the traditional directive to the Special Representative, Reynaldo Galindo Pohl of El Salvador, to report his findings to the General Assembly.

The Iranian government has taken advantage of the Gulf situation and the late appearance of the U.N. Special Representative's report on the Commission agenda to gather support for a resolution it introduced that would have brought an end to the U.N. scrutiny of its human rights situation. It was then up to the Western group, traditional sponsors of the Iran resolution, to cobble together an alternative that would continue the investigator's mandate. As late as two days before the session's end its fate remained uncertain.

The severity of the human rights abuses in Iran had been well documented in the report by the Special Representative that was presented to the 1991 Commission [E/CN.4/1991/35], reflecting his second visit to Iran and the data supplied by many witnesses. Yet the offer to end the Representative's mandate in 1992 holds out the clear possibility that the Commission will ignore Iran's human rights violations in the future, even if such practices as torture, summary executions, political imprisonment, persecution of Baha'is, and a disregard for even the minimal requirements of a fair trial continue. The Canadian government's public statement that "progress" must be interpreted as *real* progress with respect to the International Covenant on Civil and Political Rights was an important attempt at damage-limitation. At the spring meeting of ECOSOC the United States cautioned that "process" should not be confused with "progress," and called for continuing the scrutiny of Iran absent real progress.

Kuwait

Both the 45th General Assembly and the 47th Commission adopted resolutions about the human rights situation in occupied Kuwait. Most of the early drafts and Kuwaiti complaints dealt with various violations of the laws of war—treatment of civilians, bombing, looting, and visits to prisoners of war. But the Commission also cited such "grave" human rights violations as torture, arbitrary arrests, summary executions, and disappearances and approved the appointment of a **Special Rapporteur "to examine the human rights violations committed in occupied Kuwait by the invading and occupying forces of Iraq."** In June 1991, Walter Kalin of Switzerland, a professor of public and international law, received the appointment and journeyed to Kuwait on June 12.

Iraq is a member of the Commission, and barbs and charges were exchanged throughout the 47th session. After the ground war ended and news reports from Kuwait alleged summary executions of non-Kuwaitis by Kuwaitis, Iraq introduced an amendment to the resolution on Iraqi-occupied Kuwait that condemned new "acts of revenge and torture" against Palestinians, Sudanese, and Iraqis at the hands of Kuwaitis and the "occupying powers." The vote of 2–33–5, with only Cuba and Iraq in favor, defeated the amendment.

In a rare show of unanimity, the Commission approved the establishment of the special investigator of Iraqi atrocities in Kuwait by a vote of 41–1–0, with Iraq the sole dissenter. And when the appointment was challenged again at the May session of ECOSOC, the vote was 50–0–0. Four countries—Algeria, Iraq, Jordan, and Tunisia—were "absent," however.

Iraq

The decision to begin scrutiny of Iraq—a longtime goal of nongovernmental human rights groups that had been thwarted by procedural "no-action" votes in the past—was made by a vote of 30–1–10, Iraq the sole nay-sayer. China and Cuba abstained on this occasion, but the Soviet Union voted with the majority.

Resolution 1991/74 calls for the appointment of a **Special Rapporteur "to make a thorough study of the violations of human rights by the Government of Iraq,"** supplying the 46th General Assembly with an interim report and the 48th Commission with a final one. Citing evidence from the reports of the Special Rapporteur on Torture and the Working Group on Disappearances, the resolution expresses "grave concern at the flagrant violations" in Iraq and calls for a halt to arbitrary and summary executions, arbitrary detention of political and religious opponents, enforced disappearances, the practice of torture, and forced deportations of Iraqi citizens. (The Kurds are mentioned in the preamble.) It also calls for measures to correct the damage, such as a full accounting of the "disappeared," permission for the deportees to return, and "reparation."

Cuba

A resolution calling for human rights scrutiny of Cuba has been the special target of U.S. diplomacy at the Human Rights Commission for almost a decade. In 1991 a U.S. initiative succeeded in establishing a **"Special Representative" to document and report on the Cuban situation during the year.**

Two competing drafts—a hard-hitting U.S.–sponsored one and a softer Latin one—were formally proposed. Even though the U.S. resolution (among whose 17 cosponsors were the Western group, Japan, Hungary, Czechoslovakia, and Nicaragua) was introduced first and should have been voted on first, Venezuela issued a successful call for the Latin text to be considered ahead of the other. The United States then introduced an amendment to the Latin text that would provide for a Special Representative to investigate and report back to the Commission. The amendment carried, 21–8–4, and the whole resolution was approved by a vote of 22–6–15. The negative votes were those of Cuba, China, Colombia (which has often taken Cuba's side at the Commission), Ethiopia, the Soviet Union (Cuba's longtime sponsor), and the Ukraine. Voting in favor, in addition to the Western group, were newly noncommunist Czechoslovakia and Hungary as well as the Philippines, Argentina, Senegal, Bangladesh, Morocco, Swaziland, Madagascar, and Panama.

The **United States** invested heavily in the diplomatic effort to bring about formal U.N. scrutiny of Cuba, flying former U.S. Ambassador to Venezuela Otto Reich to Geneva to join efforts with the regular delegation in working on this issue. U.S. Representative to the Commission Armando Valladares, a poet and former political prisoner in Cuba, had resigned before the start of the 1991 session.

Significantly, the final text requests the U.N. Secretary-General, "after consultation with the Chairman and the Bureau, to appoint a special representative . . . to maintain direct contact with the Government and citizens of Cuba" on the issues that arose in connection with the report of the **U.N. mission to Cuba in 1988.** Such language requiring the Secretary-General to get approval from the "Bureau"—the Commission's geographically balanced roster of top officers—before acting seems unprecedented.

The U.S. effort was not helped along by the report on Cuba of the Secretary-General [E/CN.4/1991/28], which was requested in the Commission's 1990 resolution and had been the subject of considerable controversy [see *Issues Before the 45th General Assembly of the United Nations*, pp. 149–51]. The report had only seven substantive paragraphs [6–12] in which the Secretary-General provided the sought-after explanation of the specific nature of his contacts with the government of Cuba following the 1988 Cuba mission, adhering to the letter of earlier Commission resolutions. These contacts, he reported now, had to do with political prisoners detained in connection with their testimony before Commission personnel during the 1988 mission. The remainder of his efforts on Cuba, the Secretary-General declared, were carried out under his regular "good offices" function and had to remain confidential. Appended to the text were an exchange of letters between the Secretary-General and the Cuban government and the names of 22 people whose cases had been raised with the Cubans. Uncommonly, the report was drafted in New York, not at the Geneva headquarters of the Human Rights Centre, where all other human rights documentation is prepared. Further, its shape and tone were of different quality from the human rights reporting of the Geneva secretariat.

At the ECOSOC meeting in May, Cuba tried, but failed, to reverse the Commission's action. Backing Cuba in its quest were Algeria, Burkina Faso, China, Iran, Iraq, Malaysia, Somalia, Syria, Zambia, the Soviet Union, and the Ukraine.

Advisory Services: Haiti and Guatemala

Criticism of Haiti and Guatemala were more muted at the 1991 Commission, and efforts to monitor conditions in the two countries will continue under the U.N. Advisory Services program in human rights. The gentle treatment was meant to signify a vote of confidence in the newly elected governments in each country. Many NGOs publicly criticized this use of the technical assistance program, which offers an alternative to the direct scrutiny of violations. They argue that this can be interpreted as a "promotion" of the government, releasing it from consideration under the "gross violations" item whether or not real progress has been made in halting human rights abuses.

In response to requests from the interim President of Haiti, the United Nations provided technical assistance during 1990 to draw up election security plans and monitor their implementation [A/Res/45/2]. This marked the second occasion on which the United Nations has assisted a sovereign state in conducting elections. The Commission had earlier appointed an **Expert on Haiti,** Philippe Texier of France. In 1991 his report (based on a mid-1990 visit) and addendum (based on a post-election visit in late January 1991) were considered under item 12, **"gross violations,"** for the first time.

The Texier report [E/CN.4/1991/33] detailed once again a wide range of structural obstacles to improving human rights: an ineffective judicial system, the considerable military presence in rural areas, nonseparation of the army and military, and impunity for those responsible for the massacres of 1987 and 1988. These, he stated at the 47th Commission, remain the "principal obstacles" to "real improvement" in the human rights situation in Haiti.

In the report's addendum [E/CN.4/1991/33/Add. 1], he spoke of the fragility of the situation and the violence that continued to erupt from many quarters, the violence attendant on land disputes, and the attempts to overthrow the democratic process—notably the failed post-election coup attempt by Roger Lafontant. The Expert was able to report that, "despite the imperfections of the electoral process . . . the result of the presidential election is beyond question," but he expressed less certitude about Haiti's ability to strengthen respect for human rights in view of current economic and social conditions and the endemic violence.

During the Commission debate Texier spoke of the progress made during the year and called on the Commission to "help to stabilize the democratic process." He noted that the government and judicial authorities had not yet taken "effective measures to investigate past and present violations of human rights and to bring the guilty to justice," and he recommended continued reporting by an expert and greater use of technical assistance. The Commission resolution [1991/77], adopted by consensus, noted the problems that had been described by the Expert and recommended continued dialogue between the Expert and the government, to be conducted under the Advisory Services program.

Reporting on **Guatemala** in 1990, the soon-to-retire **Expert,** Hector Gros Espiell, presented a highly pessimistic picture of the situation in the country—explaining that "events have not justified the relative and cautious optimism felt in 1987 and 1988," citing the government's "contempt for pluralism," and providing a long account of atrocities [E/CN.4/1990/45 and Add. 1]. The 46th Commission's resolution [1990/80] "deeply deplore[d]" the many human rights violations in Guatemala, expressed "profound concern at the **resurgence of the so-called death squads**," and called upon the Guatemalan government "to initiate or intensify . . . investigations" aimed at bringing to justice "those responsible for disappearances, torture, murder and extra-legal executions," and "to promote any measures necessary to identify and punish the members of death squads." The resolution went on to request the next independent Expert "to examine the human rights situation in Guatemala" and to continue offering advice and assistance. It left open the question of the agenda item under which the report would be discussed in 1991, whether "advisory services" or "gross violations," making this dependent on the report itself. In a roll-call vote in 1991 in which the Latin American group prevailed, the decision was made not to consider Guatemala under the **"gross violations"** item.

The new Expert, Christian Tomuschat of Germany, likewise presented a dismal picture—of **continued disappearances** and of **summary executions after torture.** He recommended that the new government affirm its authority over the armed forces, strengthen its "almost meaningless" past attempts to investigate and prosecute perpetrators of human rights abuses, halt compulsory drafting and the militarization of the indigenous communities, adopt a new law on indigenous rights, and provide guarantees of economic and social rights for all. He called for intensifying and enlarging the democratic process so as to include those now disenfranchised and for extensive training in human rights for officials and others. And he insisted that the government put an end to the operations of **paramilitary groups** and **clandestine prisons.**

Examining allegations that the armed forces or police were responsible for disappearances, torture, and killings, the Expert came to the conclusion that with the clear exception of "the recent **mass killing in Santiago Atitlan**," for which the military was responsible, the evidence of military responsibility in other cases was "only circumstantial."

Mr. Tomuschat called for varying forms of support from the international community, and went so far as to argue that the new "policy orientation" of the elected government was doomed to fail without international aid and cooperation. The guarantees of human rights he urged the government to make, the Expert said, were in the interests of the people of Guatemala as well as of the state.

Many speakers, including NGO representatives, deplored the massive violations of human rights in Guatemala. The Commission, by consensus, deplored the continuance of serious rights violations but said that it welcomed the new government's commitment, on taking office in

January 1991, to guarantee full enjoyment of human rights and take immediate measures to that end. Its resolution calls on the government to pay special attention to the Expert's recommendations, to ensure that its security forces respect human rights, and to bring those responsible for human rights abuses to justice. The Commission directed the Expert to continue to report on the situation in Guatemala and to provide advisory services.

China

The **Tiananmen massacre** and other actions by China led the **Subcommission on Prevention of Discrimination and Protection of Minorities** to adopt a resolution condemning such developments in 1989. When the Subcommission—a subordinate expert body of the Human Rights Commission—met in 1990, the atmosphere had changed, and now it was the Iraqi invasion of Kuwait that occupied center stage. China's support for or refusal to block Security Council actions in the **Gulf crisis** deflected the introduction of any resolution critical of its human rights policies. New and detailed information had been submitted by NGOs and experts alike, but the passage of time, and a more sophisticated diplomatic effort by China, killed chances of a resolution critical of its actions and policies.

In the 45th General Assembly, China put its Gulf cooperation to use once again, managing to offset most criticism. The Swedish, Australian, Norwegian, and Canadian governments, and the Italian government speaking on behalf of the European Community ("the 12"), offered some comments about the human rights situation in China in their general statements about human rights violations. (They were criticized in turn by China's delegates, mostly in private.)

China used the Third Committee as a forum to advance its view that **noninterference in the internal affairs of states** is a guiding principle of the United Nations, applying equally to U.N. human rights activities; that attention by U.N. human rights bodies to **violations by member states** exceeds the U.N. Charter's provisions; and that **collective, economic, and social rights** have preeminence over civil and political rights. China's efforts to alter the structure and terms of reference of the 1992 World Conference on Human Rights to accord with this view received little support in the end. The Chinese delegation also participated vigorously in the Third Committee and, ultimately, the Fifth (Financial) Committee debate about financing the U.N. Human Rights Centre, attempting to alter its plans and even decrease the resources made available. Again, China was not successful, but it has firmly established itself as an anti–human rights force at the United Nations.

The Gulf crisis continued at center stage as the Commission on Human Rights gathered for its 47th session in February, and not a single resolution on China was introduced at the Commission. Ironically, it was just at meeting time that China began its **trials of prodemocracy activists,** and Western governments, prominently the United States, strongly criticized China in the public debate. China's delegates were moved to offer several detailed statements in rebuttal. Arguing that the human rights of all citizens were fully respected, they renewed the charge that the pro-democracy activists were creators of "turmoil."

South Africa

Changes in South Africa's political and human rights scene in the months before and since the 45th General Assembly have brought some changes in the language of resolutions aimed at **isolating the South African government and dismantling the system of apartheid.** In the instance of the 47th Commission on Human Rights, the moderation of language allowed a new and notable consensus on a traditionally contentious resolution.

The 45th General Assembly adopted eight related resolutions on South Africa and apartheid [A/Res/176A–H], "a crime against the conscience and dignity of humankind and a threat to international peace and security." The first of these resolutions, welcoming indications of movement toward negotiations with the African National Congress while again calling upon the international community to keep up its pressure on the government to eradicate apartheid, was adopted without a vote; and so too the last, which affirmed support for the **U.N. Trust Fund for South Africa,** one of the U.N. bodies dealing directly with apartheid. On the remaining six resolutions—ranging from an affirmation of the wisdom of **comprehensive and mandatory sanctions against South Africa,** to an expression of concern about states that collaborate with South Africa in military matters, to a demand that Israel terminate its nuclear and other collaboration with Pretoria, to an affirmation of support for the **Commission Against Apartheid in Sports**—the United States offered a negative vote, sometimes in the company of traditional allies, less often alone or with the United Kingdom.

The 47th Commission on Human Rights, meeting between February and March 1991, remained critical of Pretoria's practices on human rights but managed for the **first** time to achieve a **consensus text** as its major resolution on the human rights situation in South Africa. This resolution [1991/21] began traditionally enough. It called upon the South African government "to fulfill the commitment to release all political prisoners and detainees [and] to permit the unconditional return of political exiles; urged the repeal of all discriminatory and repressive legislation without delay; recommended further action to end the "intercommunal violence aggravated by elements opposed to the dramatic transformation of South Africa"; and expressed grave concern over the "continued detentions without trial, the continued possibility of executions of political prisoners, and the widespread violence aggravated by elements of the security organs and political activists." The same resolution also called for the **continuance of sanctions** against South Africa, but **abandoned the adjective "mandatory,"** which previously had seemed writ in stone. This paved the way for acceptance of the text by the United States, under the leadership of chief delegate Kenneth Blackwell, and by others of the Western group. The Frontline states found it "regrettable," said Zambia's delegate, that the resolution "reflected the lowest common denominator," producing an "unrealistic" text that "fell far short of the expectations of the oppressed people of South Africa" [E/CN.4/1991/SR.48]. But another African delegate, the Ambassador of Senegal, looked at the matter differently: The fact of consensus on this resolution, he said, is "a significant step forward in [the Commission's] approach" [ibid.].

The Western governments voted against, or abstained from, some other Commission resolutions on South Africa that continued the call for mandatory sanctions, whether by governments or by transnational corporations; described apartheid as akin to genocide; or used other formulations they have long opposed [see Res. 1991/9, 10, and 17]. The German and other Western delegations expressed extreme displeasure at the language used in a resolution on the **Racism Decade** [1991/11], but the resolution was finally approved by consensus: The United States had refused to participate in the voting in any way. However, the traditional resolution calling for **self-determination for South Africans** was dropped altogether—a significant concession to the Western group.

At the Commission, country resolutions on **Romania, Albania,** and **Israel** were also approved publicly.

In a notable 1991 decision that was vigorously opposed by Cuba, the 47th Commission, and later ECOSOC, approved **secret balloting** when votes are taken on country-situation resolutions at meetings of the Subcommission. This will have the effect of restoring a measure of independence to the work of the Subcommission in identifying countries in which there are gross patterns of human rights violations.

On April 5, 1991, came yet another sign of a new venue for addressing serious rights violations that affect large numbers of people. The U.N. **Security Council,** meeting on this day, condemned the **mass killings in Iraq** that had caused almost a million of its Kurdish and Shiite Muslim citizens to flee to neighboring countries. Resolution 688 called the repression against the Kurds "a threat to international peace and security," demanded that Iraq desist and seek dialogue "to ensure that human and political rights of all Iraqi citizens are respected," and insisted that Iraq "allow immediate access by international humanitarian organizations to those in need of assistance."

The question of whether the Security Council should confront massive violations of human rights is a long-standing one. For years, India and China led Third World nations in opposing consideration of the subject, making an exception only in the cases of South Africa and Palestine. In fall 1990, during the debates and resolutions on occupied Kuwait, the Security Council had made another exception by agreeing to hear eyewitness testimony about **Iraqi atrocities against residents of Kuwait.**

2. Refugees

For the destitute people fleeing conflict in the Gulf, civil war and famine in the Horn of Africa, and war in Southeast Asia and elsewhere, the year marking the 40th anniversary of the **U.N. High Commissioner for Refugees (UNHCR)** was one of enormous turmoil. This anniversary year was also a time of great strain for UNHCR, whose role in the U.N. system is being redefined.

There are an estimated **16 million refugees in the world,** and perhaps an equal number of internally or externally displaced people who are not technically "refugees." Yet at a time when the U.N. political machinery was working effectively, able to confront Iraq's aggression head on, the parallel system for providing humanitarian aid was unable to respond with similar speed and coherence. UNHCR and the other aid agencies can be faulted for their performance, but much of the problem derives from the cutbacks forced on them by donor countries. UNHCR's primary mandate is to protect refugees; it also provides a channel for raising money from member governments, establishing programs in the field and monitoring their implementation by governmental and nongovernmental organizations.

Over the past 40 years UNHCR has expanded from a tiny entity into a large organization with a staff of over 1,500 and an annual budget of $550 million. Among the world's refugees, approximately 2 million are in North America, 6.2 million in Southwest Asia and the Middle East, 590,000 in Asia and Oceania, 4.8 million in Africa, and 1.2 million in Latin America. Some 3 million Palestinians live in camps that are administered by the U.N. Relief and Works Agency. At the height of the Gulf crisis, over a million Kurds made their way to Iran and 416,000 to the Iraq/Turkey border. Many millions of other people have been forced from their homes but have not crossed an international border; these are the so-called **internally displaced,** and in Africa alone the estimate goes as high as 13 million: 1.1 million in Angola, 2.5 million in Mozambique, 3.5 million in South Africa, 2–3 million in Sudan, 1 million in Ethiopia, 800,000 in Liberia, and several hundred thousand each in Somalia, Uganda, and Chad [International League for Human Rights, "Internally Displaced People Need Human Rights Protection," *In Brief* 33, 10/90].

During 1990–91, refugee problems in the **Horn of Africa** grew steadily worse. Conflict and famine in Ethiopia brought some 1.2 million people to the brink of starvation. UNHCR, which maintains over 100 staff members in the country, had to deal with the upheavals of war while attempting to get food to starving people. Armed bandits looted and burned health centers and warehouses, and at one stage, refugees crossing from Ethiopia to Sudan were bombed by Sudanese planes while a U.N. mission was in the area. In Liberia intensification of the civil war brought a refugee exodus that, until overshadowed by the Gulf crisis, was rated the fastest in recent years. By now more than 500,000 Liberians have sought asylum in neighboring Côte d'Ivoire, Guinea, Sierra Leone, and Ghana. Even as this crisis was unfolding, however, UNHCR was being forced to cut its programs by 25 percent and its staff by 15, closing 19 offices worldwide [A/45/12/Add. 1].

Repatriation is widely seen as the best solution for refugees, but plans for carrying out the process can be controversial, as in the case of the 54,500 **Vietnamese boat people** crowded in squalid Hong Kong camps. A Comprehensive Plan of Action adopted in Geneva in 1989 established a **"screening" process** throughout Southeast Asia in the hope that the majority of boat people denied refugee status would return home voluntarily. Great Britain reached an agreement with Vietnam on the **forcible repatriation** of boat people in the Crown Colony; and despite U.S. opposition, 51 of those "screened out" were sent home from Hong Kong in 1989, raising a public outcry. Of the camps' population, only 10,529 have qualified as political refugees—defined by the **1951 Geneva Convention Relating to the Status of Refugees** as someone with "a well-founded fear of being persecuted in his country of origin for reasons of race, religion, nationality, membership of a particular social group or political opinion." To date, UNHCR has assisted in the **voluntary repatriation** of 8,000 boat people, but there remains a distinct possibility of additional forcible repatriations.

At the onset of the **Gulf crisis**, UNHCR—then under the leadership of Thorvald Stoltenberg of Norway—was accused, along with the other U.N. humanitarian agencies, of being slow in aiding the hundreds of thousands of **foreign workers** who streamed out of Iraq and occupied Kuwait after the August 2, 1990, invasion. Grim television pictures of the dispossessed, many of whom had spent weeks crossing the desert on foot, coupled with warnings that their number could reach well over a million, spurred UNHCR to begin mobilizing help for the returning migrant workers, who were not technically "refugees" with a claim to international protection but, rather, evacuees.

UNHCR drew up a comprehensive plan of action for Turkey, Syria, Jordan, and Iran in anticipation of receiving 400,000 refugees from Iraq once hostilities began. By mid-March 1991 only 65,000 Iraqis had fled the country and there was talk of U.N. "overkill" in its postwar preparations. It was only after the **Shiite and Kurdish revolts** against Saddam Hussein's regime were crushed that the real dimensions of the refugee problem could be seen. In the event, more than 1.5 million Kurds fled over the mountains into Iran and to the Turkish border, while some 53,000 Shiites fled to the areas of southern Iraq then under allied military control and still others to southern Iran.

The scale and suddenness of the flight of frightened Kurds from northern Iraq posed an acute logistical problem for UNHCR, which was complicated by Turkey's adamant refusal to grant the Kurds asylum on its own side of the border. Living in misery and squalor on mountain slopes, Kurdish refugees were dying from exposure at the rate of 1,000 a day. There was a public outcry in the West, and Great Britain proposed the establishment of **safe havens for the Kurds within Iraq** as a means of encouraging them to come down from the mountains and return home. The United States, Britain, France, and the Netherlands plunged into uncharted diplomatic waters by sending in military forces to provide emergency aid, build camps, and provide security for the flood of returning refugees. This U.S.–led humanitarian relief mission, called **Operation Provide Comfort**, began encouraging the refugees to return to the "safe havens" in Iraq, and it prompted the new High Commissioner, Sodako Ogata, to warn on May 3, 1991, that her organization was unable to guarantee the safety of Kurds who ventured back into northern Iraq. "I trust that all precautions are being taken to ensure that no forcible relocation takes place and no undue pressure is exerted on the refugees," she said, making clear her unease at the U.S. policy of immediate repatriation and Turkish reluctance to admit the Kurds as refugees [Reuters, 5/3/91].

This highly publicized refugee crisis made obvious the **limitations of international humanitarian law** in dealing with those caught up in war. Refugee status does not automatically apply to those who have run away from the threat of war or insurrection or from war's cataclysmic aftermath—which, in the case of the Gulf, included burning oil wells as well as sudden unemployment and lack of basic necessities or expulsion. There was a breakthrough, of sorts, on May 18, when a memorandum of understanding was negotiated with the Iraqi government [S/2663, 5/31/91] granting the United Nations unrestricted access to the border regions and inviting it to set up suboffices and Humanitarian Centres (UNHUCs). The landmark agreement gave UNHCR and other U.N. agencies the authority they needed to conduct operations inside Iraq.

Some four months after the invasion of Kuwait, High Commissioner Stoltenberg had resigned suddenly from his post to take up duties as Foreign Minister of Norway. There was an immediate scramble to name a replacement to a post that has become a highly sensitive one. Many of UNHCR's major donors believe that the refugee agency has fulfilled its primary role, that of aiding refugees from communism, and they now want a reluctant UNHCR to help stem the flood of migrants from formerly communist countries and elsewhere. U.N. Secretary-General Javier Pérez de Cuéllar offered the job to his Chef de Cabinet, Virendra Dayal, and was immediately accused of "cronyism" by Washington [*The New York Times*, 11/12/90]. Dayal, an Indian national, withdrawing his name from consideration, accused the donor countries of racism in trying to deny him the post.

At the same time, John R. Bolton, the U.S. Assistant Secretary of State for International Organization Affairs, circulated an extraordinarily candid document aimed at ensuring that the donor countries "get control" of the selection process and setting out the criteria by which the next High Commissioner should be judged. Bolton stated that there should be close consultation between the Secretary-General and key donor and asylum countries; that Douglas Stafford, an American, should be retained as Deputy High Commissioner; and that a senior U.S. official should "interview" the various declared candidates for the job. Washington's approach to the process angered the Secretary-General, who eventually proposed—and succeeded in appointing—**Sadako Ogata** of Japan as the new High Commissioner, the first woman to lead the agency. A professor of international relations at Sophia University in Tokyo, Mrs. Ogata had written a report for the United Nations on the human rights situation in Burma, had served in the late 1970s as Chairman of UNICEF's Executive Board, and was the first Japanese woman to hold the rank of ambassador at the United Nations, serving there from 1978 to 1979. Ogata, 63, was appointed by the General Assembly for a three-year term, effective February 1, 1991.

The new Commissioner was immediately confronted with the problems of **Kurdish and Shiite refugees.** Turning to the refugee problem in the south of Iraq, she persuaded Saudi Arabia to accept an estimated 53,000 Shiite refugees living under allied military control. Iran also agreed to accept Shiites with family links in the country, averting a possible human tragedy after the U.S. military pulled its forces from the area and the U.N. Iraq-Kuwait Observer Mission took up its post in the narrow demilitarized zone.

UNHCR remains in the throes of an **institutional crisis** brought about by the upsurge of refugee movements in the 1980s and a series of dramatic events that were touched off by the donor governments' insistence on major cuts in program and staff. In October 1989 then High Commissioner Jean Pierre Hocké resigned in a cloud of scandal that ended UNHCR's unique relationship with the United Nations—a relationship that has enabled all previous High Commissioners to keep one foot inside the U.N. system and one foot outside it [Lawyers Committee for Human Rights, "The UNHCR at 40: Refugee Protection at the Crossroads," 2/91].

Thorvald Stoltenberg used his management skills to implement the cuts demanded by donor countries, but he stimulated controversy within UNHCR by promoting the view that the agency can hope to protect "genuine refugees" only if it also takes up the cause of **all uprooted people,** whether or not they come under the 1951 Convention on Refugees. Speaking to the Executive Committee (EXCOM) on October 1, 1990, he said: "It is, in my view, increasingly evident that the issues of refugees and migration at large is bound to be one of the threats to the broad concept of international, regional and national security in the decade ahead of us." EXCOM, the agency's advisory body, is composed of 44 governments—including donor, asylum, and refugee-exporting countries—some of which have not ratified the Convention. Insisting that there was a clear human need, Stoltenberg overruled dissenters in UNHCR to offer services to all those displaced by the Gulf crisis.

Responding to the rising chorus of complaints from Europe about economic migrants who were abusing asylum procedures, Stoltenberg told EXCOM that UNHCR would also work to prevent future flows and would be attentive to "early warning" signs to help stave off emergencies. "What is needed," he said in summation, "is a clear policy of asylum for refugees and a firm commitment to development aid for the impoverished world" [ibid.].

Stoltenberg had begun to attract praise for his work as High Commissioner when he resigned the post to return to politics. In one of his final addresses to EXCOM, he spoke bitterly of the agency's unstable and unpredictable **fund-raising mechanisms.** "Living almost on a month-to-month, sometimes week-to-week basis is not only uneconomic—and may I say not very dignified—but it also makes UNHCR a much less responsive and effective organization," he stated. High Commissioner Ogata has had to deal with the legacy of poor funding at a time when the demands on the agency are growing.

3. Health

The U.N. health-giving community, led by the World Health Organization (WHO), is looking ahead to new programs that build on past successes and benefit from new technologies. At the same time, its zero-growth budgets strain to meet present commitments and to avert catastrophe in fast-developing emergency situations. The spread of acquired immune-deficiency syndrome (AIDS) into new sectors of the population, war in the Gulf, a natural disaster in Bangladesh, and an epidemic in Latin America are just a few of the situations that are commanding attention at present.

In May 1990 the **World Health Assembly,** WHO's governing body, held a "special session" within its regular annual session to consider the means of bringing health issues to the forefront of the world economic debate, in recognition of the role of health in optimizing human resources and social benefits across generations [press release WHO/6, 5/9/90]. In the course of this annual session, the Assembly agreed that WHO would add yet another goal to its special program agenda: the elimination of **iodine deficiency disorders.** The ease of preventing these disorders—which threaten an estimated 1 billion people and are the cause of mental retardation, still births, and infant deaths—and the progress already achieved in individual countries promised an easy victory by the year 2000 [*WHO Features*, 6/90].

WHO has looked forward to putting its expertise to work in the newly democratizing countries of **Central and Eastern Europe,** and in

August 1990 it held an informal consultation with UNDP representatives and World Bank officials to discuss the establishment of a special task force that would recommend ways to assist the region in financing and reforming **national health care systems.** Ministerial delegations from Bulgaria, the Czech and Slovak Federal Republic, Hungary, Poland, and Romania were in attendance [press release WHO/39, 8/3/90].

Early in the new year came confirmation of a victory that WHO and UNICEF, the major forces in the **Expanded Programme on Immunization (EPI),** had confidently predicted for months: By the end of 1990, 80 percent of the developing world's children were being immunized against six "killer diseases" [The InterDependent 17, no. 2, 1991]. The special targets of EPI have been measles, diphtheria, tuberculosis, polio, tetanus, and whooping cough.

Progress is also being made in the fight against diarrheal and acute respiratory diseases, aided by the establishment of national diarrheal disease-control programs in 100 developing countries and respiratory infection-control programs in 50. WHO estimates that in 1988, the deaths of 1.1 million children under the age of five were averted through the use of oral rehydration salts, whose development owes much to the organization. For the rest of the decade, WHO advises that it will continue to educate the populations of developing countries about the dangers of these common diseases, train health care personnel, and provide access to appropriate treatment, calling this a "formidable" task [WHO Press, 9/90]. Progress on yet another front—the eradication of screw-worm, a larval disease carried by flies that can be deadly to both humans and animals—has also been noted. The eradication process has few precedents: Sterile flies are dropped from aircraft and mate with fertile flies to produce an ever-larger population of infertile flies [U.N. press release FAO/3512, 4/11/91].

The U.N. family of development agencies was involved in the special programs of the **International Drinking Water Supply and Sanitation Decade, 1981–90.** A General Assembly resolution, characterizing the decade as a success, urged member governments to give priority to water supply and sanitation in bilateral aid projects and to provide the sort of financial and technical aid that will help developing countries stretch their resources in making further efforts in this area [A/Res/45/181]. Indications of a resurgence of **cholera in Latin America** came not many weeks later, and in April, WHO organized a global task force to counter the spread of the disease within the hemisphere, and beyond [The Financial Times, 4/26/91].

The prevention and control of **AIDS** continues to occupy a high place on the General Assembly's health agenda. Responding to the 44th

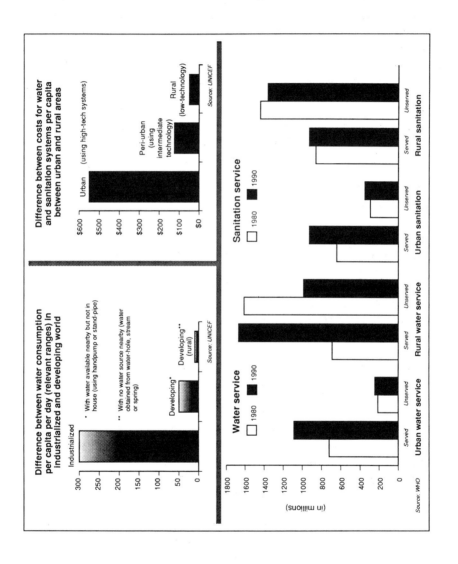

Difference between water consumption per capita per day (relevant ranges) in industrialized and developing world

Industrialized

* With water available nearby but not in house (using handpump or stand-pipe)

** With no water source nearby (water obtained from water-hole, stream or spring)

Developing*

Developing** (rural)

Source: UNICEF

300
250
200
150
100
50
0

Difference between costs for water and sanitation systems per capita between urban and rural areas

Urban (using high-tech systems)

Peri-urban (using intermediate technology)

Rural (low-technology)

$600
$500
$400
$300
$200
$100
$0

Source: UNICEF

Water service

☐ 1980 ■ 1990

Served Unserved Served Unserved
Urban water service   Rural water service

Sanitation service

☐ 1980 ■ 1990

Served Unserved Served Unserved
Urban sanitation   Rural sanitation

(in millions)

1800
1600
1400
1200
1000
800
600
400
200
0

Source: WHO

Assembly's request for a global AIDS strategy, the Director-General of WHO outlined the activities undertaken by the organization—many in tandem with U.N. development agencies—to help establish national AIDS programs, secure their financing, and disseminate information on preventing and treating the disease [A/45/256, E/1990/58]. The 45th General Assembly called upon the U.N. Secretary-General, the Director-General of WHO, the administrator of UNDP, and the heads of the World Bank, the U.N. Population Fund, UNICEF, and all other relevant U.N. organizations to intensify their efforts to combat the spread of AIDS, and urged member states to do so as well. The Secretary-General was requested to help the information process along by making the very best use of existing U.N. public information systems [A/Res/45/187].

WHO courts the public's attention on **World AIDS Day** each December. The third such observance, in 1990, took as its theme "Women and AIDS," with the aim of raising awareness that more and more women are being infected with the human immunodeficiency virus (HIV), a precursor to AIDS. WHO estimates there are 3 million HIV-infected women to date and predicts that by the year 2000 the number of new AIDS cases reported annually will show an even division between men and women [*United Nations Focus*, 2/91].

Under the leadership of Dr. Michael H. Merson, Director of WHO's **Global Programme on AIDS (GPA)** since March 1990, WHO continues to monitor the AIDS situation throughout the world, focusing in 1990–91 on the rapid spread of the disease among women and children. WHO estimates that 500,000 children five years of age or younger are now suffering from AIDS itself, 90 percent of them in sub-Saharan Africa where the childhood mortality rate may rise as much as 50 percent. Among adults, WHO estimates the worldwide AIDS population at more than 1 million [press release WHO/UN 37, 5/2/91].

In most countries of the world, HIV infection is more and more apt to be spread by the heterosexual population and by mothers to offspring during pregnancy, birth, and infancy. The number of HIV-positive adults is estimated at 8 to 10 million and the number of HIV-infected infants at 1 million, with indications that the total could surpass 10 million by the decade's end [ibid.]. The increase in pediatric AIDS, notes WHO Director-General Hiroshi Nakajima, threatens the progress achieved through the world organization's child survival programs. The new figures on women and AIDS threaten yet another goal of U.N. programs: that of halving the maternal mortality rate by the year 2000 [UNICEF, *The State of the World's Children*, 1991].

With the cessation of hostilities in the Gulf, Dr. Nakajima and

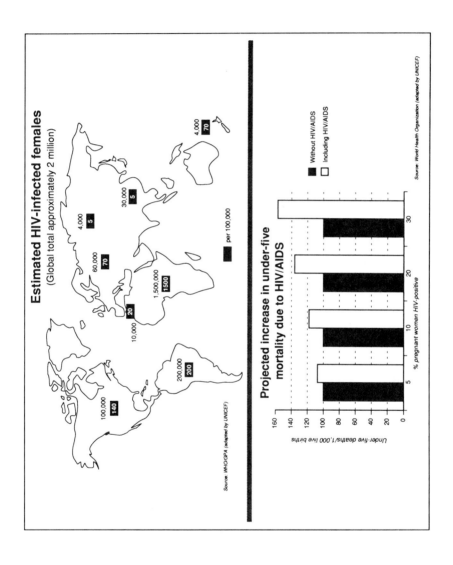

Estimated HIV-infected females
(Global total approximately 2 million)

4,000 · 70

30,000 · 5

4,000 · 5

60,000 · 70

1,500,000 · 1500

10,000 · 20

200,000 · 200

100,000 · 140

per 100,000

Source: WHO/GPA (adapted by UNICEF)

Projected increase in under-five mortality due to HIV/AIDS

■ Without HIV/AIDS
□ Including HIV/AIDS

Under-five deaths/1,000 live births

160 140 120 100 80 60 40 20 0

% pregnant women HIV-positive

5 10 20 30

Source: World Health Organization (adapted by UNICEF)

UNICEF's Executive Director, James Grant, dispatched a seven-member WHO/UNICEF **humanitarian mission to war-torn Iraq.** The five-day mission—launched at the request of Secretary-General Javier Pérez de Cuéllar and consisting of agency officials and public health and nutrition experts—entered Iraq on February 16 to deliver emergency medical supplies to children and mothers and to assess the country's essential health care needs [press release WHO/UN 11, 2/14/91].

A month later, Dr. Nakajima himself visited Iran's Khuzestan province and took samples of the black rain that resulted from the burning of Kuwait's oil wells. He expressed concern that such pollution, and the solid and chemical wastes now pouring into the region's lakes, rivers, and seas as a result of the destruction of sanitation and water-treatment facilities, would "further damage the already fragile ecosystem, with serious consequences for health" [press release WHO/20, 3/19/91]. Burns, diarrhea, and the lack of adequate water, sanitation, and health care facilities became immediate concerns as vast numbers of Iraqis made their way to the south of Iran. Water purification and sanitation equipment, medicines and hospital supplies, including ambulances, were rapidly deployed by WHO and just as rapidly depleted [press release WHO/21, 3/19/91]. Western officials estimated that over a million refugees had entered Iran by early May [*The New York Times*, 5/5/91].

On the World Health Assembly's agenda for its annual session in May 1991 was a resolution calling for an international program to investigate the health effects of the **Chernobyl nuclear accident** and the establishment of an international radiation research and treatment center in the Soviet Union [press release WHO/6, 1/25/91]. Also considered was a **proposed program budget of $763,760,000** for 1992–93, representing a zero rate of growth in real dollar terms for the fifth consecutive biennium.

4. Drug Abuse, Production, and Trafficking

Trafficking and consumption of illegal narcotic drugs have assumed global proportions, and virtually no nation is immune. At the start of 1990, this $500-billion-a-year business was being fought in the United Nations by three drug units and two supervisory bodies, armed with a mere $7.4 million in regular-budget funds [E/1991/42/Add.1]. The voluntary contributions of a dozen or so nations totaled an additional $69.3 million [U.N. press release SOC/NAR/574, 4/24/91]. By the close of 1990 there was no better news on budgetary fronts, but there had been three developments that enhanced the prospects for international drug control: the entry into force of the comprehensive 1988 **Convention against Illicit Traffic in Narcotic Drugs and Psychotropic Substances;** agreement by governments at the **General Assembly's Special Session on Drugs** in February 1990 to a **Global Programme of Action** that links demand-reduction in consuming countries with fostering economic development in producing countries; and the unification of three drug units into a new **United Nations International Drug Control Programme (UNDCP)** with an Under-Secretary-General as its full-time head.

The **International Narcotics Control Board (INCB)**—a body of experts that monitors legal drug production and the movements from source to consumer in order to trace illegal diversions—will retain its independent status. It will decidedly have a role in implementing the 1988 convention's provision for the control of substances frequently used in the manufacture of illicit narcotic drugs or psychotropic substances (the so-called precursor chemicals). This long-anticipated convention also obliges adhering states to provide legal assistance to a state that is investigating the laundering of drug profits, obliges a state harboring an accused trafficker to extradite him to the country that has made the indictment or to prosecute him in its own courts, and establishes jurisdiction in interdiction cases involving vessels flying a foreign flag. Meeting for its 48th session, October 8–25, 1990, the INCB considered the means of improving compliance with all such international drug-control treaties and used the occasion to state "emphatically" that it rejects the suggestion that drugs, such as marijuana, be legalized; this, it said, would "lead to an explosion in abuse-related deaths and health care costs" [E/INCB/1990/1].

The drug units that the General Assembly agreed to integrate in the name of efficiency, "co-ordination, complementarity and non-duplication of activities across the United Nations system" [A/Res/45/179] are the **secretariat of the INCB,** the **Division of Narcotic Drugs,** and the **U.N. Fund for Drug Abuse Control,** which provides the United Nations with the extrabudgetary resources needed to implement special technical assistance programs in the field. Each of the three has had its own structure and lines of authority. The Special Session on Drugs in February 1990 had called for a study of ways to enhance the efficiency and stature of U.N. drug activities, and the Secretary-General met this call by appointing a group of experts from 15 countries, each serving in his own capacity. Under its chairman, Jorge Montaño, Mexico's Permanent Representative to the United Nations, the group made recommendations, reported in July 1990 [A/45/652/Add.1], which formed the basis of the restructuring proposal that the Assembly adopted at its regular session in 1990. Giorgio Giacomelli, previously Commissioner-General of

UNRWA, has been named to head the integrated Drug Control Programme, to be based in Vienna.

Concurrently, the General Assembly asked ECOSOC's **Commission on Narcotic Drugs (CND)**—the main policy-making organ for international drug control—to consider at its 34th session "ways and means of improving" its own functioning and to pass such recommendations along to ECOSOC for consideration in 1991 [A/Res/45/179]. At its April 29–May 9, 1991, session, CND recommended that its membership be increased to 50 and designated a regional distribution of the ten new seats [U.N. press release SOC/NAR 586, 5/7/91]. Sitting on the commission, by tradition, are states with a particular interest in drug control, either because drug substances are produced, refined, or manufactured within their borders or because the country suffers the effects of drug abuse or trafficking. Other self-improvements recommended by CND are the scheduling of regular sessions and the creation of a subsidiary body to take up technical issues before or during these regular sessions, allowing the commission to begin focusing on priority themes [U.N. press release SOC/NAR/589, 5/9/91].

Guiding U.N. efforts in the drug field is the **Comprehensive Multidisciplinary Outline of Future Activities in Drug Abuse Control,** which emerged from 1987's **International Conference on Drug Abuse and Illicit Trafficking;** the **Global Programme of Action** of February's Special Session on Drugs; and the Declaration of the **World Ministerial Summit to Reduce the Demand for Drugs and to Combat the Cocaine Threat,** held in London in April 1990. The last of these recommended that particular efforts be made to prevent and reduce demand at the community and neighborhood levels, and at the level of the individual family. The governments represented also pledged an increase in technical cooperation, bilaterally or through the United Nations, to assist developing countries in devising and implementing demand-reduction programs [U.N. press release SOC/NAR/557, 4/17/90]. Late in 1989 the 44th General Assembly [A/Res/44/141] requested the Secretary-General to "coordinate at the inter-agency level the development of a **United Nations system-wide action plan** aimed at the full implementation of all existing drug abuse control mandates" [A/44/536]. That plan, endorsed by the Economic and Social Council in July 1990, "indicates what each part of the system . . . is doing in response to mandates given by Member States through various intergovernmental bodies; the funds available to them for that purpose; what they have been asked to do, but are unable to do for lack of resources; and an estimate of the resource gap to be filled if the United Nations is to fulfil all its existing mandates" [A/45/542]. Called a "vital new instrument," it is intended to help avoid duplication and enhance coordination within the U.N. system [ibid.]. The plan will be updated annually and reviewed by the General Assembly.

An ECOSOC resolution, drafted at its spring 1991 session, gives the CND responsibility for reviewing the progress of the Global Programme and of the United Nations system-wide plan. CND would also be directed to provide policy guidance to the newly integrated Drug Control Programme in Vienna and to monitor its activities [U.N. press release SOC/NAR/ 585, 5/7/91].

A proposal for an **international court to try drug traffickers**—the first tribunal in which global authorities would be able to hold individuals responsible for violations of international law—was referred to the International Law Commission (ILC) by the 44th General Assembly [A/Res/44/ 39]. The notion of such a tribunal raises questions not only of national sovereignty but of an exceedingly practical nature as well: What nation would have custody of the defendant until the end of the proceeding and who would get custody after conviction; where would the trial be held; and, ultimately, who would pay for any of these functions? Some have argued that a court for narcotics crimes should have a role limited to determining which nation's courts take the case—and to serving as a court of appeals after the trial [*Breaking the Drug Chain*, by Jeffrey Laurenti (New York: United Nations Association of the USA, 1990)]. As the 46th General Assembly approached, the ILC was discussing a proposal for a broader international criminal court, envisioning its use in terrorism cases and in cases involving environmental damage across national borders. The Sixth (Legal) Committee will be considering the ILC's report, with the hope—if not the expectation—of reaching agreement on a resolution to submit to the General Assembly in 1991 [interviews with *A Global Agenda: Issues Before the 46th General Assembly of the United Nations*].

Joining the network of **heads of regional drug law-enforcement agencies (HONLEAs)** is a newly established HONLEA for Europe, which held its first meeting in Moscow in November 1990 [A/Res/45/149]. These subsidiary bodies of the CND are recommending measures to counter the traffic in illicit drugs. These efforts too, participants say, will take more money than is available at present [Division of Narcotic Drugs, *Information Letter*, 1/91].

5. Crime

Cuba served as host for the **Eighth Congress on the Prevention of Crime and the Treatment of Offenders,** which met in Havana from

August 27 to September 7, 1990. These "crime congresses," organized by the United Nations every five years since 1955, have taken the lead in formulating and implementing many of the U.N. declarations and agreements that offer standards, norms, and codes to guide legislators, law enforcers, and judiciaries throughout the world. In 1990 the theme was "International Cooperation for Crime Prevention and Criminal Justice for the 21st Century." This lofty goal was given concrete form in 46 instruments and sets of guidelines—many emphasizing practical measures to improve law enforcement and information-gathering—that were approved as resolutions by the government representatives in attendance. The very number of resolutions—more than all previous congresses combined—prompted comment. Speaking in the General Assembly's Third (Social, Humanitarian, and Cultural) Committee during the 45th Session, the Italian delegate remarked that "the exceptionally high number of resolutions adopted in Havana showed the success of the congress and the weakness of the [U.N. Crime Prevention and Criminal Justice] programme," which lacks adequate funds and resolve to carry out such a broad mandate [A/C.3/45/SR.24, para. 48]. Secretary-General Pérez de Cuéllar's report on the congress took up a similar cry, noting the "futility of piecemeal measures" and stressing the need to develop a coherent strategy for combating the increasingly sophisticated forms of international crime [A/45/629]. He also spoke of the "chasm that still exists between declared precepts and even widely accepted United Nations norms and the actual practice," echoing an earlier report of the Vienna-based Committee on Crime Prevention and Control (CCPC) that addressed the "gap between mandates and resources" in the United Nations' burgeoning criminal justice program [E/1990/31].

The crime congress, noting the CCPC report's addendum devoted to "The Need for the Creation of an Effective International Crime and Justice Programme" [E/1990/31/Add. 1], had recommended that the General Assembly establish an intergovernmental working group to elaborate proposals for an effective crime prevention and criminal justice program and to suggest how that program could be implemented. The General Assembly accepted the recommendation [A/Res/45/108], and a 29-member Working Group, chosen along geographical lines [A/45/973 and Add.1], will meet in Vienna between August 5 and 9, 1991. Its proposals will be reported to a ministerial summit scheduled for Paris in November before being transmitted to the General Assembly for consideration and action late in the 46th Session.

A spokesman at the U.S. Mission to the United Nations reiterated the Bush administration's policy of "zero real growth" in the U.N.

budget [interview with *A Global Agenda: Issues Before the 46th General Assembly of the United Nations*] and, referring to the intergovernmental Working Group, expressed concern that so much consultation was being crammed into so little time. The United States did not send a delegation to the congress in Cuba (calling it a country that "flouts" international norms in such areas as human rights [*Issues Before the 45th General Assembly of the United Nations*]) but is a member and full participant in the Working Group.

One resolution recommended by the congress and passed by the 45th General Assembly dealt uniquely with crime in the context of development [A/Res/45/107 and Annex]. Building on the principles and objectives of the Seventh Congress's Milan Plan of Action (1985) [E/86/IV.1] and the Sixth Congress's Caracas Declaration (1980) [35/171], the resolution recommends international cooperation in crime prevention and, in an annex, outlines cooperative efforts to bolster the morale and fortify the economies of developing countries, the better to resist criminal activity within and beyond their borders. It goes on to advocate a "systematic approach to crime prevention planning . . . to provide for the incorporation of crime prevention policies into national development planning."

Reaffirming resolutions it had approved on the recommendation of past crime congresses, the Assembly went on to approve four sets of rules and guidelines recommended by the delegates at Havana: the "Tokyo Rules" on noncustodial measures of punishment and rehabilitation [A/Res/45/110]; on the treatment of offenders [A/Res/45/111]; the "Riyadh Guidelines" on the prevention of juvenile delinquency [A/Res/45/112]; and the United Nations Rules for the Protection of Juveniles Deprived of Their Liberty [A/Res/45/113]. An annex to each supplies the rules and guidelines themselves, and member states are requested to inform the Secretary-General of progress in implementing these at home.

The General Assembly also approved by consensus two new model treaties and two new model agreements intended to strengthen bilateral and multilateral cooperation between and among member states. The models—on Extradiction [A/Res/45/116], Mutual Assistance in Criminal Proceedings [A/Res/45/117], Transfer of Criminal Proceedings [A/Res/45/118], and Transfer of Offenders Conditionally Sentenced or Conditionally Released [A/Res/45/119]—are supplied in an annex.

Practical measures to improve law enforcement and information-gathering were a leitmotiv of the congress, and the General Assembly responded by approving a recommended resolution on the computerization of criminal justice systems [A/Res/45/109]. It requested the Secretary-General to investigate sources of funding from the governmental, non-governmental, and private sectors to aid this effort and to ensure the long-term viability of the new Global Crime and Criminal Justice Information Network—one of the mechanisms mandated in Resolution 107, which linked crime prevention with development. Resolution 109 also calls for the establishment of an international group of experts to assess national experiences with computerization, to monitor the exchange of know-how, and to inform member states of the funds available for this purpose from various sources. The United Nations' proposed medium-term plan for the Crime Prevention and Criminal Justice Programme 1992–97, recognizing that "the application of computer technology . . . can help to streamline procedures and increase the system's capacity to deal with new and sophisticated forms of crime," also speaks of the need to enhance data collection and exchange in crime prevention and draws attention to the Fourth World Crime Survey, to be launched in 1992 [A/45/6 (Prog. 29)].

As part of this urgent effort to improve international cooperation in crime prevention and control, the General Assembly issued a call for greater collaboration between member states and between criminal justice agencies and educational authorities; it also suggested the possibility of including information supplied by national correspondents in the U.N. Criminal Justice Information Network, with the aim of increasing the flow of information to the criminal justice community [A/Res/45/122]. The process of strengthening cooperation among the criminal justice systems of member states will continue at the U.N.–sponsored **International Seminar on Organized Crime Control,** to be convened in Moscow in October 1991. Calling attention to this event, the 45th General Assembly requested the CCPC to take a look at organized crime and its prevention through cooperative activities and report its finding to the CCPC's own 12th session in early 1992 [A/Res/45/123].

In the Assembly resolution entitled "Eighth United Nations Congress on the Prevention of Crime and the Treatment of Offenders," the Secretary-General is requested to review the resources available to the CCPC, which must now act on the broad agenda set by the crime congress [A/Res/45/121]. He is also requested to consider including in the proposed program budget for the 1992–93 biennium "resource proposals . . . to assist with the long-term solution of the problems posed by the implementation of existing mandates." Sides began to form when the subject of funding was discussed in the Third Committee: On one side was the British delegate, who advised "tailor[ing] the programme to the existing resources"; on the other was the Costa Rican delegate, who warned that the Eighth Congress would be "a mere exercise in rhetoric" unless the U.N. Secretariat was "provided with the resources which were indispensable for the accomplishment of the mandates adopted by consensus" [A/C.3/45/SR.27, para. 30, 47]. The resource issue, at the heart of all plans and hopes for the U.N. Crime Prevention and Criminal Justice program, will be at the top of the agenda for the intergovernmental Working Group and Paris ministerial summit in the fall and winter of 1991.

Decisions taken at these meetings will determine the items considered by the 46th General Assembly under the rubric "Crime Prevention and Criminal Justice." When the CCPC gathers for its 12th session, it will examine the implications of those priority and funding decisions for the United Nations' newly expanded crime prevention and control agenda and will report its findings to ECOSOC at the first regular session of 1992.

6. The Status of Women

In the winter preceding the 45th General Assembly, **ECOSOC's Commission on the Status of Women** held a prolonged 34th session to take stock of the progress made in carrying out the Forward-Looking Strategies for the Advancement of Women to the Year 2000—the declaration of the world conference in Nairobi that capped the U.N. Decade of Women 1975–85 and shortly became the official U.N. guide for national and international action in this sphere [A/Res/40/108]. Reviewing the record of five years, the Commission noted generally "slow progress" in implementing the Strategies [E/CN.6/1990/14], and the 45th Assembly went on to "reaffirm" the Commission's conclusion "that the pace of implementation of the Strategies must be improved in the crucial last decade of the twentieth century since the cost to societies of failing to implement the Forward-Looking Strategies would be high in terms of slowed economic and social development, misuse of human resources and reduced progress for society as a whole" [A/Res/45/129]. The Secretary-General will be reporting to the 46th Assembly on further developments in this area.

On the agenda of the Commission's 35th session, February 27 through March 8, 1991, were measures to bolster the Strategies' three interrelated goals or "priority themes"—equality, development, and peace—with a focus on particular subthemes under each category. When the Commission gathered in Vienna, the Gulf war was at its height, lending special immediacy to the subthemes chosen for the members' attention: vulnerable women, with a focus on the young, the old, the disabled, and migrants (equality); national, regional, and international mechanisms for integrating women in the economic and political policy-making process (development); and refugees and displaced women and their children (peace). Among the seven draft resolutions the Commission recommended for consideration at ECOSOC's spring session, one called upon the international community to extend legal and physical protection to refugees and displaced women (80 percent of the world's 15 million refugees) and to ensure their full integration into assistance programs [E/CN.6/1991/L.11/Rev.1]; and another noted the urgency of establishing the international, regional, and national machinery that allows women a direct role in shaping the policies that affect their lives, with technical assistance to be provided when necessary [E/CN.6/1991/L.10/Rev.1; U.N. press release WOM/611, 3/8/91]. A third resolution urged member states to adopt, strengthen, and enforce legislation prohibiting violence against women, and called upon the Council to recommend that a framework be developed—in consultation with CEDAW—for an international legal instrument that would explicitly address violence against women [E/CN.6/1991/L.11/Rev.1; U.N. press release WOM/607, 3/8/91]. The Division for the Advancement of Women is planning to convene a meeting of experts in November 1991 to explore the possibilities of preparing such an instrument.

To ensure equal status and legal rights for women migrants, the Commission adopted a resolution inviting member states to sign and ratify the International Convention on the Protection of the Rights of All Migrant Workers and Members of Their Families, which was adopted by the General Assembly and opened for signature on December 18, 1990 [E/CN.6/1991/L.18/Rev.1; A/Res/45/158, 12/18/90].

Education—whether on the subject of women's rights or in the form of schooling for women themselves—remains an important ingredient of the United Nations' approach to enhancing the status of women. With the pronouncement of "slow progress" in implementing the Strategies, ECOSOC called upon the U.N. **Department of Public Information (DPI)** to launch a "world education campaign" aimed at increasing awareness of the obstacles to de facto equality in education, employment, and health. Since no additional funds have been earmarked for the campaign, DPI has had to make do with existing resources, focusing its activities related to the status of women on this single area. Describing the communications issue as "complex," the 35th session of the Commission on the Status of Women decided to defer discussion of a draft resolution on this subject until its 36th session, in 1992 [U.N. press release WOM/611, 3/8/91]. For its part, the 45th General Assembly had called upon member states to "work towards the elimination of illiteracy of women of all ages," requested the Secretary-General to examine "the relationship between the literacy of women and their economic and social advancement" when preparing the next quadrennial update of the *World Survey on the Role of Women in Development* in 1994, and commended the efforts of International Literacy Year 1990 in this area [A/Res/45/126].

Women's crucial role in breaking the cycle of undereducation and poverty was recognized by the heads of state who gathered in September 1990 for the **World Summit for Children.** The plan of action they approved calls for national policies that would not only provide girls with equal access to education but also reduce by half in a single decade the number of adult illiterates, two-thirds of whom are women [A/Res/45/ 625 Annex]. The 45th General Assembly seconded the motion and directed the Secretary-General to report to the 47th Assembly on the progress made in implementing these and other features of the World Summit's action plan [A/Res/45/217].

During the **International Year of the Family, 1994,** some of the spotlight will fall on the status of women in the home and, inevitably, on domestic violence—a matter of concern to U.N. bodies that deal with human rights; to bodies that deal with crime-prevention policies; to the Commission on the Status of Women, which offered a recommendation on the subject following its five-year review of the Strategies; and to the General Assembly, which in 1991 requested the Secretary-General to convene a working group of experts "to formulate guidelines or a manual for practitioners concerning the problem of domestic violence," to be considered at the **Ninth U.N. Crime Congress in 1995** [A/Res/45/114]. Discussion of women's (and girls') status in the home will also raise such issues as the distribution of responsibility for child-rearing and other household duties. (One nongovernmental organization representative at the 35th Commission noted that the word "father" was not taken up at the World Summit for Children—save for the British Prime Minister's charge that Summit participants had reduced the male role in the family to that of breadwinner, if they mentioned the male role at all [U.N. press release WOM/597, 3/1/91].)

The 35th Commission called for stronger efforts by parties to the Convention on the Elimination of All Forms of Discrimination Against Women [A/Res/35/3] to implement the convention's provisions [E/CN.6/1991/ L.8]. (During the nine months preceding the Commission session, the number of ratifiers increased marginally, from 102 to 104.) After considering a report that "[highlighted] the double discrimination faced by African women on the basis of both race and gender" but also "[indicated] considerable changes relating to the elimination of *apartheid*" in the previous year, the Commission for the first time recommended that

220 • *A Global Agenda: Issues Before the 46th General Assembly*

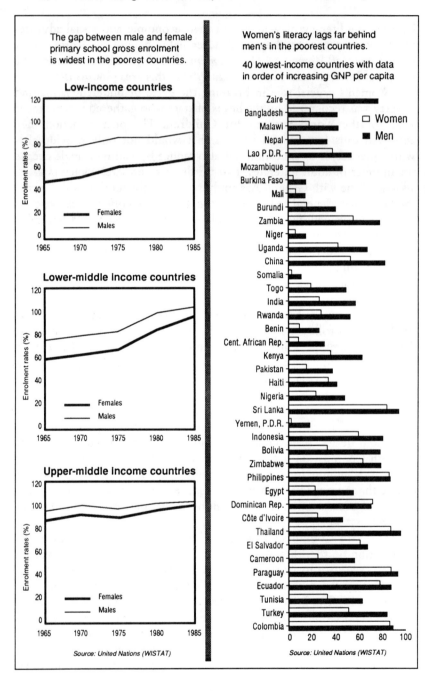

The gap between male and female primary school gross enrolment is widest in the poorest countries.

Women's literacy lags far behind men's in the poorest countries.

40 lowest-income countries with data in order of increasing GNP per capita

Source: United Nations (WISTAT)

ECOSOC urge South Africa to sign and ratify the convention—a step up from that country's pariah status. The United States was the sole dissenter in a vote on this proposal; its representative stated that the proposal was not consistent with the omnibus resolution of the 45th General Assembly acknowledging the progress made in dismantling the system of apartheid and that this would send conflicting signals to the Pretoria government, possibly discouraging further progress [U.N. press release WOM/611, 3/8/91].

The Commission again noted its concern for **women with AIDS** and their families. It continued to make plans for the **1995 World Conference on Women**—a suggestion of the 44th General Assembly [A/Res/44/77]—and assigned its formal title: "The Fourth World Conference on Women: Action for Equality, Development and Peace" [U.N. press release WOM/611, 3/8/91]. Austria and China had volunteered to host the conference, and the 45th Assembly directed the Commission to announce its choice by the group's 36th session in 1992 [A/Res/45/129].

The 44th General Assembly had endorsed the convening of an interregional consultation on women in public life, and the 45th "invited" governments to provide "extrabudgetary resources to facilitate preparations for the consultation" [A/Res/45/127]. In preparation for the consultation—scheduled for September 10–12, 1991, in Vienna—a meeting of a group of experts convened in Vienna from May 21 to 24 to explore the reasons for the low rate of participation by women in politics and decision-making at both national and international levels, to examine issues that could encourage women to become more active in public affairs, and to consider the desirability of a convention on Women in Public Life [U.N. press release WOM/594, 2/22/91; WOM/614, 5/1/91]. Days after the expert meeting, the September consultation was canceled due to a lack of funds to cover conference service costs and the travel costs of participants from developing countries.

The "potential experience of double discrimination" was explored at the first U.N. **Seminar on Women and Disability**, held in Vienna between August 20 and 24, 1990 [*Women 2000*, no. 1, 1991]. Such issues as reduced access to rehabilitation and education, social isolation, discrimination in employment, and vulnerability to violence were among the agenda items for the score of experts (all of them women and most of them disabled) brought together on this occasion. The experts made 77 recommendations, which were considered at the 35th session of the Commission on the Status of Women when attention turned to the theme of "equality." Under the terms of the Commission's draft resolution on disabled women, ECOSOC would request its ad hoc open-ended working group (established to elaborate standard rules on the equalization of opportunities for disabled children, youth, and adults [E/1990/26]) to pay attention to the particular needs of disabled women [U.N. press release WOM/607, 3/8/91].

The **U.N. International Research and Training Institute for the Advancement of Women (INSTRAW)**—the world body's center of specialized research, training, and information for and about women—joined with the International Fund for Agricultural Development and the Mediterranean Institute of Management to offer rural financial institutions a two-week training seminar on "How to Improve Banking for Rural Women" [*INSTRAW News* 15, Winter 1990]. The November 1990 workshop, held in Cyprus, recognized that credit programs have made it possible for women to make a greater contribution not only to the family's economic welfare but to national development as well. The host government presented an overview of its own banking systems and procedures, and INSTRAW (headquartered in Santo Domingo) offered three case studies on credit for women in the Dominican Republic ["Women's Access to Credit in the Dominican Republic," adapted from the longer report, is available as a supplement to *INSTRAW News* 15].

Helping to support such activities that "increase the visibility of women"—"a bridge between the needs and aspirations of women and the resources, programs, and policies for their economic development," in the words of the General Assembly—is the **U.N. Development Fund for Women (UNIFEM)**. The 45th Session welcomed the "development of new strategies for the programme management of the Fund based on long-term and short-term priorities" [A/Res/45/128]. A report on the activities of this voluntary fund, prepared by the administrator of UNDP, is transmitted to the General Assembly each year.

The Nairobi Forward-Looking Strategies' goal for the improvement of the status of professional women in the U.N. Secretariat—30 percent by December 31, 1990—fell short, by 27 women, at the target date [U.N. press release WOM/595, 2/28/91]. The Secretary-General's report to the 45th General Assembly called attention to the appointment of a woman as the U.N. High Commissioner for Refugees, but noted that no woman holds the rank of Assistant Secretary-General [A/45/125]. The 45th General Assembly urged the Secretary-General to increase the number of women in the U.N. system, "particularly in senior policy-level and decision-making posts," and set a goal of 35 percent by 1995 [A/Res/45/125]. When it considers the Forward-Looking Strategies, the 46th Session will have before it the Secretary-General's report on the progress made in, and future strategies for, carrying out these in-house goals.

June 1991 saw the release of a long-awaited statistical report on "The

World's Women 1970–1990," prepared by the Programme to Improve Gender-Specific Statistics of the Statistical Office of International Economic and Social Affairs, in collaboration with the Division for the Advancement of Women in Vienna, UNICEF, the U.N. Population Fund, and UNIFEM. Participants in the 35th session of the Commission on the Status of Women were apprised of its findings: "The majority of women still [lag] behind men in terms of power, wealth and opportunity," although "some improvements" had been noted "over the past 20 years" [U.N. press release WOM/595, 2/28/91].

7. Other Social Issues

Youth

The world's young took the limelight in September 1990, when 71 heads of state, and another 88 delegations led by ministers and ambassadors, journeyed to U.N. Headquarters in New York for the first **World Summit for Children** [E/ICEF/1991/12]. Summit participants adopted a **World Declaration on the Survival, Protection and Development of Children** as well as a **Plan of Action** for carrying it out. The guidelines for implementing the Declaration and monitoring its progress are supplied by the **Convention on the Rights of the Child,** which entered into force on September 2, 1990, less than ten months after adoption by the General Assembly.

The World Declaration outlines opportunities for reducing threats to the world's children (poverty, malnutrition, discrimination, disease, lack of education, and exploitation) through international cooperation and sets immediate goals for improving their lot (among them, lowering the infant, childhood, and maternal mortality rates and providing adequate drinking water, sanitation, health care, and education). In signing the Declaration, the heads of government agreed to "take political action at the highest level" and "to give high priority to the rights of children, to their survival and to their protection and development," aware that this will help to ensure "the well-being of all societies."

UNICEF will promote the Summit's health, sanitation, education, family planning, and economic goals through its normal country programming and monitoring [E/ICEF/1991/12]. In April 1991, UNICEF and WHO, close collaborators in an **Expanded Programme on Immunization,** confirmed the achievement of a goal they had set for the year 1990: innoculation of 80 percent of the world's children against six "killer diseases." At the urging of the 45th General Assembly, UNICEF will be working with the U.N. Secretary-General to protect children's rights in the criminal justice system. "Juveniles deprived of their liberty, under arrest or awaiting trial," it was noted, are "highly vulnerable to abuse, victimizing, and the violation of their rights" [A/Res/45/113].

James Grant, Executive Director of UNICEF, and Hiroshi Naki- jima, WHO's Director-General, sent a joint humanitarian **mission to Iraq** shortly after the cease-fire, at the request of the Secretary-General, to assess immediate needs of civilians in the area [press release WHO/UN 11, 2/14/ 91]. UNICEF and WHO also responded quickly to the devastation wrought by the **cyclone in Bangladesh** in spring 1991. UNICEF ad- vanced $1 million from its Emergency Reserve Fund for such survival supplies as food, medicines, and water purification tablets and launched an appeal for $5 million more to restore destroyed water systems [UNICEF press release PR/18/91, 5/3/91]. WHO's Emergency Relief Operations dispatched emergency health kits, which reached the region on May 3 [press release WHO/UN 40, 5/7/91].

The World Declaration of September 1990 made reference to "the current moves towards disarmament" and the release of "significant resources . . . for purposes other than military ones," stating that "improving the well-being of children must be a very high priority when these resources are reallocated." That hoped-for peace dividend has proved elusive. Equally elusive may be achievement of the goal of radically reducing maternal and infant deaths as pediatric AIDS cases continue to climb, totaling 500,000 in early 1991. The problem appears most acute in sub-Saharan Africa, where the HIV virus is being transmit- ted from mothers to their unborn or infant children in approximately one-third of all pregnancies [press release WHO/UN 37, 5/2/91].

By May 1991, 157 countries had signed the Convention on the Rights of the Child, and 79 countries had taken the further step of ratifying it. (Not yet among the signatories to the Convention is the United States, although it joined the consensus on the Declaration and Plan of Action at the Summit. The latter documents were initialed by Secretary of Health and Human Services Louis W. Sullivan on behalf of President George Bush.) The Convention established a ten-member committee—men and women of "high moral character" and "recognized competence in the field"—to "examine progress made by States Parties in achieving the realization of the obligations undertaken in the . . . Convention." The parties began the selection process at an open meeting on February 27, at which time it was decided to call a three-week session in September and a second session in 1992. Taking their committee seats

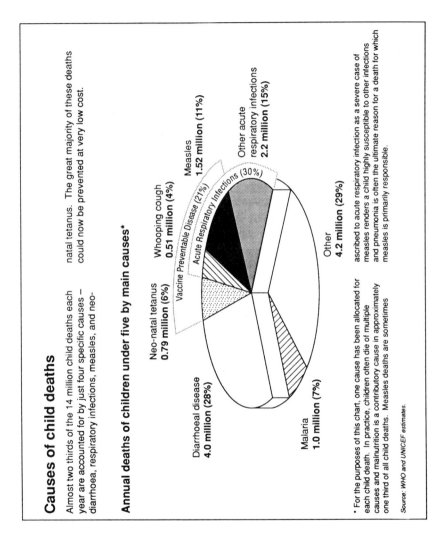

Causes of child deaths

Almost two thirds of the 14 million child deaths each year are accounted for by just four specific causes – diarrhoea, respiratory infections, measles, and neo-natal tetanus. The great majority of these deaths could now be prevented at very low cost.

Annual deaths of children under five by main causes*

Neo-natal tetanus
0.79 million (6%)

Whooping cough
0.51 million (4%)

Vaccine Preventable Disease (21%)

Acute Respiratory Infections (30%)

Measles
1.52 million (11%)

Other acute respiratory infections
2.2 million (15%)

Other
4.2 million (29%)

Diarrhoeal disease
4.0 million (28%)

Malaria
1.0 million (7%)

* For the purposes of this chart, one cause has been allocated for each child death. In practice, children often die of multiple causes and malnutrition is a contributory cause in approximately one third of all child deaths. Measles deaths are sometimes ascribed to acute respiratory infection as a severe case of measles renders a child highly susceptible to other infections and pneumonia is often the ultimate reason for a death for which measles is primarily responsible.

Source: WHO and UNICEF estimates.

Saving 100 million children from malnutrition

Prevalence of malnutrition* in children under five, developing world (excluding China)

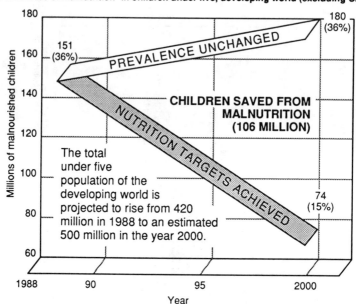

PREVALENCE UNCHANGED

151 (36%)

180 (36%)

NUTRITION TARGETS ACHIEVED

CHILDREN SAVED FROM MALNUTRITION (106 MILLION)

The total under five population of the developing world is projected to rise from 420 million in 1988 to an estimated 500 million in the year 2000.

74 (15%)

Year

* Malnutrition is here defined as more than two standard deviations below the desirable weight for age.

Source: The State of the World's Children Report 1990, p. 30.

Number of children malnourished by region

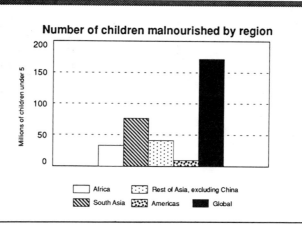

☐ Africa   ▨ Rest of Asia, excluding China
▧ South Asia   ▨ Americas   ■ Global

in September will be several social workers, doctors, and legal figures, a former teacher-turned-nongovernmental organization leader, and a consecrated bishop who helps lead a major religious charity.

Reporting in the annual *State of the World's Children* for 1991, James Grant sought to bring into perspective the cost of reaching the World Summit's goals. A "best guess," he said, is $20 billion over a decade— "approximately one eighth of one percent of the world's annual income," "half as much as Germany will find for the process of national reunification in 1991," and "as much as the world spends on the military every 10 days."

Toledo, Spain, was the site of the Centre for Social Development and Humanitarian Affairs' June 1990 **International Symposium on the Integration of Young People into Society.** The meeting was organized as a precursor to the 32nd session of the Commission for Social Development, which was to consider this issue when it met in Vienna, February 11–20, 1991. The Symposium's final report emphasized the importance of defining the concept of "integrating young people into society," and it recommended a focus on education, training, and employment problems, and the identification of needs and ways to meet those needs.

The work of the Symposium proved critical to the outcome of the Commission's deliberations: On February 20 the Commission adopted by consensus a draft resolution, cosponsored by 22 countries, entitled "Integration of Young People into Society: Participation, Development, and Peace" [E/1991/26, E/CN.5/1991/9]. The resolution commits the Commission to create at its 33rd session an "open-ended ad hoc working group," responsible for assessing and facilitating the objectives of the **International Youth Year 1985;** calendaring activities to commemorate its tenth anniversary in 1995; and preparing the first draft of the **World Youth Programme of Action Toward the Year 2000 and Beyond.** Representatives hope that the resolution will lead to greater identification of future strategies for youth integration.

In May 1991 the Vienna-based Centre convened a three-day youth forum in order to strengthen channels of cooperation and communication between the United Nations and youth organizations and to examine how youth organizations could contribute to the preparation of proposals that would serve as a basis for a World Youth Programme of Action Toward the Year 2000 and Beyond. The Centre for Social Development and Humanitarian Action is expected to prepare the first draft of the World Youth Programme and submit it to the General Assembly at the 46th Session [A/Res/45/103].

Aging

In 1990, as the U.N. **International Plan of Action on Aging** was approaching its tenth anniversary, Secretary-General Pérez de Cuéllar called for "renewed momentum" in carrying out the plan through the year 2000 and beyond, envisioning an "exchange of information within and between global networks" to spur the process. For 1992, the anniversary year itself, he recommended the publication of numerous volumes that would provide technical guidelines for setting up programs for the aging and enable nations to share experiences in providing for graying populations [A/45/420]. There was also the suggestion of a "walkathon" to publicize the fact that by the early decades of the 21st century 1 billion of the earth's inhabitants will be over 60 years of age—13 percent of the population—and that by far the largest percentage will make their homes in the developing world. However, even such modest undertakings as exchanges of information and publications that anticipate the problems and possibilities of such a world may be stalled by funding problems.

The 45th General Assembly noted that resources now assigned to the subprogram on aging, located in the **Centre for Social Development and Humanitarian Affairs (CSDHA)** of the U.N. Office in Vienna (UNOV), were insufficient to carry out the plan and that voluntary contributions to the **U.N. Trust Fund for Aging** "have steadily declined since 1982," jeopardizing the technical assistance offered to developing countries. Nonetheless, the Assembly endorsed the Secretary-General's recommendations and urged the community of nations, all pertinent government bodies, and intergovernmental organizations to cooperate in carrying them out [A/Res/45/106]. UNOV is preparing a calendar of activities for the anniversary year and will attempt to distribute it widely. The 46th General Assembly will have before it a progress report by the Secretary-General when it considers its agenda item on the Question of Aging.

In 1990–91, when the Centre for Social Development and Humanitarian Affairs biennium budget was $12.3 million, aging received $787,000; in the first six months of 1990, the Fund for Aging received new donations of $44,680 [A/Conf.150/2]. The Centre's provisional budget for the 1992–93 biennium is $14 million. The newly established **Banyan Foundation** will attempt to secure additional extrabudgetary funds from corporations, nongovernmental organizations, and governments. Named for the tree that is a symbol of endurance and longevity, the foundation held its first meeting in January 1991.

A review of the Plan of Action is conducted quadrennially; the last was in 1989. The Plan is still in its second phase, with emphasis placed on developing national infrastructures for dealing with the needs of an aging populace. Stage three will consider the human resource potential of the elderly in the national development process. In the words of the Plan, "as the elderly are enabled to be more active, self-reliant, self-determining and contributing members of society, they will become healthier and less isolated and economically dependent" [U.N. Department of Public Information/932]. According to the Secretary-General, the goal of the 1990s is to ensure that the elderly enjoy the "independence," "care," "self-fulfillment," and dignity they deserve [A/45/420].

In February 1991, ECOSOC's **Commission on Social Development** proposed for adoption by the 46th General Assembly a draft resolution VI entitled "Implementation of the International Plan of Action on Aging and Related Activities," by which the United Nations would define targets on aging issues in order to provide a pragmatic focus for the broader goals of the Plan. The Assembly would launch a global information campaign on the Action Programme on Aging for 1992 and beyond, and would also adopt the **U.N. Principles for Older Persons,** annexed to the draft. The Principles are based on the International Plan under the general headings of independence, care, self-fulfillment, and dignity, and governments are encouraged to incorporate the Principles into their national programs [U.N. press release ECOSOC/5270, 5/10/91].

The body of the resolution recommends that in 1993 the General Assembly devote four plenary sessions to aging, and that it spell out the activities to be undertaken by the CSDHA, including the formulation of global targets on aging and the issuance of a special U.N. stamp to mark the tenth anniversary of the adoption of the International Plan. It also asks the Secretary-General to explore the feasibility of launching a service composed of experts who are elderly, modeled on the U.N. Volunteers Programme [conversation with *A Global Agenda: Issues Before the 46th Session of the General Assembly of the United Nations*].

The Disabled

For the final years of the **Decade of Disabled Persons (1983–92),** the Centre for Social Development's subprogram on the disabled has been attempting to make do with the same small budget as the subprogram on the aging, although voluntary contributions to the Voluntary Fund for the U.N. Decade of Disabled Persons ($237,000 in the first six months of 1990 [A/Conf. 150/2]) are currently running well ahead of contributions to its counterpart. The Fund finances technical assistance programs in developing countries, where 80 percent of the world's half-billion disabled persons live. Aiding in publicizing program goals and raising funds is Hans Hoegh, Special Representative for the Promotion of the Decade, himself a disabled person.

With the end of the Decade approaching, the General Assembly sought a fitting conclusion to the observance, hoping to further the aims of the U.N. **World Programme of Action Concerning Disabled Persons** [A/Res/43/98]. The group of experts asked to explore the matter met in Järvenpuää, Finland, in May 1990. Reaffirming the validity and value of the action program and calling attention to the failure of many nations to respond to the special problems of the disabled, the experts recommended that the Decade be capped by the sort of basic international, regional, and national activities that will heighten awareness of the needs of the disabled [A/C.3/45/7].

The Secretary-General relayed these findings and recommendations to the General Assembly, noting that the world had become more sensitive to the needs of the disabled since the action program got under way but that the years 1981 to 1987 had actually seen a decline in the number of national committees dealing with the disabled. He called on the Centre for Social Development and Humanitarian Affairs (CSDHA) to disseminate the message of the action program in an effective fashion—first by providing all member states with a straightforward explanation of the program and also by regularly reporting on actions taken around the world to implement it—and he urged member states to hold national and other conferences to exchange information about problems that had been encountered and projects that had proved successful [A/45/470]. The 45th General Assembly endorsed the Secretary-General's recommendations and "invited" governments to sensitize their populations to the difficulties encountered by the disabled [A/Res/45/91].

To ensure the implementation of the World Programme of Action Concerning Disabled Persons beyond the Decade's close, the Commission for Social Development submitted a draft resolution to the Economic and Social Council in the spring of 1991, proposing that the Council invite member states to review their policies and programs and design long-term strategies for national action. Nations would also be invited to contribute financial and technical support to the efforts of the Secretary-General to pursue and develop an international information network at the U.N. Office in Vienna [U.N. press release ECOSOC/5270, 5/10/91]. The draft recommended further that ECOSOC call upon member states, regional commissions, and other intergovernmental bodies to adopt an integrated policy approach to disability issues. The CSDHA would be requested to support pilot projects aimed at designing integrated disability policies in developing countries, and would be authorized to seek voluntary contributions for that purpose.

The calendar of **international conferences** provides some indication of a new awareness of the need for cooperation in addressing the problems of the disabled. One such gathering in **Beijing** in November 1990 focused on the establishment and strengthening of the institutional framework for national disability programs [U.N. press release DIS/26, 11/6/90]. Sweden and Austria helped to fund this effort, and additional conferences are scheduled for Germany, Canada, Brazil, Hong Kong, and Japan during 1991. The first U.N. Seminar on Women and Disability, held in **Vienna** in August 1990, took up such issues as social isolation and discrimination in employment [U.N. press release WOM/607, 3/8/91]. Other cooperating bodies within the U.N. system are UNESCO, which sponsors the development of educational materials, seminars, and workshops about and for disabled children; and UNICEF, which has as a priority the detection and prevention of childhood impairments.

The 45th General Assembly requested the Secretary-General to report to the 46th on the implementation of the recommendations for disseminating information about the World Programme of Action. This program, and plans for the penultimate year of the Decade of Disabled Persons, will be taken up at the 46th Session.

The Homeless

The **U.N. Centre for Human Settlements (HABITAT)** calculated in 1989 that "nearly every government, 25 organizations of the United Nations system, several bilateral agencies and multilateral financial institutions, and more than 1,000 nongovernmental organizations" already had some role in carrying out the national shelter strategies developed during the **International Year of Shelter for the Homeless (1987)** [HS/170/89E, "Shelter: From Projects to National Strategies"]. These strategies are an important component of the **Global Strategy for Shelter to the Year 2000,** which was drafted by HABITAT and carries the endorsement of the intergovernmental U.N. Commission on Human Settlements and the General Assembly [A/Res/43/171]. The aim is to launch a collective and sustainable self-help effort among the people most affected by poor housing conditions [HS/185/90E, "The Global Strategy for Shelter to the Year 2000"]. Reporting to the Commission in 1990, HABITAT noted the "positive beginning" but advised that "in the majority of the developing countries much greater efforts need to be made to apply the guidelines for national action provided in the Strategy" [HS/C/13/3, p. 20].

HABITAT, which coordinates the U.N. system's shelter programs and monitors the progress made in implementing the Global Strategy, confirms that voluntary contributions have been rising but that its resources are still "inadequate to deal effectively with the complex and enormous problems concerning human settlements" [HS/C/13/9]. "Severe staff cuts" have been one result. At present, 115 technical cooperation projects to assist national efforts at developing shelter strategies and policies are awaiting funding. HABITAT currently supports some 270 such projects in over 100 countries. Fifty-six others were completed in 1990 [HS/C/13/2].

HABITAT's **eight program areas**—global issues and strategies, national policies and instruments, integrated settlements management, financial resources, land management, infrastructure development and operation, housing production, and construction—capture the essentials of the development process. Indeed, the United Nations proposed medium-term plan for the period 1992–97 suggests that "sound management of rural and urban settlements can be the vehicle for overcoming many of the economic problems faced by developing countries" [A/45/6 (Prog. 22)].

At the Commission's behest, and with the support of the Netherlands and the four Nordic countries, HABITAT organized an Intergovernmental Meeting on Human Settlements and Sustainable Development in The Hague, November 5–9, 1990. Its recommendations—relating to land-resource management, water-supply policies, sanitation and waste water, solid waste disposal, energy systems, and transport and construction policies [HABITAT: *People, Settlements, Environment and Development*, n.d.]—were to be the foundation of the Commission's contribution to the 1992 U.N. Conference on Environment and Development in Brazil [HS/C/13/14/Add.1].

At its 13th biannual session, held in Harare, April 29–May 8, 1991, the Commission again took up the sustainable development theme, this time focusing on the use of energy "by households, in construction and in production of building materials, with emphasis on the use of energy sources which are new and renewable and that minimize pollution problems" [HS/C/13/7]. A report on the Commission session—the first to have available a summary of the actions taken by individual countries to implement the national shelter strategies [HS/C/13/3]—will be reviewed by ECOSOC, which may choose to transmit the report directly to the 46th General Assembly [E/1991/1].

"Shelter and Urbanization" was the theme of World Habitat Day 1990, an annual event celebrated on the first Monday in October. With predictions that nearly half of the developing world's population will be living in urban areas by the end of the decade and that the public sector will not be able to meet the increased demand for safe and sound shelter, HABITAT's Executive Director, Arcot Ramachandran, spoke of the need for "more realistic and pragmatic measures," which "build on the self-help shelter construction efforts of the urban poor and include mobilization and strengthening of the private construction sector, both formal and informal, for that purpose" [World Habitat Day 1990 Information Kit].

The theme of World Habitat Day 1991, "Shelter and the Living Environment," looks ahead to the 1992 Conference in Brazil. A new HABITAT Goodwill Ambassador, actress Polly Bergen, will help to "promote United Nations goals and activities in alleviating homelessness and other human settlement problems throughout the world" [*Habitat News*, 8/90].

VI
Legal Issues

The General Assembly remained on the sidelines of the most striking legal and political development of the year: the reactivation of enforcement action under Chapter VII of the U.N. Charter. Nonetheless, the Assembly and the U.N. organs reporting to it undertook a variety of actions that demonstrate the increasing internationalization of areas once considered the prerogative of domestic, especially criminal, law. In a year in which the U.N. Security Council authorized the use of force to preserve the "rule of law," other U.N. bodies sought to advance the rule of law in a variety of less spectacular ways. The United Nations considered the possibility of establishing an international criminal court and of endorsing a proliferating body of "soft law" norms on issues as diverse as the treatment of prisoners and computerized data files, and it quietly released a number of texts designed to prevent the escalation of disputes into threats to international peace. Among these were a handbook to promote the peaceful settlement of disputes, model treaties in international criminal law, and guidelines on U.N. fact-finding. Yet in 1991, the second year of the **U.N. Decade of International Law**, a number of East/West and North/South differences continued to prove intractable in various U.N. bodies that consider legal issues.

1. The International Law Commission

The International Law Commission (ILC), established in 1947 by the General Assembly, consists of 34 individuals serving in their personal capacities, not as representatives of their governments, whose task it is to assist the General Assembly in codifying and encouraging the progressive development of international law. Gathering for its 42nd session from May through July 1990, the ILC devoted 16 meetings to the Draft Code against the Peace and Security of Mankind; eight to the law of non-navigational uses of international watercourses, state responsibility, and international liability for injurious consequences arising out of acts not prohibited by international law, respectively; six to jurisdictional immunities of states and their property; and five to relations between states and international organizations.

The ILC's efforts with respect to a **Draft Code of Crimes Against the Peace and Security of Mankind** date to 1947, when the General Assembly directed the Commission to "formulate the principles of international law recognized in the Charter of the Nurnberg Tribunal and in the Judgement of the Tribunal" and "prepare a draft Code . . . indicating clearly the place to be accorded to the principles" [A/Res/177 (II)]. Long delayed because of difficulties in reaching an agreed definition of aggression, the ILC resumed work on this topic in 1981 [see A/Res/36/106]. Through 1989 the Commission had provisionally adopted 15 articles outlining, inter alia, general principles; the obligation to try or extradite; a prohibition on statutory limitations; minimum judicial guarantees; limitations on double jeopardy, retroactive application, and "official position" immunity; and responsibility for acts of subordinates, and defining as crimes against peace "aggression," "threat of aggression," "intervention," and "colonial domination and other forms of alien domination" [for discussion of the last three articles, provisionally adopted in 1989, see *Issues Before the 45th General Assembly of the United Nations*, pp. 193–95].

During its 42nd session, the ILC discussed the eighth report of its special rapporteur [A/CN.4/430 and Add. 1] and, on the recommendation of the Drafting Committee, provisionally adopted three new "crimes."

Article 16, on **"international terrorism,"** defines as a crime against peace "the undertaking, organizing, assisting, financing, encouraging or tolerating by the agents or representatives of a State of acts against another State directed at persons or property and of such a nature as to create a state of terror in the minds of public figures, groups of persons or the general public" [A/45/10, p. 62]. Article 16 also extends individual liability for acts within this definition. According to the ILC's commentary, this crime, adapted from the Commission's previous 1954 draft Code, is designed to distinguish state-sponsored terrorism organized and carried out by one state against another from non-international or "internal" terrorism (not encompassed as a crime against peace) organized and carried out by nationals within a state. (The commentary notes that "internal terrorism" is governed by "internal law, since it does not endanger international relations.") Thus, the defined crime is limited to acts undertaken by or with the conscious acquiescence of state agents and directed at "public figures," which is intended to include both political leaders and "other eminent persons who play an important part in the economic or social life of a country." Although the inclusion of terrorism as a crime drew wide support, many states were critical of these limitations, since the defined crime excludes, in the words of one state, "the majority of terrorist acts" committed by individuals [see comments in the Sixth Committee by the United Kingdom and Israel, A/C.6/45/SR.35, p. 8; and A/C.6/45/SR.36, pp. 5–6]. Some states argued that "internal" terrorist acts should also be defined by the Code as crimes against humanity, whether or not they threaten international relations [A/CN.4/L.456, pp. 17–18]. Other states criticized Article 16 for failing to distinguish "freedom fighters" or for failing to clarify the overlap between Article 16 and the separate crimes of "aggression" and "intervention" [see A/CN.4/L.456, pp. 18–19].

Article 18 defines as a crime against peace the **"recruitment, use, financing and training of mercenaries,"** drawing from the General Assembly's 1989 international convention on the same subject [see *Issues/45*, pp. 202–203 and A/Res/44/34]. Although this crime had not been included in the ILC's 1954 draft Code, Article 18 draws heavily from the 1989 Convention, with some differences. The article defines as a crime the acts of "recruiting, using, financing or training," not the activities of the mercenaries themselves if these acts can be attributed to the agents or representatives of a state. In a further refinement, the acts must be either "directed against" another state or for the purpose of "opposing the legitimate exercise of the inalienable right of peoples to self-determination." Additional paragraphs define "mercenary" in terms of Article 1 of the 1989 Convention, to include persons recruited to fight in an armed conflict or those recruited to participate in a "concerted act of violence" aimed at overthrowing a foreign government or otherwise undermining another state's constitutional order or territorial integrity. Critics of Article 18 included those who had been opposed to provisions in the 1989 Convention [see *Issues/45*, p. 203]. Others argued that the acts covered are not of sufficient gravity to justify their inclusion in the Code [see A/CN.4/L.456, p. 20].

Article "X," on **"illicit traffic in narcotic drugs,"** is the first "crime against humanity" to be recognized and adopted by the ILC as part of the Code. Borrowing from the language on "international terrorism," this crime is defined as the "undertaking, organizing, facilitating, financing or encouraging by the agents or representatives of a State, or by other individuals, of illicit traffic in narcotic drugs on a large scale, whether within the confines of a State or in a transboundary context." Unlike Article 16 on international terrorism, however, this crime extends to acts by private individuals so long as these are not "isolated or individual activities of small dealers, but, rather . . . large-scale, organized operations" [Commentary, A/45/10, p. 69]. In addition, unlike terrorism, Article X extends to drug trafficking within the territory of a single state if on a large scale. These extensions are attributable to the ILC's desire to stress that these activities present "a danger for all mankind" and pose a "threat not only to the public order of the country where it occurs, but also to the international community" [ibid., p. 68]. Paragraph 2 of Article X offers some examples of what it means by "facilitating" and "encouraging," making it clear, for instance, that money laundering is covered but is restricted to those with knowledge of such dealings. Finally, paragraph 3 adopts a definition of "illicit traffic" that parallels the one contained in the 1988 Convention against Illicit Traffic in Narcotic Drugs, which includes psychotropic substances but not drugs that are lawful under domestic or international laws. Much of the debate in the ILC concerned the proper classification of this crime, whether a crime "against peace" because of the threat drug trafficking poses to the stability of states and international relations or, as ultimately adopted, a crime "against humanity" because, like genocide, it poses a universal threat and the state element is superfluous [see proposed Article Y at A/45/10, p. 35].

The matter of classification was not the only contentious issue. The ILC and the Sixth Committee were both divided on the wisdom and practicality of making these actions international crimes, with some suggesting that international efforts are better focused on encouraging international cooperation and domestic enforcement. At least one representative suggested that the ILC had exceeded its mandate, since the General Assembly mandate to the ILC had referred to "persons engaged in illicit trafficking in narcotic drugs across national frontiers" [A/Res/44/39; see discussion at A/CN.4/L.456, p. 21]. Colombia argued, on the other hand, that Article X did not go far enough, since neither it nor Article 16 covered "narco-terrorism," which it regarded as a clear "crime against peace" [A/C.6/45/SR.34, pp. 5–7].

Divisions proved insurmountable when it came to the Rapporteur's draft articles on "complicity," "conspiracy," and "attempt," and these were not adopted at the 42th session. At least three positions emerged on this subject: (a) these were not separate offenses but should be defined as part of the Code's general principles; (b) none of these could be defined in the abstract but had to be discussed in terms of their applicability to each crime in the Code; and (c) these could be accepted, as was the case with the Rapporteur, as self-contained separate offenses [see discussion at A/45/10, pp. 15–30, and draft articles 15–17 contained therein].

ILC representatives also held irreconcilable positions with respect to the possibility of including, as a separate offense in the Code, "breach of a treaty designed to ensure international peace and security." Some believed that the code had to cover the breach of such significant treaties as those on arms control and disarmament, especially when relatively less important "crimes" had been included. Others contended that such an offense, unless restricted to treaties with universal participation, would apply only to state parties and would violate the principles of universality upon which the Code was based. It would also, in the views of some, raise difficult treaty law issues, since, for example, nonparties to a treaty could presumably invoke its breach [see, for example, A/CN.4/L.456, p. 37].

The United States had even more fundamental problems with the entire exercise in the Sixth Committee, refusing to approve the ILC's work on the Code to date. It said that the 42nd session of the ILC merely confirmed its opinion that Code provisions would not command the universal acceptance required, that the attempt to "codify the whole field of international criminal law was over-ambitious and premature," and that the ILC could spend its time on "more useful endeavors" [A/C.6/45/ SR.36, pp. 12–13]. Nonetheless, the United States joined the consensus approving the annual General Assembly resolution accepting the Report of the ILC. That resolution endorses the ILC's current identification of topics, including the Commission's goal of completing a first reading of the draft articles of the Code during its 43rd session [A/45/10, para. 540; A/Res/ 45/41].

The United States took a different tack on another subject that received considerable ILC attention: the possibility of an **international criminal court**. To the United States, "[a] Code without a court would seem unhelpful, but a court might be of some use without a Code" [A/C.6/45/SR.36, p. 13]. That comment was made in the Sixth Committee in the course of a wide-ranging discussion about the practical problems involved in establishing an international criminal court.

In May 1990 the ILC had set up a separate working group pursuant to the General Assembly's request [A/Res/44/39] that the Commission establish a subgroup to study the matter of an international criminal court and issue a report to the 46th General Assembly [A/Res/44/39; see *Issues/ 45*, p. 195]. The General Assembly had asked the ILC to consider the establishment of such a court "or other international criminal trial mechanism" with jurisdiction to consider cases involving persons charged with violating the Code of Crimes against the Peace and Security of Mankind. The ILC's and the Sixth Committee's discussion of this issue, although preliminary, was wider than this mandate would suggest. The Commission not only discussed the prior U.N. efforts to establish an international criminal court (including a 1951 draft statute for such a court), but also complex issues of subject matter competence and jurisdiction, alternatives for instituting proceedings and institutional structure (including options for composition, election of judges, and financing), and possibilities for implementing judgments (including permissible penalties and even the notion of an international detention facility for those convicted). The Commission's report to the General Assembly identified two other options on jurisdiction other than competence over all Code offenses: The court could exercise jurisdiction over only some of the crimes defined in the Code or over all crimes in respect of which states would confer competence upon it.

Although the range of opinions was extremely diverse on all issues and no conclusions were reached on any point, delegations generally supported continued study of an international criminal court—albeit with varying degrees of enthusiasm. Many strong supporters of the Code of Crimes Against the Peace and Security of Mankind argued that it would not make sense to elaborate a code without establishing a mechanism for implementing it; an international criminal court would "revolutionize" international law by helping to ensure obedience and uniformity of application. According to this view, many disputes concerning the specific Code provisions would evaporate because an international court would make specificity unnecessary. The new international court would be entrusted with the adoption of non-unilateral, acceptable interpretations of Code provisions and would also guarantee against the partisan interpretations of the Code that could be expected of domestic courts if they were charged with enforcement. It would also permit the enforcement of laws against some crimes, such as large-scale drug trafficking, that some domestic court systems cannot handle at present. Enthusiastic support for a criminal court independent of the present International Court of Justice also came from members outraged by numerous alleged violations of the present Draft Code of Offenses by Iraq [see summary of views at A/CN.4/L.456, pp. 38–41; see also, for example, the views of Kuwait, A/C.6/45/SR.28, p. 2; Jamaica, A/C.6/45/SR.31, p. 17; and Australia, A/C.6/45/SR.32, p. 5]. Even those who encouraged further examination of the criminal court were skeptical, however, that complex issues, such as whether the court would have exclusive or concurrent jurisdiction with domestic courts, could be resolved. Others contended that discussion of the topic was premature, since they doubted that states, which had never conferred on the International Court of Justice a true sanctions power, would now relinquish sovereignty to an international criminal court [see, for example, A/CN.4/L.456, p. 41].

The General Assembly resolution approving the ILC's report invited the Commission to give continued attention to this issue [A/Res/45/41]. In addition, the ILC Rapporteur's ninth report to the ILC offered two draft provisions of a statute for an international criminal court "as a basis of discussion." One of the articles would give the court jurisdiction to try individuals accused of Code crimes, while another provides that in the case of certain Code offenses, such as crimes of aggression or the threat of aggression, criminal proceedings would be subject to a prior determination by the Security Council [E/CN.4/435/Add.1]. It appears likely that this topic will continue to occupy the ILC's attention.

The ILC's general plan for its work on **state responsibility,** originally adopted in 1975, called for draft articles on (1) the origin of international responsibility; (2) the content, forms, and degrees of international responsibility; and (3) the settlement of disputes and implementation. Part 1 of the draft articles was provisionally adopted in 1980, and the ILC began work on Parts 2 and 3. At its last session the ILC referred to the drafting committee two articles in Part 2, but basic disagreements emerged concerning the organizing scheme, which divides topics into "delicts" and "crimes" [see *Issues/45,* pp. 195–96].

At its 42nd session, the ILC examined the Rapporteur's second report, concerning remedies for internationally wrongful acts (delicts), and referred three articles—concerning pecuniary damages (called "reparation by equivalent" by the Rapporteur), interest, and satisfaction/guarantees of nonrepetition—to its drafting committee. Discussion during the session and in the Sixth Committee revealed basic support for all three types of remedies but widely divergent views on specifics as well as on the general approach. For example, many agreed with one of the Rapporteur's alternative formulations for pecuniary damages, which provided that injured states are entitled to claim from the state that has committed an internationally wrongful act pecuniary compensation "for any damage not covered by restitution in kind, in the measure necessary to re-establish the situation that would exist if the wrongful act had not been committed." But at least one state found this principle objectionable, since it assumed that all states were equal, thereby putting developing states at a disadvantage vis-à-vis richer ones. Others focused on ambiguities in the text, such as the meaning of "damage not covered by restitution" and the nature of the damages ("economically assessable"? "moral" damages?) to be covered. Similarly, while most generally agreed that interest is part of the compensation legally due, members differed on the need for a separate provision to this effect as well as on such details as the date from which interest should accrue, applicable rates, and the appropriateness of compounding. Finally, with regard to satisfaction as a remedy, many states opposed the Rapporteur's suggestion that "punitive damages" could sometimes be appropriate [see, generally, discussion in A/45/10, pp. 179–221; see also, for example, comments by Bahrain in A/C.6/45/Sr.31, pp. 2–3].

Members also expressed widely divergent views on another issue raised by the Rapporteur: whether fault (or willful intent or negligence) on the part of an offending state should play a role in determination of reparations and, if so, how fault should be attributed to a sovereign. These disagreements, as well as the glacial pace of the ILC's progress on the topic (only five articles in Part 2 have been provisionally adopted to date), led to proposals that the ILC provide a clearer survey of its work here. Nonetheless, many states stressed the importance of the topic, since many of the other ILC topics (such as the Code of Crimes) depend on the resolution of such basic issues of state responsibility, and they urged the ILC to finish its draft on the topic before the end of the U.N. Decade of International Law (1999) [see A/CN.4/L.456, pp. 97–105].

The Commission began work on draft articles for a general convention on **International Liability for Injurious Consequences Arising Out of Acts Not Prohibited by International Law** in 1978. Since that time the Commission has received ten reports from the two rapporteurs who have served on the topic. In 1988 the Commission referred ten articles, containing general provisions as well as principles, to its drafting committee. Many of these articles have proved controversial, and 1989 ended without the ILC approving a single one [see Issues/45, pp. 196–97].

At its 42nd session, the ILC considered the present rapporteur's sixth report, which, in reaction to prior discussions, offered a view of the subject that can only be called panoramic, both in terms of its schematic outline and by dint of the fact that it introduces 33 articles, including revisions to one of the 10 articles previously submitted. The report examines further the possibilities of separating obligations involving risk from those with harmful effects, attempts anew to clarify the concept of activities involving risk, introduces revised procedural rules for activities with harmful transboundary consequences, and proposes a complete set of substantive rules on the question of liability. In particular, drawing from draft rules on environmental protection promulgated by other bodies, the new draft articles incorporate in a single regime activities that involve risk as well those that, even if they do not involve risk as such, nonetheless cause transboundary harm. These two types of activities are further defined in the newly revised article 2: "Activities involving risk" are those, inter alia, involving the handling of dangerous substances and with technologies that produce hazardous radiation, or that introduce into the environment dangerous genetically altered organisms and dangerous micro-organisms; activities with harmful transboundary effects are those that cause "appreciable" or "significant" physical damage in the territory of another state, whether to persons, property, or the environment. The concept of "transboundary harm" now takes into account the cost of preventive measure taken by affected states [see article 2, A/45/10, pp. 251–52]. The regime envisions that the responsible state of origin will pay for necessary measures to restore conditions to what they were prior to the harmful occurrence. The draft continues to impose obligations on states to take actions to cooperate and prevent transboundary harm, as well as to assess, notify, and inform—although the extent of these duties, and the penalties for failure to comply (if any), remain in dispute [see draft articles 7, 8, and 9, and Chapter III on "prevention," A/45/10, pp. 257, 260].

The new draft articles contain many innovative and controversial provisions, among them a provision requiring nondiscriminatory application of domestic laws on point, designed to permit nondiscriminatory access by foreign individual claimants to the domestic courts of the offending state [article 10, p. 258]. Another provision details hortatory "balance of interests" guidelines for states to consider in negotiating applicable regimes [article 17, p. 264]. And an entirely new chapter, on "civil liability," attempts "to ensure a minimum degree of uniformity in the treatment of claims . . . by national courts" [p. 279].

The new provisions gave rise to numerous controversies, particularly with respect to the proposed rules of liability, with divergent views expressed on whether any obligation for reparation should arise in the absence of any breach of international law, on whether states of origin or the operator should be presumptively liable, on the meaning or applicability of "full compensation," and (a continuing controversy) on whether any concept of strict liability should apply [see, generally, A/45/10, pp. 242–82]. The Rapporteur's report also contained, in response to comments during the previous session, discussion of myriad issues that would arise were the convention to include harm to the "global commons," but it proposed no draft provisions on the subject [ibid., pp. 282–85; see *Issues/45*, pp. 196–97].

Given the multitude and complexity of the topics raised, discussions of the draft articles were merely tentative, and no articles were adopted provisionally. Some members urged that the ILC give priority to this topic in view of the 1992 U.N. Conference on Environment and Development, while others urged caution, given the ambitiousness of the undertaking. The ILC resolved merely to continue to discuss the Rapporteur's sixth report at its next session, although at least one member suggested that the topic had become so wide in scope that the Sixth Committee should have the opportunity to take a fresh look at the ILC's work to see whether members agreed with its direction or whether there were specific aspects of the topic that ought to be given priority in light of the international community's current needs [A/CN.4/L.456, p. 112; and see, for example, comments by the United Kingdom, A/C.6/45/SR.30, p. 16]. The ILC took one step in this direction by inviting comments on two specific subjects: (a) the desirability of providing in the Convention a list of substances so inherently dangerous that activities relating to them risk causing transboundary harm; and (b) whether the state of origin should be liable for transboundary harm caused by private parties within its jurisdiction or control [A/45/10, p. 285].

During its 42nd session, the ILC also examined the third report of its rapporteur on **Jurisdictional Immunities of States and Their Property,** a topic on the ILC's agenda since 1978. In 1989, the ILC referred to the drafting committee draft articles 1–11 *bis,* including provisions on scope, definitions, state immunity regarding commercial contracts, and segregated state property. At its 1990 session, the Commission discussed and referred yet another set of articles, 12–28, to that committee. While the debate in the Sixth Committee again reflected divisions among states about the legality of absolute or restrictive theories of sovereign immunity, the discussion in the ILC focused instead on the possibility of forging pragmatic consensus resolutions on the types of state activity that should enjoy immunity without getting embroiled in irreconcilable doctrinal issues. The states that pressed this discussion believe that the applicable legal regime should strike a balance between efforts to seek fair and reasonable settlement of disputes and the need to give sovereign governments adequate protection from abusive domestic judicial proceedings [see A/CN.4/L.456, pp. 54–55]. Others, however, expressed qualms about the compromise limitations on state immunity in the draft articles, on the grounds that these reflect only "the legislative practice of some states" and not general practice [ibid., p. 58].

The articles include proposed exceptions to sovereign immunity in cases involving contracts of employment; personal injuries and damage to property; ownership, possession, and use of property; patents, trademarks, and intellectual or industrial property; fiscal matters (such as duties and taxes); participation in companies or other collective bodies; state-owned or state-operated ships engaged in commercial service; arbitration agreements; and nationalization. Additional articles provide for "measures of constraint" (such as attachment, arrest, and execution) and detail rules on service of process, default judgments, immunity from measures of coercion (specific performance), and immunity from certain procedural measures (such as the requirement to provide security, bond, or deposit). The final article discussed, Article 28, is a general non-discrimination guarantee as between all parties. All 28 articles were adopted during the ILC's 43rd session in late spring 1991.

Despite limited time allocated to the topic, the ILC made significant progress in its consideration of a "framework agreement" concerning the **Law of the Navigational Uses of International Watercourses,** a subject on its agenda since 1971. At its 1990 session, the Commission renewed its discussion of the fifth and sixth reports of the Rapporteur on the topic, provisionally adopting six new articles proposed therein to join the 21 articles the Commission had adopted through 1988 [see *Issues/45,* pp. 198–99]. The new articles concern the protection and preservation of ecosystems; the prevention, reduction, and control of pollution; the introduction of alien or new species; the protection and preservation of the marine environment (including estuaries); the prevention and mitigation of harmful conditions whether resulting from natural causes or human conduct; and the duty to notify and take all practicable measures in cases of emergency situations, such as floods. Other proposed articles, including one on the status of international watercourses and water installations in time of armed conflict, including provisions on implementation, were discussed but not adopted [see A/A/45/10, pp. 113–78]. Representatives did agree, however, that the framework agreement contemplated could reflect rules of customary international law and was not merely hortatory [ibid., p. 116].

The Commission made some progress on the second half of the topic **Relations between States and International Organizations,** dealing with the privileges and immunities of international organizations, including their property, premises, and personnel. It has taken up this topic only intermittently and enjoyed at best a mixed reception for its treatment of the first part of the topic—the controversial 1975 Vienna Convention on the Representation of States in Their Relations with International Organizations [see *Issues/45,* p. 199]. The 1990 session of the ILC managed to discuss the Rapporteur's fourth report containing 11 draft articles for a second convention on the subject—including definitions and a consideration of the relationship with existing multilateral treaties or constituent instruments, of legal personality, of treaty-making power, of immunities for assets, of inviolability of premises, and of the use of premises for refuge—without, however, adopting any of them. Serious differences emerged on general issues—the need for the exercise, given existing conventions—as well as on particulars—whether international organizations should enjoy absolute or merely functional immunity [see A/ 45/10, pp. 225–41]. Among the many other unresolved issues is whether the topic will embrace regional organizations as well as those with universal membership.

The controversy over further U.N. action with respect to the ILC's **Draft Articles and Draft Optional Protocols One and Two on the Status of the Diplomatic Courier and Diplomatic Bag Not Accompanied by Diplomatic Courier** [see Issues/45, pp. 192–93] was not resolved. Although informal consultations were held during the 45th Session of the General Assembly, no decision was taken on whether to convene a plenipotentiary conference to seek acceptance of the draft articles and protocols. Instead, the Assembly merely resolved, at the recommendation of the Sixth Committee, to resume informal consultations during the 46th Session [A/Res/45/43].

2. Peace and Security

The Security Council was, of course, the U.N. organ responsible for the historic resolutions designed to restore **international peace and security in the Persian Gulf.** Council Resolution 660 of August 2, 1990, an unequivocal Security Council determination under Charter Articles 39 and 40 of a "breach of international peace and security," as well as an official U.N. condemnation of Iraq's invasion of Kuwait, began the series. In prompt succession there followed an affirmation of Article 51 rights of self-defense and a legally binding "decision" under Chapter VII calling on all states to impose economic sanctions on Iraq and a protective freeze over Kuwaiti assets (Resolution 661); a declaration that the Iraqi annexation of Kuwait was "null and void" and of "no legal validity," and a call to all states to refuse to recognize that annexation (Resolution 661); a demand that Iraq respect diplomatic immunity and respect the human rights of foreign nationals (Resolutions 664 and 667); a call on all states to impose a maritime embargo using such measures "commensurate to the specific circumstances as may be necessary" (Resolution 665); an affirmation of the continued application of humanitarian law, including the Fourth Geneva Convention, to both Iraq and the U.N. (Resolution 666); authorization for the U.N. Sanctions Committee to assist states facing problems in the implementation of trade sanctions, as anticipated in Article 50 of the Charter (Resolution 667); another Chapter VII decision imposing an air embargo and reminding Iraq that it is liable for breaches of humanitarian law (Resolution 670); and the climactic authorization under Chapter VII to use "all necessary means" to implement these resolutions as of January 15, 1991 (Resolution 678). After the war, the Security Council took the stage once again to impose the terms of the peace (see, for example, Resolution 686).

That the Security Council was able to take effective action, including resort to the use of force, despite the formerly paralyzing effect of the permanent member veto, is the most publicized aspect of these events. Perhaps no less important in terms of long-term significance is the flexibility with which the Security Council applied Chapter VII, taking advantage of ambiguities in Charter provisions about the implementation of economic and military sanctions. Thus, the Security Council was not deterred by the ostensible need for "special agreements" to secure armed forces (Article 43) or by the Charter's anticipation of military coordination through the Military Staff Committee (Articles 45, 46, and 47). The result was the ultimate "authorization" to unnamed member states "cooperating with Kuwait" to use force, invoking the spirit of Article 42 military action but in a context that suggests Article 51 collective self-defense licensed by the Security Council. The hybrid Council actions— binding decisions on all U.N. members to take certain actions (presumably pursuant to Articles 48 and 49) and sweeping authorization for collective self-defense actions by members without coordination through the Military Staff Committee—proved effective. Whether these actions herald a permanently reinvigorated Security Council, making resort to the General Assembly's Uniting for Peace Resolution unnecessary, remains to be seen, but the Persian Gulf resolutions have left in their wake a host of tantalizing legal issues that will likely keep legal scholars busy for some time.

Among the broader questions is the meaning of Article 51, which acknowledges "the inherent right" of individual and collective self-defense "until the Security Council has taken measures necessary to maintain international peace and security." A lively academic debate promptly arose as to whether the United States (or any other state acting at the request of Saudi Arabia) continued to have the right to act unilaterally in the absence of Security Council authorization or whether, once the collective security mechanism of Chapter VII was triggered, states lost the right to act unilaterally [see, for example, L. S. Damrosch and D. J. Scheffer, eds., *Law and Force in the New International Order*, forthcoming from Westview Press, 1991]. There have been similar debates concerning the permissible range of U.N. actions once it calls for the use of force and thereafter. Where does the Security Council acquire the authority to delegitimize a government, as it purported to do in Resolution 662, and what consequences follow from this action? Can the Security Council replace a sitting government, establish a war crimes tribunal, or itself act in violation of humanitarian law? Are there meaningful limits on a determination of "breach of the peace," or can the Security Council call for economic sanctions should, for example, a civil war threaten the stability of neighboring states through the influx of refugees? Disputes also emerged within the United States concerning the interplay between the U.S. Constitution's grant of authority to the U.S. Congress to "declare war" and the United States' legal duty to use force if required to do so by the Security Council. These issues, dormant since the Korean War, may arise with renewed vigor in the future—particularly if the Security Council is urged to act in controversial cases.

The General Assembly's actions regarding peace and security necessarily took a back seat to the more momentous actions of the Security Council. With the completion in 1989 of the **International Convention against the Recruitment, Use, Financing and Training of Mercenaries** [see *Issues/45*, pp. 202–3], the General Assembly limited its activity on this issue to the annual resolution on the **use of mercenaries as a means to violate human rights and to impede the exercise of the right of peoples to self-determination** [A/Res/45/132]. This resolution urges all states to accede to the new Convention, condemns South Africa for "its use of armed mercenaries," and denounces "any state that persists in the recruitment, or permits or tolerates the recruitment, of mercenaries and provides facilities to them for launching armed aggression against other states." It goes on to reaffirm the "legitimacy of the struggle of peoples and their liberation movements for their independence . . . from colonial domination, *apartheid* and foreign intervention and occupation," advising that "their legitimate struggle can in no way be considered as or equated to mercenary activity." As in the past, most industrialized states either voted against the resolution or abstained.

Less controversial was a resolution to implement the **Declaration of the Right of Peoples to Peace** [A/Res/45/14]. This resolution, adopted in light of a report of the Secretary-General on the implementation of the Declaration on the Right of Peoples to Peace [A/45/546] and reminiscent of a similar resolution adopted during the prior session [A/Res/44/21], asks states to "respect the principles of sovereign equality, political independence and territorial integrity of States and non-intervention in internal affairs" and to refrain from the threat of use of force inconsistent with the Charter. Another resolution, regarding **the situation in Central America: threats to international peace and security and peace initiatives,** was also adopted by consensus. In this instance the General

Assembly endorsed the intermediary role played by the Secretary-General in connection with various regional accords aimed at addressing ongoing threats to the peace in Central America, calls on the Secretary-General to submit a report to the 46th Assembly, and calls for the implementation of various agreements recently concluded in the region [A/Res/45/15].

Other Assembly action, with respect to peace and security issues in the Middle East, drew dissenting votes from Israel and the United States. These two states voted against a resolution calling for the convening of an **International Peace Conference on the Middle East** "under the auspices of the United Nations, with the participation of all parties . . . including the Palestine Liberation Organization, on an equal footing, and the five permanent members of the Security Council" [A/Res/45/68]. They also voted against the Assembly's condemnation of Israeli "policies and practices" that "violate the human rights of the Palestinian people in the occupied Palestinian territory." This resolution, on **the uprising** (*intifadah*) **of the Palestinian people,** also demands that Israel, as "occupying power," abide by the 1949 Geneva Convention relative to the Protection of Civilian Persons in Time of War and reaffirms that Israeli occupation of "Palestinian territory since 1967, including Jerusalem, and of the other Arab territories, in no way changes the legal status of those territories" [A/Res/45/69].

3. Administration of Justice

The 45th Session of the General Assembly adopted a range of resolutions, some of considerable detail and substance, concerning **crime prevention and criminal justice.** The range of topics, which includes but is not limited to terrorism (the criminal activity with which the Assembly has been preoccupied for many years), as well as the ongoing nature of the activities involved, suggests that these topics may become perennial Assembly agenda items. At its 45th Session, the General Assembly adopted some 17 resolutions on the subject of crime prevention and criminal justice, most of them at the recommendation of the Eighth U.N. Congress on the Prevention of Crime and the Treatment of Offenders [see Report of the Third Committee, A/45/756].

The Assembly endorsed by consensus **Standard Minimum Rules for Non-custodial Measures,** promulgating basic principles to encourage the use of alternatives to imprisonment, including legal safeguards to protect defendants' rights, examples of alternatives to prison and post-sentencing dispositions, and recommendations on how to implement these measures [A/Res/45/109]; **Basic Principles for the treatment of prisoners** and **Rules for the Protection of Juveniles Deprived of Their Liberty,** an elaboration of basic human rights principles to facilitate the full implementation of the United Nations' Standard Minimum Rules for the Treatment of Prisoners [A/Res/45/111 and A/Res/45/113]; **Guidelines for the Prevention of Juvenile Delinquency (The Riyadh Guidelines),** articulating standards to assist the implementation of the 1985 Standard Minimum Rules for the Administration of Juvenile Justice [A/Res/45/112]; and **Model Treaties on: Extradition** [A/Res/45/116], **Mutual Assistance in Criminal Matters** [A/Res/45/117], the **Transfer of Proceedings in Criminal Matters** [A/Res/45/118] and the **Transfer of Supervision of Offenders Conditionally Sentenced or Conditionally Released** [A/Res/45/119]. More generally, the Assembly took note of the proliferating guidelines, model treaties, and principles designed to protect **human rights in the administration of justice,** most the product of the Seventh or Eighth U.N. Congresses on the Prevention of Crime and the Treatment of Offenders, and called on all states to

> pay due attention to those norms and standards in developing national or regional strategies for their practical implementation and to spare no effort in providing for effective legislative and other mechanisms and procedures, as well as for adequate financial resources to ensure more effective implementation of these norms and standards [A/Res/45/166].

The Assembly also took note of child exploitation resulting in the **instrumental use of children in criminal activities** and requested that the Secretary-General report on the phenomenon to the Ninth U.N. Crime Congress [A/Res/45/115]. The Assembly took similar action with respect to **domestic violence,** requesting that the Secretary-General convene a working group of experts to formulate "guidelines or a manual for practitioners" concerning the problem for consideration at the Ninth Congress [A/Res/45/114]. It also adopted detailed recommendations on **international cooperation for crime prevention and criminal justice in the context of development,** urging states to give priority attention to the development of international criminal law through the promulgation and implementation of laws, including comprehensive model codes at the regional and subregional levels, to combat such transnational crimes as those involving narcotics or the destruction of the environment. The resolution went on to urge concerted efforts to exchange information and ratify relevant international instruments on transnational crime, including crimes that, like computer fraud, make extensive use of advanced technology [A/Res/45/107].

In a related resolution, the Assembly established an intergovernmental working group and called for an early ministerial meeting on the subject of such crimes [A/Res/45/108]. It also asked the Secretary-General to establish a technical cooperation program and undertake other efforts on behalf of the **systematization and computerization of criminal justice,** expected to be on the agenda of the Ninth U.N. Crime Congress [A/Res/ 45/109]. At the same time, the Assembly showed sensitivity to the privacy problems raised by computerized information files, adopting **guidelines for the regulation of computerized personal data files** [A/Res/45/95; Guidelines (as revised) at E/CN.4/1990/72]. The guidelines, a combined effort of the Commission on Human Rights, the Economic and Social Council, and the Sub-Commission on the Prevention of Discrimination and Protection of Minorities, may be useful to governments in developing domestic legislation and to organizations in devising administrative regulations.

These Assembly actions suggest an international readiness to go beyond the condemnation of reprehensible activity, such as terrorism, to address matters related to the actual administration of justice—this despite possibly significant repercussions for domestic legislation and practice. The degree to which members adhere to the standards they have affirmed here so ringingly will indicate the impact and influence of what has been called institutional "soft" law. The Organization's attention to these criminal justice issues may also have an impact on customary international human rights norms regarding the treatment of prisoners and juveniles. In addition, it confirms standard bilateral treaty practices in specialized areas, such as the rules of specialty and dual criminality in extradition, while attempting to steer clear of evident controversies. Thus, the United Nations' model treaty on extradition does not attempt to define the "political offense" exception to extradition. (The model treaty does suggest, as an alternative to the standard political offense exception clause, that parties can opt out of the exception by mutual agreement, and it also notes that parties may agree to prosecute or extradite in the case of certain offenses, when provisions have been made for such an option in multilateral agreements.) Less obviously, U.N. action with regard to "transnational crimes" may make it difficult to claim that members' actions in these areas, whether unilateral or in concert, when taken in accordance with U.N. recommendations, violate traditional jurisdictional doctrines to prescribe or enforce law. These consensus-based resolutions also suggest that such transnational crimes are matters of "international concern" and thus worthy of U.N. General Assembly, and perhaps Security Council, action in the future.

With regard to terrorism, the International Civil Aviation Organization (ICAO) held an International Conference on Air Law from February 12 to March 1, 1991, to consider a draft **Convention on the Marking of Plastic Explosives for the Purpose of Detection**, prohibiting the manufacture, importation, or exportation of unmarked plastic explosives. The Convention, which had been prepared by the Legal Committee of ICAO in response to Security Council Resolution 635 [(1989); see *Issues/45*, p. 201], was adopted at the end of the Conference and signed by the United States and 40 other countries. A Technical Annex describes the plastic explosives the Convention seeks to regulate and describes as well the agents that can be introduced into the explosives to render them detectable; and the Convention establishes an International Explosives Technical Commission, appointed by the Council of ICAO, to evaluate technical developments relating to the manufacture, marking, and detection of these explosives and to recommend amendments to the Technical Annex as appropriate [see Final Act of International Conference on Air Law, Montreal, 3/1/91, and Convention].

4. Effectiveness of the Organization

The **Special Committee on the Charter of the United Nations and on the Strengthening of the Role of the Organization**, established in 1975, has completed its work on three pending projects: (1) a declaration on U.N. fact-finding to aid in the maintenance of international peace and security, (2) a handbook on the peaceful settlement of disputes, and (3) a document on rationalization of existing U.N. procedures [see A/45/33; A/Res/45/44; and A/Res/45/45].

At its sessions in 1990 and 1991, the Special Committee discussed revised proposals on **U.N. fact-finding** originally submitted in 1989 by Belgium, the Federal Republic of Germany, Italy, Japan, New Zealand, and Spain, as well as revisions to proposals submitted in 1989 by Czechoslovakia and the German Democratic Republic. The Committee divided these two proposals into topic "clusters" and hammered out a single declaration, adopted by consensus, to be submitted for approval at the 46th Session of the General Assembly. The final declaration, as yet unavailable, is a hortatory guide intended to encourage the use of fact-finding by the Security Council, General Assembly, and Secretary-General to defuse situations likely to lead to breaches of international peace and security. The draft under discussion in 1989, entitled "Fact-Finding by the United Nations in the Field of the Maintenance of International Peace and Security," distinguishes more formalized fact-finding from the information-gathering capabilities of the Secretary-General; says that fact-finding should be comprehensive, objective, and impartial; encourages states to admit U.N. fact-finding missions into their territory and asks that refusals be accompanied by reasons "when appropriate"; specifies some of the "freedoms and facilities" that states should accord fact-finders (including privileges and immunities, freedom of communication and movement, and confidentiality); and encourages the Assembly, Council, and Secretary-General to make use of fact-finding [A/45/33, pp. 30–34].

The 46th General Assembly will also have before it for approval the **Handbook on the Peaceful Settlement of Disputes Between States,** prepared by the Secretary-General in consultation with a special Consultative Group on the Handbook drawn from the members of the Special Committee. The 185-page Handbook, reviewed by the Sixth Committee as well as by the Special Committee during its 1990 and 1991 sessions, is designed to help increase compliance with international law by providing information on the established procedures for dispute settlement between subjects of international law, such as states and international organizations [see draft text contained in Progress Report by the Secretary-General, A/AC.182/L.68; final not yet in print]. It begins with a survey of a variety of international instruments containing the principle that states should settle their disputes by peaceful means [Chapter I]; enumerates the different methods of peaceful settlement (among them, negotiation/consultation, inquiry, good offices, mediation, conciliation, arbitration, judicial settlement, and regional agencies or arrangements [Chapter II]; describes the relevant procedures under the U.N. Charter [Chapter III]; and surveys the procedures envisaged in other international instruments, whether or not these instruments create a permanent dispute-settlement institution [Chapter IV].

During its 45th Session, the Assembly approved, with one abstention (Cuba), the conclusions of the Special Committee on **the rationalization of existing United Nations procedures,** incorporating the text of this document as an annex to its Resolution 45. This annex encourages informal consultations and the avoidance of roll-call votes in the General Assembly, recommends that related topics be grouped or merged to facilitate discussion, urges that before establishing subsidiary organs the Assembly consider the usefulness of existing bodies, and suggests other methods to avoid duplication of efforts [A/Res/45/45, Annex].

The Assembly also requested, on the recommendation of the Sixth

Committee, that the Secretary-General circulate for comment **draft conciliation rules of the United Nations** [A/45/143 and Corr. 1; Decision 45/413; and see *Issues/45*, pp. 204–5]. The Secretary-General is scheduled to report on this at the 46th Session, and the rules will be examined as part of the program of the U.N. Decade of International Law and by the Special Committee [Decision 45/413].

With three of its major tasks now completed, the Special Committee on the Charter is likely to turn to other methods of encouraging the peaceful settlement of disputes—a task with which it was charged by the Assembly [Decision 45/412] and the subject of working papers on "new issues for consideration" submitted by the Soviet Union in 1990. These "other methods" include cooperative efforts between the United Nations and regional organizations, expansion of the Secretary-General's role, a general instrument on the settlement of disputes, and implementation of Charter norms through provisional measures or other enforcement actions [see *Issues/45*, p. 205, and A/45/33, pp. 5–7, 35–36].

5. International Organizations and Host Country Relations

In 1990, as in years past, the General Assembly discussed the report of the Secretary-General regarding **Respect for the Privileges and Immunities of Officials of the United Nations and the Specialized Agencies and Related Organizations** [A/Res/45/241]. This resolution, adopted by consensus, reminds members of their legal duties to U.N. officials and representatives under Articles 100 and 105 of the Charter as well as under various multilateral conventions, deplores violations of these duties and the illegal detention of U.N. staff members, and welcomes the International Court of Justice's affirmation of these legal obligations in its advisory opinion in Applicability of Article VI, Section 22, of the Convention on the Privileges and Immunities of the United Nations [see *Issues/45*, p. 216]. The Secretary-General also filed with the Assembly, as requested in the 43rd General Assembly's Resolution 167, an annual report on members' views relating to **consideration of effective measures to enhance the protection, security and safety of diplomatic and consular missions and representatives** [A/45/455 and additions]. Resolution 167 had requested states to report to the Secretary-General on alleged violations of their international obligations concerning the protection of missions or the security of U.N. representatives or officials, and the 1990 report suggested an increase in the number of incidents. Discussion of this report in the Sixth Committee led many members to denounce Iraq for what were considered "unprecedented" violations of diplomatic and consular immunities in Kuwait in both their scope and deliberateness. Iraq's response was that no violations had taken place, since, "as a result of the unification which had taken place, there was no justification for the existence of diplomatic missions in Kuwait City" [see comments made during the sixth meeting of the Sixth Committee, A/C.6/45/SR.6]. Iraq's treatment of diplomats in Kuwait also led to Security Council denunciation (see Peace and Security section above). In related action, the Assembly endorsed a proposal to include on the agenda of its 46th Session a study of an **additional protocol on consular functions to the Vienna Convention on Consular Relations** [A/Res/45/47; see also comments in the Sixth Committee's 22nd meeting, A/C.6/45/SR.22].

The **Committee on Relations with the Host Country,** established in 1971 to deal with the security of missions and the safety of their personnel, dealt with complaints about demonstrations at or near mission premises, heard complaints from the Palestine Observer Mission concerning the issuance of entry visas, and heard various complaints relating to travel restrictions and other problems encountered by the Iraqi Mission to the United Nations. The Committee also gave more extensive attention to complaints by various states, including Canada, Spain, the United Kingdom, and France, relating to alleged problems in obtaining an exemption from taxes within local jurisdictions in the United States or in their dealings with such large enterprises as hotel and rental car chains in the United States. United States representatives promised to take practical steps to improve the situation.

The ongoing controversy relating to U.S. travel restrictions on members of missions and U.N. personnel from certain member states [see *Issues/45,* pp. 206–7] eased somewhat with the lifting of travel restrictions on certain states that had been members of the Eastern bloc. The United States, however, adhered to its position that such restrictions are justified by national security concerns and do not interfere with U.S. obligations under the Headquarters Agreement with the United Nations. The United States claimed that its current lifting of the restrictions merely represented a change in the "objective situation" [A/45/26, pp. 8–9]. The General Assembly took note of the report of the Host Country Committee and endorsed its recommendations by consensus [A/Res/45/46].

The Secretary-General's report on the **current financial crisis of the United Nations** painted a picture of an organization tasked with new challenges but unable to convince member states to contribute financially to them. Thus, the Secretary-General reported that the financial prospects of the Organization remain a source of "grave concern" since, as of

November 1990, $290 million, or 35.1 percent of the year's total regular budget assessments, remained unpaid; when added to prior years' unpaid assessed contributions, the Organization was owed $407.3 million [A/45/ 830]. Perhaps more disturbing than the amounts owed was the pattern of payments: Fewer member states paid their assessments on time than was the case in 1989. The Secretary-General also reported that the Organization has had to rely on the Working Capital Fund to finance unforeseen peacekeeping expenses, concluding that

> the only real solution . . . is the payment by all Member States of their assessed contributions in full and on time. Unless and until this basic legal obligation under the Charter of the United Nations is honoured by all Member States without exception, the threat of financial collapse will continue to haunt the United Nations [A/45/830, p. 3].

The Assembly struck a similar note of urgency in its resolution reiterating the "legal obligation" to pay the expenses of the Organization as apportioned by the General Assembly [A/Res/45/236] and in many of its resolutions on the financing of particular peacekeeping forces and observer missions [see A/Res/45/243–247]. The Assembly continued to implement the management and financial reforms called for in the 41st Session's Resolution 213 and continued to adopt budgetary resolutions by consensus [see A/Res/45/254 and A/Res/45/255]. Among the staffing reforms sought is an increase in the number of women in the U.N. Secretariat, particularly in senior policy-level and decision-making posts [see A/Res/45/125].

A more recent Secretariat report on the **status of contributions** as of March 31, 1991, suggests that the financial problem continues, with 90 members in arrears with respect to the regular budget at the end of 1990 [ST/ADM/SER.B/354, Annex XI]; the United States was still the leading U.N. debtor, owing $678.7 million as of mid-1991. The Bush administration plan to pay most arrearages over a five-year period [see *Issues/45*, p. 207] has been held back by congressional sequestration of foreign affairs programs. A first payment of $36.1 million toward arrearages to the U.N. regular budget was made in July 1991 [see Chapter VII for more detailed consideration of the subject].

Pursuant to the recommendation of the Security Council, as required by Article 4 of the Charter, the Principality of Liechtenstein was admitted to U.N. membership [A/Res/45/1]. The International Committee of the Red Cross was granted observer status in the General Assembly [A/Res/45/6]. Far more controversial was the Assembly's attempt to urge states to abide by the **1975 Vienna Convention on the Representation of States in Their Relations with International Organizations of a**

Universal Character [A/Res/45/37]. That Convention, which has not been accepted by most of the states that are host to international organizations, would grant observers to these organizations, including the observer for Palestine, functional privileges and immunities. At the 45th Session, this attempt by the Assembly to extend these privileges to observers drew the dissenting or abstaining votes of 35 states, including Western industrialized states and Japan.

6. Economic Relations

Under the rubric of the Programme of Action for the Least Developed Countries for the 1990s and related U.N. development efforts, the General Assembly passed with only one dissenting vote (Cuba) an unusual resolution encouraging all member states to develop "entrepreneurship" and to "enhance their institutional, legal and regulatory frameworks to ensure greater consistency with market approaches" [A/Res/435/188]. The **"Entrepreneurship"** resolution, which would surely have failed to enlist the support of the General Assembly majority only a few years back and would appear at odds with programs for development endorsed by the General Assembly in the past, "acknowledges" the "important rule of entrepreneurship, notably in small and medium-sized enterprises, in mobilizing resources and in promoting economic growth and socio-economic development"; calls for "international support for specific programmes for private enterprise development in the least developed countries, which should address, inter alia, the promotion of domestic and foreign direct investment"; and recognizes development efforts focused on "free enterprise, decentralized decision-making, deregulation, demonopolization of economic activities, simplification of administrative procedures, market opportunities, structural adjustment and market-oriented reforms." Although the resolution does not endorse any specific legal reforms designed to enhance market mechanisms or foreign investment, it signals a departure from traditional positions on the **codification and progressive development of the principles and norms of international law relating to the new international economic order,** a subject that has been on the General Assembly's agenda since 1974 and is scheduled to be reviewed by the 46th Session of the Assembly [see, e.g., *Issues/45*, p. 208].

The long-standing negotiations on a **Code of Conduct on Transnational Corporations** were reviewed at a symposium of international lawyers gathered in The Hague in September 1989 and by the enlarged

Bureau of the Special Session of the Commission on Transnational Corporations in January 1990. Although participants endorsed the validity of the Code exercise and even suggested that current trends reinforced the need for an international framework for the operation of transnational corporations, their summary of outstanding controversial issues included the question of a reference to international law, noninterference in national affairs, respect for national sovereignty, provisions on nationalization and compensation due the investor in such circumstances, dispute settlement, and national treatment [E/1990/94 and 96]—questions on which the developing and the developed countries remain divided. Nonetheless, the 45th General Assembly called on the President of the Assembly to arrange for intensive consultations with the aim of adopting the Code during the Assembly's 46th Session [A/Res/45/186]. The Assembly also asked the Secretary-General of the U.N. Conference on Trade and Development (UNCTAD) to report at that time on consultations conducted on another long-standing negotiation effort of interest to multinational corporations and their lawyers: the **code of conduct on the transfer of technology** [A/Res/45/204]. Negotiations on this code, initially mandated by the General Assembly in 1977 and conducted under UNCTAD auspices, have been protracted and difficult, uncovering sharp divisions in such key areas as restrictive practices and applicable law [see, e.g., A/45/588].

As every year, the Assembly also considered the report of the **U.N. Commission on International Trade Law (UNCITRAL)** on the work of its previous session. The Assembly approved the report of UNCITRAL's 23rd session, held June 25–July 6, 1990, and invited states to accede to conventions elaborated under the Commission's auspices. UNCITRAL, established in 1966 and with a present membership of 36 states elected by the Assembly, is charged with removing obstacles to international trade arising from disparities in national law. UNCITRAL has produced major conventions or uniform rules on the international sale of goods, the international transport of goods, international commercial arbitration and conciliation, and international payments (most recently, the United Nations Convention on International Bills of Exchange and International Promissory Notes [1988]). The Commission also organizes regional seminars to promote the adoption and use of UNCITRAL texts by developing countries. UNCITRAL reports annually on the status of conventions adopted under its auspices [see A/CN.9/ 337, which reports, for example, that the U.N. Convention on Contracts for the International Sale of Goods (Vienna, 1980) received seven additional ratifications or accessions over the past year].

The 44th General Assembly had called for an international conference in Vienna in April 1991 to consider the last UNCITRAL effort, the

Convention on the Liability of Operators of Transport Terminals in International Trade [see *Issues/45*, p. 209]. The Convention was adopted at the end of the three-week conference by a vote of 31–0 with 7 abstentions (Belgium, Indonesia, Libya, Netherlands, Saudi Arabia, Turkey, and the United Kingdom) [L/TR/218, 4/19/91]. The 25-article Convention governs liability for loss of, and damage to, goods involved in international transport while they are in a transport terminal, and for delay by the terminal operator in handing over the goods. It will remain open for signature at the United Nations until April 30, 1992, entering into force on the first day of the month following the expiration of one year from the date of deposit of the fifth instrument of ratification or accession.

Among UNCITRAL's ongoing projects is a **Legal Guide on Drawing Up International Countertrade Contracts** (that is, trade that consists of the direct exchange or barter of goods without the use of currency). During UNCITRAL's 23rd session, representatives made technical suggestions about the draft provisions proposed so far. There was general agreement that such a Guide is necessary, since states need advice on contractual issues that arise in such arrangements, and that the Guide could focus on issues involved in drawing up countertrade agreements without indicating approval of countertrade itself. Some states consider countertrade both inefficient and detrimental to developed and developing countries alike, charging that it distorts competition in international markets and distorts the terms of trade between participants. Others, particularly developing countries, urge that priority be given to this project, since developing countries are driven to countertrade by the lack of hard currency and weak competitiveness resulting from the shortage of hard, freely used foreign currency [see, e.g., comments in the Sixth Committee, A/C.6/45/SR.3, 9/24/90, and by China, Press Release GA/L/2648, p. 3]. Representatives agreed that the effort did not duplicate a similar effort of the Economic Commission for Europe (ECE), since the UNCITRAL Guide was considerably more detailed. Nonetheless, it was agreed that the Guide would take the ECE's solutions into account and would discuss the applicability of the United Nations Convention on Contracts for the International Sale of Goods. The Commission has generally approved the draft chapters of the Guide, which have been prepared to date by the Secretariat, and it has agreed that the draft Guide, once completed, should be submitted to the Working Group on International Payments. The Working Group meets next in September 1991 [see A/45/17, pp. 4–5 and Annex I; for sample chapters see A/CN.9/332 and Add. 1–8].

A full draft text of UNCITRAL's **Model Law on International Credit Transfers** is expected to be considered for approval at the Working

Group on International Payments' 23rd session in 1991. The Working Group had adopted, by the end of its December 1990 session, 18 articles of the Model Law, which would apply to credit transfers between sending and receiving banks located in different states. Among the agreed provisions are definitions and rules establishing the duties of the parties (including the sending and receiving bank); revocation; the consequences of failed, erroneous, or delayed credit transfers; completion of credit transfer and discharge of obligation; and conflict of laws [see A/CN.9/344 (22nd session); A/CN.9/341 (21st session)]. The topic has been on the Commission's agenda since 1986.

In the same year, UNCITRAL's Working Group on the New International Economic Order was entrusted with drafting a **Model Procurement Law** to assist both developed and developing countries in restructuring or improving the rules governing transactions involving governmental agencies and thus reduce the costs of procurement by countries that adopt the law. Such transactions constitute a significant portion of the trade between Third World and developed countries. The Working Group began by discussing a study of national procurement policies, laws, and practices prepared by the U.N. Secretariat. At its 12th session in Vienna in October 1990, the Working Group had before it draft revisions of 42 articles and considered the first 27 of these. At its sessions in 1991, the Working Group will continue to study these provisions. Among the issues are whether states should be free to exclude procurement involving national defense or national security, how best to accommodate procurement by government organs in a federal state, and how to resolve conflicts between the model law and a state's international obligations [A/CN.9/343, reporting on the Working Group's 12th session]. The Working Group has decided to include the procurement of goods and construction but not of services (except where services are incidental to the goods or construction being procured) in deference to the ongoing GATT Uruguay Round that is addressing trade in services [ibid., p. 6].

UNCITRAL's project on a **Uniform Law on Guarantees and Stand-By Letters of Credit** resulted from its consideration in 1988 of a report by the Secretary-General concluding that greater certainty and uniformity was desirable in this area [A/CN.9/301]. Since 1989, UNCITRAL's Working Group on International Contract Practices has been attempting to provide a basic framework for such guarantees to fill existing gaps in national law and contractual practice. To date the Working Group has received various reports from the Secretariat on such issues as conflict of laws and jurisdiction, party autonomy and its limits, rules of interpretation, fraud and other objections to payment, and injunctions and other court measures. At its September 1990 session, the Working Group commented on the Secretariat's first draft set of seven articles, including critical definitional issues, and discussed more generally other technical questions, such as the requisites for amending a guaranty letter [see A/CN.9/342]. Regarding the substantive issue of whether traditional (commercial) letters of credit will be covered by the uniform law, the Working Group reaffirmed its prior decision "that the uniform law should focus on independent guarantees, including stand-by letters of credit, and that it should be extended to traditional letters of credit where that was useful in view of their independent nature and the need for regulating equally relevant issues" [ibid., pp. 5–6]. The draft now under consideration takes the form of a model national law; a multilateral treaty is a possible alternative. In either case, it is expected that UNCITRAL's text will have an impact on the development of national letter of credit laws as well as on commercial banking practices. The Working Group's 15th and 16th sessions in 1991 will revisit the Secretariat's draft articles and continue to discuss, in particular, definitional difficulties arising from differences in national practice.

In 1988 the Commission requested the Secretariat to prepare a preliminary study on the need for uniform legal principles to guide the formation of international commercial contracts by electronic means. During its 23rd session the Commission studied this report on legal problems of **electronic data exchange,** which, among other things, summarized developments in the European Community and in the United States and, drawing from ICC experience, suggested the possibility of a written model "communications agreement" [A/CN.9/333, 5/18/90]. The Commission requested that the topic remain under study [A/45/17, p. 10].

During its 23rd session, UNCITRAL also had before it a report of the Secretary-General on **current activities of international organizations related to the harmonization and unification of international trade law** [A/CN.9.336, 4/23/90], an annual report requested by the General Assembly in 1979. The latest offers an invaluable guide to the internationalization of a multitude of activities increasingly requiring harmonization efforts—and serves as a reminder of the increased need to coordinate the often overlapping efforts of myriad international organizations. The report deals with activities of international organizations under the following headings: international commercial contracts in general (including procurement, countertrade, commercial agents and distributorships, and franchising), commodities, industrialization (including trade in services, investment insurance, and joint ventures), transnational corporations, transfer of technology, industrial and intellectual property law, international payments, international transport (including charter parties, marine insurance, maritime fraud, and multimodal transport), international commercial arbitration, private international law (including negotiable instruments and studies of contract practices), trade facilitation, and such other topics of "international trade law" as restrictive business practices, securities regulation, insider trading, and international aspects of bankruptcy. Among the U.N.–related developments summarized in the report are the activities of UNCTAD (including a survey of countertrade policies around the world, the establishment of the Common Fund for Commodities in Amsterdam, and recent developments in commodity agreements), the U.N. International Institute for the Unification of Private Law (including consideration of a draft Convention on Contracts of Commercial Agency in the International Sale of Goods), and the World Intellectual Property Organization (including study of revision of the Paris Convention) [see ibid.].

7. Space Law

The General Assembly endorsed the 1990 report of the Committee on the Peaceful Uses of Outer Space [A/45/20], including the report of the 29th session of the Legal Subcommittee on its ongoing threefold agenda: elaboration of draft principles on the use of nuclear power sources in outer space, consideration of the definition and delimitation of outer space and the character and utilization of the geostationary orbit, and discussion of the legal ramifications of applying the principle that exploration and utilization should be carried out for the benefit of all states, especially developing countries [A/Res/45/72].

Regarding the **use of nuclear power sources in outer space,** a Working Group of the Legal Subcommittee continued to review draft principles submitted primarily by Canada. The Working Group had reached consensus last year on Principle 3, entitled "guidelines and criteria for safe use," which seeks to minimize the quantity of radioactive material and the use of nuclear power sources in space and offers criteria for the operation of nuclear reactors and radio-isotope generators [see *Issues/45*, pp. 211–12]. At the end of its 1991 session the Working Group reported progress toward consensus on Principle 8, which proclaims that

> States shall bear international responsibility for national activities in outer space involving the use of nuclear power sources, whether such

activities are carried on by governmental agencies or by non-governmental entities, and for assuring that such national activities are carried out in conformity with (the Treaty on Principles Governing the Activities of States in the Exploration and Use of Outer Space, including the Moon and Other Celestial Bodies) and the recommendations contained in these principles.

Principle 8 also provides that this responsibility will be borne by international organizations that conduct such activities as well as by members participating in the activity.

The Group continued to discuss Principles 2 (requiring notification of the Secretary-General of the existence and generic classification of nuclear power sources), 4 (requiring safety assessments prior to launch), and 9 (requiring compensation for damage caused). Among the controverted issues that emerged are the relationship between the proposed principles and existing treaties, questions concerning which states involved in a launch would be responsible for undertaking required safety assessments, and the extent of liability for damage [A/45/20, pp. 16–18; A/AC.105/457, Annexes I and III].

Discussion of the **definition and delimitation of outer space** consisted of reiterations of positions taken in previous sessions of the Legal Subcommittee, with as yet no prospect of agreement between the diametrically opposed views of those advocating a clear distinction between the legal regimes for airspace and outer space and those denying the need for such a boundary [see *Issues/45*, p. 212]. As in the past, there was no agreement on whether the stalemate should lead the Subcommittee to drop the topic from its agenda [A/45/20, pp. 18–20; A/AC.105/457, Annex II].

There was similar lack of progress concerning the **character and utilization of the geostationary orbit.** Some delegations contend that the geostationary orbit is a "limited natural resource" that is in danger of saturation because of the large number of satellites placed in orbit by (largely) developed countries, and they argue the need for a *"sui generis* legal regime, supplementing the existing space law, to regulate equitable access . . . and rational utilization" [A/AC.105/457, pp. 26–27]. Others opposed the formulation of a separate legal regime on the grounds that regulation of the orbit is being "adequately resolved" through the work of the International Telecommunications Union (ITU). Yet others contend that there is no scientific basis for worry that the orbit is being saturated or contend that the orbit is already an integral part of the existing treaty regime for outer space [ibid.]. At its 1991 session, the Legal Subcommittee discussed a "working non-paper," circulated by a number of Group of 77 countries, containing proposed principles on the subject, but reached no consensus on any of the proposed principles or on the need for legal norms or principles on point [A/AC.105/C.2/L.181/Add. 2. See also *Issues/45*, pp. 212–13]. The topic continues on the agenda of the Legal Subcommittee.

In 1989 the General Assembly requested the Legal Subcommittee to consider the **application of the principle that the exploration and utilization of outer space should be carried out for the benefit and in the interests of all states** [A/Res/44/46]. The Subcommittee considered responses to the Secretary-General's 1988 note verbale inviting members' views of priorities under this topic and requesting information on national legal implementation of Article 1 of the 1967 Treaty on Principles Governing the Activities of States in the Exploration and Use of Outer Space, including the Moon and Other Celestial Bodies [A/AC.105/C.2/L.181/ Add. 3]. (Article 1 of that treaty provides that the exploration and use of outer space "shall be carried out for the benefit and in the interests of all countries . . . and shall be the province of all mankind." It also provides for nondiscriminatory access to all celestial bodies, freedom of scientific investigation, and facilitation and encouragement of "international cooperation" [610 U.N.T.S. 205].) Delegations, particularly those from the Group of 77 countries, saw a need to "fill in lacunae in the existing legal regime applicable to the use of outer space" through legal principles that provide for the equitable distribution of the benefits gained from the exploration and use of outer space, including hardware, launching, the training of technical experts, and access to data banks [A/AC.105/457, pp. 10–12]. Others contended that the new agenda item did not provide a mandate for the negotiation of a new international legal framework [ibid., p. 14]. It appears likely that the Legal Subcommittee will devote a greater proportion of its time to this topic in coming sessions.

The 45th General Assembly's Resolution 72 also endorsed the agenda of the **Scientific and Technical Subcommittee** of the Committee on the Peaceful Uses of Outer Space, whose topics overlap to some extent those being considered by the Legal Subcommittee. The agenda for the 28th session of the Scientific and Technical Subcommittee, February 19–March 1, 1991, was as extensive as in prior years but focused largely on improving international cooperation regarding the benefits of space activities, including sharing the benefits of airborne and satellite remote sensing with developing countries [see *Issues/45*, p. 213]. Like the Legal Subcommittee, it is examining such issues as the physical nature and technical attributes of the geostationary orbit and the use of nuclear power sources in space [see report, A/AC.105/483].

The Committee on the Peaceful Uses of Outer Space will, of course, also be involved in a variety of activities resulting from the 1989 General

Assembly's designation of 1992 as **International Space Year** (ISY) [A/Res/ 44/46]. The United Nations published a proposed program of activities for ISY, all dependent on voluntary contributions [see *Guide to the Participation of the United Nations in the International Space Year (ISY) 1991* (1990)].

As in the two previous sessions, the 45th General Assembly passed, 149–0–1 (United States), a resolution on the **prevention of an arms race in outer space** [A/Res/45/55/A]. The resolution "recognizes" that the existing legal regime for space "by itself does not guarantee the prevention of an arms race in outer space." Seeing a "need to consolidate and reinforce that regime and enhance its effectiveness," it encourages bilateral negotiations between the Soviet Union and the United States as well as multilateral negotiations under the Conference on Disarmament. The item is continued on the agenda for the 46th Assembly.

The question of which U.N. body should take further initiatives to preserve outer space for peaceful purposes proved a contentious one at the 45th session of the Committee on the Peaceful Uses of Outer Space, which had been urged to consider the subject by the 44th General Assembly [A/Res/44/46]. Some delegations to the Outer Space Committee sought Committee involvement in the work of the Conference on Disarmament, while others opposed the introduction of such "extraneous and divisive topics" into the work of the Outer Space Committee [A/45/20, pp. 4–5]. The 45th Assembly renewed its request that the Outer Space Committee consider the subject "as a matter of priority" and report on it for the Assembly's 46th Session [A/Res/45/72].

8. International Court of Justice

In accordance with the Statute of the Court and the procedural rules of the Assembly and Security Council, five members—three of them new— were elected to the World Court effective February 6, 1991: Andres Aguilar Mawdsley (Venezuela), Gilbert Guillaume (France, reelected), Sir Robert Yewdall Jennings (United Kingdom, reelected), Christopher Gregory Weeramantry (Sri Lanka), and Raymond Ranjeva (Madagascar) [Decision 45/307]. On February 7, 1991, Sir Robert Jennings was elected President of the Court and Judge Shigeru Oda of Japan was elected Vice President. Their terms of office run until 1994. The Court remains engaged in a variety of cases. A summary of the status of pending cases follows.

The only case giving rise to a substantive decision over the past year was the **Case Concerning Land, Island, and Maritime Frontier Dispute**

(El Salvador v. Honduras). This dispute, pending since 1986, concerns, among other things, the interpretation of the General Peace Treaty betweeen the two states, in which they had agreed to delimit certain sections of their common land frontier but had not achieved settlement in respect of remaining land areas or in respect of the legal situation of the islands in the Gulf of Fonseca or other maritime areas. El Salvador and Honduras had agreed to submit their dispute to a chamber of three judges of the Court and two additional ad hoc judges chosen by the parties. The parties exchanged memorials, countermemorials, and replies pursuant to the Court's orders, but in November 1989 faced another challenge: Nicaragua's petition to the full court to intervene in the case. On February 28, 1990, the full court ruled, 12–3, that it was for the chamber to rule on Nicaragua's intervention request. The chamber— President José Sette-Camera, Judges Oda and Sir Robert Jennings, and judges ad hoc Valticos and Torres Bernárdez—heard oral arguments on the issue in June 1990, and on September 13, 1990, upheld unanimously Nicaragua's request to intervene but carefully delimited the nature of the intervention.

The original two parties in the case had taken different positions on Nicaragua's request, Honduras stating that it had no objection to intervention insofar as this was limited to permitting Nicaragua to state its views on the legal status of waters within the Gulf of Fonseca and El Salvador opposing the Nicaraguan intervention. The chamber's decision was sensitive to the positions of El Salvador and Honduras as well as to the legal requisites for intervention spelled out in Article 81(2) of the Rules of the Court. Under that article, a state seeking to intervene must demonstrate (a) the "interest of a legal nature" that may be affected by a decision, (b) the "precise object" of intervention, and (c) any basis of jurisdiction as between the intervenor and the parties to the case. El Salvador argued that Nicaragua had failed to establish these requisites, that its intervention request was untimely, and that its intervention ran counter to the "established rule" that court proceedings be brought to the Court only after a process of diplomatic negotiation between the parties.

In a decision that is likely to be important to future intervenors and the interpretation of Article 81, the chamber rejected these arguments, finding that Nicaragua had "convincingly" established an "interest of a legal nature which may be affected by the decision" such as to justify intervention. The chamber was confronted with disagreements between the original parties as to the proper issues to be decided on the merits and, while refusing to rule on these disagreements at this stage, nonetheless refused to find that Nicaragua could intervene in all the conceivable issues in the case. The chamber dismissed Nicaragua's argument that the chamber would have no power to render a decision without Nicaragua's participation, rejecting the suggested analogy with the interests of Albania in the case concerning Monetary Gold Removed from Rome in 1943 [ICJ Rep. 1954, p. 190]. Noting that Nicaragua was, after all, one of the three riparian states in the Gulf of Fonseca and had been a party to a 1917 Central American Court of Justice case that the chamber was being asked to interpret, the chamber upheld the intervention request insofar as the case concerned a determination of the nature of the legal regime within the Gulf of Fonseca—for example, whether or not a condominium. Over the separate opinion of Judge Oda, the chamber rejected claims that Nicaragua had demonstrated any interest in the delimitation of the internal waters of the Gulf of Fonseca or of waters outside that Gulf. The chamber also rejected claims that Nicaragua had shown an interest in the possible determination of the sovereignty of islands in the Gulf. The chamber accordingly decided that Nicaragua could intervene under Article 62 of the Statute of the Court but only to the extent, in the manner, and for the purposes set out in its opinion. It gave Nicaragua until December 14, 1990, to file a further written statement and El Salvador and Honduras until March 14, 1991, to respond. Oral arguments on the merits of this case were heard in April 1991 and a decision was pending at the time of writing.

Iran's case against the United States for compensation growing out of the destruction of Iran Air Airbus A–300B, Flight 655, by two surface–to–air missiles launched by the USS *Vincennes*, **Aerial incident of 3 July 1988 (Islamic Republic of Iran v. United States)** [see *Issues/45*, pp. 214–15], remains at the pleading stage. Iran has alleged violation of the 1944 Chicago Convention on International Civil Aviation and the 1971 Montreal Convention for the Suppression of Unlawful Acts against the Safety of Civil Aviation and is requesting damages payable directly to the government of Iran. The United States denies legal liability but has to date offered to compensate the bereaved families directly, on an ex gratia basis only. It also filed, on March 4, 1991, preliminary objections to the jurisdiction of the Court, thereby suspending proceedings on the merits under Article 79 of the Rules of the Court. Iran has until December 9, 1991, to respond to these objections. On April 9, 1991, Mohsen Aghahossein, the judge ad hoc appointed by Iran, made the solemn declaration required of all judges under the Court's Statute.

Also at the pleading stage is Denmark's proceeding against Norway concerning the **Maritime delimitation in the area between Greenland**

268 • *A Global Agenda: Issues Before the 46th General Assembly*

and Jan Mayen. That case requests the Court's intercession with respect to a disputed area of some 72,000 square kilometers in the waters between the east coast of Greenland and the Norwegian island of Jan Mayen to which both parties lay claim. Norway's rejoinder to Denmark's reply is due October 1, 1991.

In April 1991 the Court heard oral arguments in the case concerning the **Arbitral Award of 31 July 1989 (Guinea-Bissau v. Senegal).** Guinea-Bissau brought the case, seeking a determination that an arbitral award rendered in the course of a maritime delimitation dispute between the two states was void. By order of March 2, 1990, the Court had dismissed Guinea-Bissau's request for provisional measures pending consideration on the merits [see *Issues/45*, p. 218]. Shortly before the oral arguments, Keba Mbaye, Senegal's ad hoc judge and a former member of the Court (1982–91), made the solemn declaration required of all judges.

Nauru's case against Australia in respect of the rehabilitation of **certain phosphate lands in Nauru** mined under Australian administration prior to Nauruan independence remains at the pleading stage. Nauru claims that Australia breached its trusteeship obligations under the U.N. Charter and the trusteeship agreement with Nauru, as well as general international law, and it has requested restitution or "other appropriate reparation" as determined by the Court. Australia submitted preliminary objections to jurisdiction on January 16, 1991, thereby suspending proceedings on the merits. By order of February 8, 1991, the Court gave Nauru until July 19, 1991, to respond to these objections.

The Court is also handling two new disputes. The first, **concerning a territorial dispute (Libya v. Chad),** arises from separate notifications to the Court by each of the states on August 31 and September 1, 1990, that they had entered into a "Framework Agreement on the Peaceful Settlement of Territorial Dispute Between the Great Socialist People's Libyan Arab Jamahiriya and the Republic of Chad" in 1989 under which they agreed to settle their dispute within one year or thereafter submit the dispute to the ICJ. According to Chad's notification to the Court, the parties are asking the Court to "determine the course of the frontier . . . in accordance with the principles and rules of international law applicable in the matter as between the Parties." The parties have appointed their respective agents and, by order of October 26, 1990, the Court fixed August 26, 1991, as the first deadline for memorials.

The other new case is a proceeding filed by Portugal against Australia on February 22, 1991, concerning **certain activities of Australia with respect to East Timor,** with jurisdiction based on the two states' declarations under Article 36(2) of the Court's Statute. Portugal claims that

Australia, by negotiating with Indonesia an agreement on the exploration and exploitation of the continental shelf in the area of the Timor Gap, through its subsequent actions to implement that 1989 agreement, and by excluding Portugal from participation in those negotiations, caused "particularly serious legal and moral damage to the people of East Timor and to Portugal, which will become material damage also if the exploitation of hydrocarbon resources begins" [Court Communiqué, 2/22/91]. The sweeping nature of Portugal's claims are evident from its request that the Court

> adjudge and declare that, firstly, the rights of the people of East Timor to self-determination, to territorial integrity and unity . . . and to permanent sovereignty over its wealth and natural resources and, secondly, the duties, powers and rights of Portugal as the power administering the territory of East Timor are opposable to Australia, which is under an obligation not to disregard them, but to respect them.

Portugal is requesting that the Court declare Australia in breach of its international obligations under the U.N. Charter and find that Australia must pay reparations to the people of East Timor and to Portugal as a result [ibid.]. By order of May 3, 1991, the President of the Court fixed November 18, 1991, as the deadline for Portugal's memorial and June 1, 1992, as the deadline for Australia's countermemorial.

According to the latest report of the ICJ to the General Assembly [A/45/4, p. 2], 51 states have now made declarations (albeit many with reservations) recognizing the Court's "compulsory" jurisdiction under Article 36(2) of the Statute of the Court. In addition, three treaties providing for the jurisdiction of the Court in contentious cases were deposited with the Secretariat of the United Nations: the Convention on the Protection of the Marine Environment of the Baltic Sea, the Paris Act relating to the Berne Convention for the Protection of Literary and Artistic Works, and the International Convention against the Recruitment, Use, Financing and Training of Mercenaries [ibid.].

9. Other Legal Developments

In 1989 the General Assembly declared 1990–99 the **U.N. Decade of International Law**—a Decade dedicated to promoting acceptance and respect for the principles and institutions of international law, and encouraging the settlement of disputes [A/Res/44/23]. At that time the

General Assembly asked the Secretary-General to seek the views of members and appropriate international bodies on a program for the Decade, including the possibility of holding a third international peace conference at its conclusion, and to report to a Working Group of the Sixth Committee. In November 1990 the General Assembly accepted the recommendations of the Sixth Committee and adopted a program detailing actions with respect to the objectives of the Decade [A/Res/45/40; Secretary-General's Report, A/45/430 and Corr. 1 and Add. 1–3; Report of Sixth Committee Working Group, A/C.6/45/L.5].

Among the General Assembly's recommendations are that states and international organizations provide technical assistance to facilitate adherence to and implementation of multilateral treaties; that relevant organizations, states, and the Sixth Committee study and report on methods to promote use of peaceful methods for dispute settlement, including resort to the International Court of Justice; that the Secretary-General and the Sixth Committee report on existing codification efforts or identify "areas of international law which might be ripe for progressive development or codification"; that relevant U.N. organs and members undertake specific training and dissemination efforts, particularly in developing countries; and that the Sixth Committee consider various possibilities for making the judgments and advisory opinions of the ICJ available in all the official languages of the United Nations. The Assembly also urged states to establish national, subregional, and regional committees to assist the Sixth Committee's implementation of the program and strongly encouraged voluntary contributions, including the establishment of a trust fund, for the Decade.

Despite wide support for the Decade, opinions vary on its specific goals, reflecting long-standing differences about international law. Although member states tend to agree that the Decade's programs should be acceptable to all states, well defined, and action oriented, they differ on whether they should (1) seek to introduce new principles of international law or merely strengthen existing ones; (2) focus on ways to encourage resort to international tribunals or seek more effective ways to incorporate international law into municipal law as enforced by domestic courts; and (3) elaborate a new international convention that would require states to submit a wide range of disputes to peaceful settlement or utilize existing mechanisms of dispute settlement, including increased resort to the Security Council. There are also differences on the wisdom of convening a third international peace conference by the end of the Decade. Members of the European Community, for example, suggest that a decision on this is premature and recommend instead a midterm review of the Decade's program [see, generally, Secretary-General's Report, A/45/430]. Perhaps the most interesting, specific, and controversial list of priorities for the Decade was that of the International Commission of Jurists, which, in response to the Secretary-General's inquiry, suggested

> (a) the creation of a universal court and of regional courts of human rights (quite separate from the present world court); (b) support for ratification of the protocol to the International Covenant on Civil and Political Rights; (c) penal law: how to finance improvement in the conditions of detention and the reinsertion into society of convicted prisoners; (d) family law: protection of the child; (e) civil law: guarantee of housing; (f) commercial law: protection of the consumer; (g) administrative law: protection and international aid against major natural or industrial catastrophes.

The Commission also suggested holding a conference to discuss making the ICJ's jurisdiction "obligatory, as far as possible, in certain fields of international law" [A/45/430 at p. 80].

Another legal issue likely to generate controversy when addressed directly by the General Assembly is the tension between the Charter's call to advance the cause of human rights (Articles 1[3], 55, and 56) and the Charter's avowal of noninterference in matters within the domestic jurisdiction of a sovereign state (Article 2[7]). The problem was no more evident than in back-to-back, Janus-like resolutions of the 45th General Assembly [A/Res/45/150 and 151] that pointed to the need to **enhance the effectiveness of the principle of periodic and genuine elections** and to the need to **respect the principles of national sovereignty and noninterference in the internal affairs of states in their electoral processes.** Resolution 150, adopted by a vote of 129–8–9, affirmed the Universal Declaration of Human Rights' principle that "everyone has the right to take part in the government of his or her country, directly or through freely chosen representatives" and that "the will of the people shall be the basis of the authority of government . . . expressed in periodic and genuine elections which shall be by universal and equal suffrage and shall be held by secret vote or by equivalent free voting procedures." It concluded that, inter alia, apartheid must be abolished and that

> periodic and genuine elections are a necessary and indispensable element of sustained efforts to protect the rights and interests of the governed and that, as a matter of practical experience, the right of everyone to take part in the government of his or her country is a crucial factor in the effective enjoyment by all of a wide range of other human rights and fundamental freedoms, embracing political, economic, social and cultural rights.

The resolution continues this item on the agenda for the 46th Assembly— part of a growing number of U.N. efforts to provide electoral assistance when requested to do so by member states [A/Res/45/150; see also A/Res/45/2 directing electoral assistance to Haiti]. Resolution 150 drew the ire of Angola, China, Colombia, Cuba, Iran, Myanmar, Sudan, and Vietnam.

Resolution 151, adopted by a vote of 111–29–11, with a very different group in opposition, looks to Article 2(7) for the proposition that "nothing contained in the Charter shall authorize the United Nations to intervene in matters which are essentially within the domestic jurisdiction of any state." It affirms that "extraneous activities that attempt, directly or indirectly, to interfere in the free development of national electoral processes . . . violate the spirit and the letter of the principles established in the Charter." As might be expected, those opposed to this resolution included Western industrialized states and Japan.

Presumably the common ground between the resolutions is the principle, to which apparently most U.N. members now subscribe, that U.N. action directed at election assistance is possible when the government in question agrees to such assistance. Less clear, however, is the degree of unilateral action permitted or perhaps required by international human rights law, including the law of the Charter. Are U.N. members licensed to, or in fact under a legal duty to, provide assistance directed at bringing about free elections in a country? Could a U.N. organ (such as the Security Council) take action in a case in which the absence of elections breeds the sort of instability that is likely to breach the international peace, Article 2(7) notwithstanding? These questions are raised implicitly but not answered by these two resolutions and may be debated in future sessions under the "elections" agenda item.

The General Assembly also urged member states to accede to a variety of multilateral agreements, particularly in the area of human rights, including the international human rights covenants, the 1989 Convention on the Rights of the Child, and 1979 Convention on the Elimination of All Forms of Discrimination against Women [see, e.g., A/Res/ 45/135; A/Res/45/104; and A/Res/45/124]. It also adopted and opened for signature the **International Convention on the Protection of the Rights of All Migrant Workers and Members of Their Families,** the product of a special Working Group established in 1979 [A/Res/45/158].

VII
Finance and Administration

1. U.N. Finances

Evolution of the U.N. Financial Crisis

On paper, the U.N. financial situation looks a bit brighter than it did one year ago. At the end of 1990 its regular budget shortfall stood at $403 million, compared to $461 million a year earlier and $395 million at the end of 1988. Also, the United States has pledged that, beginning in 1991, it will pay its annual assessment plus a fifth of its arrears until those arrears have been fully paid.

Even in calendar year 1990, because of late payments for 1989, the United Nations collected $303 million from the U.S. treasury, more than in any previous year and more than the $234 million of its 1990 assessment. As a result, U.S. regular-budget indebtedness to the Organization dropped from $365 million on December 31, 1989, to $296 million on December 31, 1990. Assuming that the United States actually pays what it says it will, almost three-quarters of the overall U.N. shortfall—that is, most of what is attributable to U.S. withholding—will have been erased by the end of 1995.

However, in terms of cash flow, serious problems still remain. In the first place, the United States' $296 million debt, while by far the largest, is not the only big debt. Others at the end of 1990 included South Africa ($40.9 million), Brazil ($13.5 million), Argentina ($8.8 million), Iran ($6.5 million), Yugoslavia ($4.6 million), Libya ($3.9 million), Israel ($3.3 million), the Soviet Union ($2.6 million), Turkey ($2.5 million), Romania ($1.6 million), Nigeria ($1.5 million), and Hungary ($1.5 million). In all, 89 member states—more than half the membership—still owed money for their 1990 and previous-year assessments. Since many of these members now face growing shortages of foreign exchange, there is the risk that their indebtedness will tend to increase.

Some other members, in the face of serious economic reverses, may begin to fall behind in their payments.

Second, the United States has not promised to pay *all* that it owes in back dues. Moneys will still be withheld that would cover the U.S. share of the costs of activities that the government strongly opposes on grounds of principle, such as the Division for Palestinian Rights and the Office for the Law of the Sea. The U.N. Charter does not permit such withholdings, and only seven member states are now involved in this dubious practice. At the end of 1990, U.S. withholdings for such purposes amounted to only $18 million, but the total will steadily increase until the policy is changed. In addition, there is a dispute between the United Nations and the United States over the methodology for calculating the refunding of income tax to U.S. staff members in order to give them the same remuneration as their non-American colleagues; this, too, will increase the total U.S. indebtedness on the U.N. books.

Third, while member governments are supposed to pay their annual dues within 30 days, the United States, relying on the pretext that its financial year begins in October, makes its payments in the final quarter of the calendar year. Some other major contributors also tend to pay late. This gives other members that have to ration their limited foreign exchange an excuse for postponing their U.N. payments. As of the end of March 1991, only $243 million of the $963 million assessed for 1991 had been paid, and thus $720 million was overdue. In his report on the financial crisis, the Secretary-General pointed out that the pattern of payments by the membership as a whole was much less encouraging in 1990 than it had been in previous years [A/45/830, para. 4].

Fourth, the increasing reliance on the United Nations to backstop peacekeeping and to carry out a widening spectrum of other activities means that as time goes on the regular budget will probably be growing in real terms rather than remaining static as in the recent past. For example, the 1990–91 biennium budget was increased by $159 million at the 45th Session of the Assembly. The Secretary-General envisages expenditures of $2,363 million in the 1992–93 program budget that he is submitting to the 46th Session. This is $229 million more than the final appropriation for 1990–91 and $388 million more than the original budget adopted in 1989—an increase of about 0.9 percent in real terms. Unless members respond to this trend by paying more of their assessments earlier in the year, it will tend to exacerbate the Organization's already serious cash-flow problems.

Fifth, the Organization's peacekeeping operations are also financed mostly through the assessed contributions of member states. Here, too, there have been serious shortfalls, creating similar cash-flow problems. The shortfalls are shown in the following table (figures are as of December 31, 1990):

Operation	Amounts Owed (in millions of U.S. dollars)
U.N. Emergency Force and U.N. Disengagement Observer Force	$ 16.1
U.N. Interim Force in Lebanon	281.7
U.N. Iran-Iraq Military Observer Group	9.8
U.N. Transition Assistance Group (Namibia)	30.2
U.N. Observer Group in Central America	5.0
Total:	$342.8

Thus, the aggregate indebtedness of the United Nations at year-end 1990 for both regular budget and peacekeeping stood at $746 million. The Organization's Working Capital Fund of $100 million, which covers only 13 percent of this amount, has long been woefully insufficient to fill the gap. The rest has had to be provided through voluntary contributions by member states to "special accounts" ($114 million); through allowing appropriated funds remaining at the end of successive biennia to be used for payment of bills instead of being retained by governments ($199 million); through delaying reimbursements to governments that furnish peacekeeping forces ($214 million); and, as a last resort, through temporary borrowing from peacekeeping and other funds [A/C.5/44/27].

In the long run, all these devices should be done away with; the moneys owed to governments repaid; and the U.N. Working Capital Fund increased to cover the Organization's legitimate cash-flow needs. However, some fear that any increase in the Fund would encourage even greater irresponsibility among member states with "deadbeat" inclinations—in other words, that some of them would still not pay what they owe but allow even more of the financial burden to fall on the shoulders of those that have always paid their assessments in full and on time. Unfortunately, these fears are focused principally on the United States. The Congress, faced with intractable budgetary problems, tends to act erratically and to engage in last-minute cuts of appropriations for activities that have no powerful domestic constituencies, even when this means ignoring the country's legal obligations.

The Secretary-General has long held that, even if all governments were to pay their assessments on time, the Working Capital Fund is much too small and needs to be at least doubled in size. If the 1992–93 program budget is adopted at the level of $2,363 million proposed by the Secretary-General, it would cover only about 8 percent of the annual regular budget and only about 4 percent of combined U.N. expenditures on regular-budget and peacekeeping activities.

In 1989 the Secretary-General urged the Assembly to double the size of the Fund to $200 million in order to enable the United Nations to meet regular-budget cash-flow requirements and to take into account the increased demand for cash to finance the start-up costs of new peacekeeping operations. He outlined several options on how that money might be raised: by a single assessment of member states, by a series of assessments spread out over several years, or even by transferring unspent funds retained from biennial budgets to the Working Capital Fund. In the end, the Advisory Committee on Administrative and Budgetary Questions (ACABQ) proposed, and the Assembly agreed, to postpone any action on this matter until 1990 [A/C.5/44/27, A/44/873, A/Res/44/195].

In 1990 the Secretary-General again urged the Assembly to increase the Fund to a level of "not less than $200 million." He pointed out that during 1990 the Fund was utilized repeatedly to finance unforeseen and extraordinary expenses related to setting up an ever-increasing number of peacemaking and peacekeeping forces. The contingent sent to the Iraq-Kuwait border in May 1991 is the latest example of this kind. The Secretary-General added that if disbursements during 1991 follow 1990's pattern, the United Nations would probably remain solvent, but there is little or no leeway for error in these forecasts:

> Should any additional demands be placed upon these depleted reserves to meet the cash requirements for existing or new peacekeeping operations, or the negative impact of acute currency fluctuations or inflation, the financial situation of the U.N. could deteriorate rapidly and dramatically [A/45/830, para. 9].

The ACABQ fully agreed that the level of the Working Capital Fund needed to be increased but insisted that "it should be clear from the outset that an increase . . . is not occasioned or seen as a solution to the financial difficulties of the U.N." The precise amount of the increase should be determined only when the time had come to implement it. The Committee concluded that the Fund can work properly as a mechanism for ensuring an orderly cash flow only when the financial regime of the Organization is respected by member states. Thus, an increase in the size of the Fund should be contemplated only when the principle of payment by member states of their full financial obligations is honored. The

Committee did not set forth the precise criteria that would signal that this condition had been met [A/45/860].

The subsequent discussion in the Fifth (Administrative and Financial) Committee took place on the eve of adjournment and was even briefer than in earlier years. In introducing his report, the Chairman of ACABQ commented that rarely had his Committee discussed any subject at such great length, showing the intensity of feelings behind the scenes. He raised the possibility of a Working Capital Fund that would be financed partly on the main scale of assessments for regular-budget drawings and partly on the special scale of assessments established for peacekeeping forces in drawings for their start-up costs. Repayments would then be made from the respective accounts.

In the exchange of views that followed, the representative of Italy, speaking on behalf of the European Community, warned that the question was no longer a financial one but one of political will and of the United Nations having to restrict its activities at a time when ever-greater demands were being placed on its peacekeeping capacities. The EC believed that increasing the level of the Working Capital Fund, by itself, would not help much in repaying former and current troop-contributing countries the large sums owed to them. The five Nordic countries (including Iceland) called for an immediate increase in the Fund, which "everyone was aware . . . was too low." The representative of Australia also urged an immediate increase, since the failure to do so would "ignore the realities of the situation." He spoke of the anachronistic and cumbersome procedures required before procurement could begin and urged that practical steps be taken promptly to avoid such delays in the future. China and Japan, on the other hand, opposed any increase in the Fund at this time, and the representative of Japan suggested that reserve funds be set up outside the Working Capital Fund, which might be financed by voluntary cash grants or advances in anticipation of future peacekeeping operations. The discussion focused on the financing of these operations, with participants taking a wait-and-see attitude on the regular-budget problems, which they felt would be manageable if the United States kept its promise to pay most of what it owed [A/C.5/45/SR.47–49].

The resolution that emerged from these discussions was bland and unexceptionable, focusing mainly on the financing of the peacekeeping operations. As regards the Working Capital Fund, the Assembly merely noted the Secretary-General's proposal and the observations of the ACABQ and decided to revert to the matter "if necessary" at the 46th Session. It asked to be furnished with a detailed analysis of the reimbursements owed to member states for their participation in peacekeeping operations and requested the Secretary-General to try to persuade governments to pay in full all their assessed contributions still outstanding and to encourage them to come forward with additional, voluntary contributions [A/Res/45/236B].

Since most of the recent U.N. financial problems have originated in Washington, developments there deeply affect the Organization's underlying financial situation. Just as the United Nations has been suffering from its own financial woes, the United States government has been undergoing what is perhaps its worst financial crunch ever. In past years, U.S. withholdings sprang largely from anger over the steadily increasing costs of the Organization and its tendency to vote funds for purposes with which the United States disagreed. Now, with the introduction of consensus voting on financial appropriations and with the United Nations playing what seems to most Americans a more helpful role, the continuing shortfalls in U.S. payments come not so much from any lingering grudges against that Organization but from the need to rely on overall cuts to hold down its spiraling national deficit, cuts that tend to fall most heavily on items that lack powerful national lobbies to defend them.

If one takes into account not just the U.N. regular budget but the four categories of expenditures needed to support the many international entities, the sums involved have become substantial enough to weigh on an already overstrained budget. For example, one of these categories alone, that of the multilateral development banks, now requires $1.7 billion in annual appropriations, with $1.1 billion going to the World Bank and the rest going to the regional development banks. This does not include other sums needed to support the activities of the International Monetary Fund. The other categories are the assessed regular budgets of the Organization, its specialized agencies, and other international organizations of which the United States is a member (for FY 1992 $750 million has been requested); the peacekeeping forces (for FY 1992 $107 million has been requested); and voluntary contributions (for FY 1992 $250 million has been requested). If the costs of repaying arrears is added, the United States may be spending as much as $3 billion a year on regional and global organizations [UNA-USA, *Washington Weekly Report* (WWR, XVII, 5, 6, 10)].

Moreover, the U.S. budget is now stretched so tight that the slightest mishap can throw carefully made plans out of whack. For example, during 1990 the value of the U.S. dollar declined in terms of the Swiss franc and the Austrian shilling, the currencies in which some major U.N. agencies, such as ILO, WHO, IAEA, and UNIDO, have to pay their bills. This meant that the assessed contributions required from the member states of those organizations had to be adjusted upward, in the case of the United States by some $35 million. In the middle of the budget year there was no place to find this money except from another account. Thus, the money was preempted from the $93 million ear-marked to pay off U.S. arrears to the various U.N. organizations and, as a result, only about $58 million of arrears is scheduled to be paid from the FY 1991 (October 1990–September 1991) federal budget. The U.N. regular budget received $36.1 million of these funds in July 1991.

The U.S. currency crisis has thrown into doubt the complex arrange-ment by which arrears totaling $621 million owed to those organizations were to have been paid over five years. Furthermore, the administration is seeking congressional assent to such payments, especially since its policy calls for prior negotiations on the use of the funds within each organization, negotiations that would be almost sure to run into many legal and practical obstacles.

Nevertheless, in its 1991–92 federal budget (fiscal year 1992), the Bush administration is once again seeking almost full funding of annual assessments and budget authority for payment of all outstanding arrears. On February 6, 1991, Secretary of State James Baker said:

> We remain absolutely committed to full funding for U.S. assessed contributions, to the extent permitted by law, and to paying our prior year arrearages over the next four years. . . . The United States has a vital interest in strengthening this new, revitalized United Nations as a full partner in the building of a post–Cold War world where peace, stability and prosperity will prevail [ibid., XVII, 5].

The request, however, includes only $226 million for the U.N. regular budget, somewhat less than the $272 million bill submitted by the United Nations. Some $40 million of this difference stems from the fact that the budget submission was finalized before the General Assembly appor-tioned the United Nations' own exchange rate losses (it also has large units in Geneva and Vienna) of $160 million among the membership. It is understood that the administration remains ready to pay the additional $40 million that it owes and that it will work with the Congress to find a satisfactory solution to that problem. The remaining $6 million difference presumably relates to U.S. withholdings for cause [UNA-USA, *Washington Weekly Report* (WWR, XVII, 5)].

In the realm of peacekeeping, the U.S. government is requesting $69 million for the U.N. Interim Force in Lebanon, the U.N. Disengagement Observer Force on the Golan Heights, and the U.N. Observer Group in Central America. It is also seeking $38 million for payment of the country's arrears in the various peacekeeping accounts. Money will likewise need to be found for the force that is now guarding the Iraq-Kuwait border. As far as can be determined by comparing the U.N. monthly figures and the administration's request for FY 1992, if all of these requests are granted by the Congress, the United States will be paying its current dues and will be beginning to bring down the serious arrearages it also has in this area, mainly its $128 million debt for UNIFIL [ibid. and ST/ADM/SER.B/345, 1/3/91].

As of June, none of these FY 1992 budget requests had moved very far along the long chain of authorization and appropriation of funds in either of the two houses of Congress. Moreover, while international organizations' expenses are usually authorized by committees in which members are knowledgeable about, and in many cases sympathetic to, the needs (and national interests) the organizations are intended to serve, the sums actually appropriated are determined during the financial crunch that occurs just before the budget's adoption and by bodies less cognizant of these needs and interests. Their fate at that crucial time is unpredictable.

The United States also makes voluntary contributions to about 30 programs, most of which provide economic and social services on the ground in developing countries. In this area there is no legal requirement for the United States to make any specific contributions, but many of the organizations providing this assistance are highly regarded, and there is not the same difficulty in securing congressional approval of these appropriations. Indeed, in some cases, the Congress is eager to appropriate more than the administration wants. Overall, the administration is suggesting $250 million, or $35 million less than the amount approved in FY 1991 and $24 million less than that spent in FY 1990. The administration is likely to cite budgetary stringency in defending these cuts. Another reason may be the belief that legally required assessments should have priority over voluntary contributions.

The principal organizations receiving such support include UNDP ($115 million, an increase of $6 million over FY 1991); UNICEF ($55 million, a decrease of $20 million); IAEA ($25 million, an increase of $1.45 million); IFAD ($18.36 million, a decrease of $11.6 million); UNEP ($13 million, a decrease of $2.8 million); and the Development Assistance Programs of the OAS ($10 million, no change). The congressional committees have begun the process of reinstating the cuts proposed in the moneys allocated to UNICEF and UNEP.

New Scale of Assessments for Member States

In order to meet its bills, the United Nations assesses each of its member states a certain proportion of the expenses incurred under its regular budget and in carrying out authorized peacekeeping operations. Since it would clearly be inequitable and impractical to allocate these costs equally among all member states, there has to be a "scale of assessments." This is a listing of each of the 159 U.N. member states accompanied by the percentage of the Organization's expenses that it is required to pay. The three-year term of the present scale expires at the end of 1991. Accordingly, the 46th Assembly will have to agree on a new scale to take its place, an outcome likely to be preceded by loud complaints from those who feel that their assigned rate of assessment is too high.

The fundamental criterion for determining what each member state's rate should be is its "capacity to pay," a deceptively simple concept. It means nothing without a reliable statistical base that permits the member states' varying capacities to pay to be compared in a way that is widely acceptable. Furthermore, the methodology for determining relative capacity must be sensitive not just to the ups and downs of the economic cycle, which affect some member states more than others; it must also take into account the extreme poverty that pervades most of its 120 developing members, including those known as the least developed countries that are at the very bottom of the economic ladder. Thus, in fairness, the U.N. scale of assessments must be even more progressive than the tax regimes of most developed countries.

Over its 45-year existence, the United Nations has evolved its own ways of dealing with these problems. It has struggled to make an inadequate statistical base increasingly reliable. Using national income figures, it has developed a methodology by which the assessments of developing countries are greatly reduced by increments when their per capita income falls in lower categories, so that those in the lowest income categories pay, by far, the least. At the same time, it has been agreed that, regardless of what the statistics show, no member should pay less than a floor percentage (since 1978, 0.01 percent of the total), and no member more than a ceiling percentage (since 1974, 25 percent). As a consequence of this, some small developing countries pay more than their fair share, and the United States pays somewhat less.

Under the present scale, developed countries already pay for about three-quarters of U.N. expenses; the countries formerly falling within the Soviet sphere approximately 14 percent; and the 120 or so developing

countries, including China, the remaining 11 percent. Negotiations leading to a widely acceptable new scale will probably prove particularly
difficult since they are likely to be conducted against a backdrop of either
worldwide recession or tentative recovery, and a number of member
states, particularly China, the Soviet Union, Kuwait, Iraq, and many
Eastern European countries, are in economic crisis and may be seeking
substantial reductions. The only countries able to pick up these costs are
the Western developed countries and Japan, thus increasing still further
the lopsided relationship under which they pay the lion's share of U.N.
costs and expect, in return, to exercise a proportionate influence over the
Organization's financial decision-making.

Fortunately, the United Nations has long had special machinery to
help guide it through the thickets of member state assessment—its
Committee on Contributions, composed of 18 independent experts who
are familiar with the views of their own and like-minded governments
and thus can anticipate to some extent what will and will not be
acceptable to the Assembly as a whole. They meet every June to work on
improvements in the assessment system and submit their recommendations to that autumn's Assembly. Their sessions in 1989, 1990, and 1991
have been devoted to finding ways of improving the proposed new scale
of assessments that the Committee will submit to the 46th Session of the
Assembly.

At its 1990 session the Committee suggested that the threshold of
full (or highest) assessment should be raised from $2,200 to $2,600 of per
capita income. This would reduce the rates of assessment of some states
at the upper end of the developing-country spectrum. This proposal,
which mainly offsets the inroads of three years of inflation, was well
received, but the Assembly will take a final decision later in 1991 on what
the exact figure should be in the new scale. The Assembly also requested
the Committee to maintain the "debt-adjustment" approach used in the
preparation of the present scale [A/Res/45/256A]. This is a methodology for
lowering the rates charged countries whose foreign exchange is heavily
encumbered by interest and debt repayment obligations. Finally, the
Assembly decreed that no least developed country should be charged
more than the lowest rate of 0.01 percent.

At the same time, since the rates churned out on the basis of available
statistics (primarily those of the 1980s) will not compensate adequately
for the economic crises that some member states are facing in the 1990s,
there may be a need for more than the usual number of ad hoc adjustments. To this end, the Assembly requested the Committee, at its June
1991 session, to use the criteria it had developed in 1990 and to include

in the scale it submits its proposals for such ad hoc adjustments. It also left to its 1991 session the vexing question of the new scale's period of applicability; that is, whether it would continue to be three years or some shorter period.

The criteria to be applied are the following: (1) factors affecting capacity to pay but not adequately reflected in the present methodology, such as artificially high dollar/national-currency exchange rates; (2) ad hoc adjustments should not be more than 0.02 percent; (3) ad hoc adjustments should not be made for member states whose rates in the proposed scale have not been increased; (4) under certain circumstances, the present limitation on the amount of upward or downward shift in rates in successive scales might be waived; (5) a Committee member must be silent when the downward adjustment of his or her own country's rate is under review.

While the Committee on Contributions and the Assembly are likely to be preoccupied with the political and economic intricacies of introducing a new scale, long-term improvements in the methodology for determining rates are also on the table. These include: (1) a possible shortening or lengthening of the ten-year period for national income statistics on which that methodology is based; (2) correcting the distorting effects produced by the present limitation on the amount of upward or downward shift in rates from one scale to the next; (3) clarifying the methodology for downward adjustments of the rates assigned to heavily indebted countries; (4) obtaining price-adjusted exchange rates, which would get rid (at least for this purpose) of artificially fixed rates that exaggerate many countries' capacities to pay; (5) exploration of certain alternative income concepts, such as income adjusted for sustainable development and net changes in national wealth; (6) special arrangements for countries whose foreign exchange resources are dependent on the export of one or a very few commodities. These are old problems, most of which are highly resistant to solution [A/45/11, section III].

Some countries unrepresented on the Committee on Contributions have long pressed to have some form of direct access to the Committee. This has been resisted on the grounds that it would open the door for political pressures to be applied on a group whose work is supposed to be apolitical. The Assembly has now requested the Committee to hold, "on an experimental basis, one or two information meetings, in a manner to be decided by the Committee" prior to any ad hoc adjustment of the new scale. This was designed to give member states "the opportunity to provide the Committee with additional information as deemed necessary for the purpose of making the ad hoc adjustments" [A/Res/45/256C].

2. Program Planning

More important in the long run than the problems of raising the necessary funds to carry out U.N. activities are the mechanisms for ensuring that the world community uses these funds wisely and with cost efficiency in satisfying its highest-priority needs. In effect, the two tasks are linked, for governments are likely to be more generous and readier to pay if they are persuaded that their needs for international services are being met in an efficient and effective way. For example, it is not nearly as hard to raise money for peacekeeping operations now that their value is widely recognized.

But the planning and programming of future activities, whether to serve the purposes of policy-making or management, present many of the same challenges and frustrations at the international level that they do at the national and local levels of government. In some respects, the challenge is much greater because the United Nations does not have governmental powers, and the centrifugal tendencies with which it has to cope are very powerful. Countries disagree on which of its main activities should receive priority status. Very often these disagreements are based on valid assessments of their differing national interests. For example, developing countries tend to attach more importance to industrial development than to environmental protection, whereas countries whose industrial needs are no longer so pressing tend to be more concerned over their adverse environmental side-effects. On the other hand, there seems to be a consensus among all groups of countries that U.N. peacekeeping activities are of general benefit to the world community.

In an entity composed of sovereign states, the most practical way of reconciling the many differing perceptions of national interest is to provide a full spectrum of activities for all problems that each of the main groups of governments wishes to see addressed. This is, of course, expensive and makes the planning and programming of such activities a complex and somewhat disorderly process. There is the ever-present danger that, because of financial constraints, the attempt to do everything at once will result in nothing being done very well.

In order to plan U.N. activities as responsibly and effectively as possible, the General Assembly has long depended upon two specialized bodies to assist it, the ACABQ and the 34-member Committee for Program and Co-ordination (CPC). The former deals mainly with the financial aspects and the latter mainly with the program planning aspects of activities that are actually elaborated and approved by substantive organs, such as ECOSOC, and its specialized subsidiary bodies, such as the Commissions on Human Rights and on Narcotic Drugs and Social Development and the Governing Council of UNEP.

The systematic planning and programming of what the United Nations will do and how much it will cost is consolidated and reviewed primarily by means of three instruments: (a) a six-year medium-term plan (the one for 1992–97 was adopted in December 1990), which is the Organization's principal policy directive; (b) a program budget "outline" prepared a year in advance of the main document itself (the most recent one, for 1992–93, was also adopted in December 1990); and (c) a biennial program budget that mandates exactly what activities the Organization will carry out and how much may be spent on them (the one for 1992–93 is to be reviewed and adopted at the Assembly's 46th Session). This machinery has just been substantially overhauled and has now passed through its first two-year cycle in the new form. There is general agreement that the results need to be carefully assessed.

On the face of it, the purpose of a medium-term plan is to determine what the United Nations will do over the next six years to serve the needs of the world community and how it will do it. However, because these needs cannot be fully foreseen or planned for so far in advance, the U.N. medium-term plan has somewhat more modest aspirations; in the words of the Under-Secretary-General for Administration and Management, it seeks mainly to provide "a framework for policy-making and integrated management" and "a medium-term perspective at a time of rapid changes in the world and in the Organization itself" [A/C.5/45/SR.12, p. 10].

Even attaining these more modest goals has proved a tricky task. There are problems of aggregating and presenting in a digestible form the vast amounts of data generated by hundreds of program managers anxious to attract attention (and funding) to the activities that his or her unit will be carrying out. There is also the vastness of what the United Nations has been asked to do. Even though its structure was recently simplified, the plan still must cover 11 major programs, 45 programs, and 259 subprograms, since the Organization deals with a wide spectrum of political, economic, social, legal, and human rights issues. Medium-term planning involves projecting all of these activities some two to eight years into the uncertain future.

In view of all this, it is little wonder that the Secretary-General's 650-page medium-term plan did not win general plaudits. In its report on the plan, the ACABQ gave articulate expression to widely held reservations, most of which were, incidentally, shared by the plan's authors:

In the Committee's opinion, the plan must be simplified and shortened if it is to be of use; the verbosity, repetitiveness and length of the current submission undermine its usefulness. . . . Notwithstanding the improvements which have been effected since the previous plan, . . . much remains to be done if the medium-term plan is to be of real use to Member States and the Secretariat [A/45/617, pp. 2–4].

The Committee's comments were not all negative. It recognized that efforts had been made to streamline the plan's structure, for example, by reducing the number of major programs and programs. Members were also pleased that the Secretariat had had the wide-ranging and comprehensive consultations with governments and specialized intergovernmental bodies that the Assembly had requested. Indeed, 29 of the 45 programs had been reviewed by these specialized bodies, a good record considering that for some programs there is no specialized body. However, most of these reviews had been "less than exhaustive." It was understood that this was partly because these bodies were unfamiliar with this type of exercise and partly due to a lack of a "common language" and deficiencies in the texts they received. The Committee urged that some of these difficulties be corrected through the greater involvement of top management in the preparation of future plans.

The Chairman of CPC was equally reserved when he introduced his committee's report on this subject in the Fifth Committee. While welcoming the structural improvements and the reductions in the numbers of major programs, programs, and subprograms, he called for further progress in defining the sectors of activity and in the clear presentation of these activities. He also noted that the plan contained no indicative estimates of the financial resources required to carry out the various activities, as required under the regulations, and that most subprograms in the political sector did not include proposals for priorities.

The Soviet representative called for "a hard-nosed, critical examination" of the program planning process and added:

That complex, rigid process had become an end in itself and gave rise to voluminous documentation that was not only impossible to analyze in detail but impossible even to read. The medium-term plan, which had initially been designed to improve the efficiency of the Organization, had become an extremely complicated, confusing and costly bureaucratic mechanism. Additional methodological innovations would not improve matters [A/C.5/45/SR.17, p. 4].

He suggested that members explore ways to radically simplify U.N. planning activities, perhaps through focusing more on the approach of the plan's introduction. The Japanese delegate thought that the plan should be a strategic and pragmatic document for guiding U.N. program activities. He urged that it should be "bold and action-oriented" and would have preferred a shorter text. The U.S. representative, supporting this idea, suggested that the plan be no more than 50 to 100 pages in length. He added that the plan's present format encouraged delegations to address its narrower technical elements, such as legislative mandates and the detailed activities being carried out under each program. He also suggested that low-priority subprograms, as well as high-priority ones, be identified. Other speakers backed the ACABQ's comments, which jibed with their own frustrations in grappling with a long and inevitably complex document.

The problems of priority setting received a good deal of attention in the Fifth Committee's discussion of the plan. Seventy of the 259 subprograms had been proposed for high-priority designation by the Secretariat. Wide agreement emerged that priority setting should focus primarily on the subprograms within each broad program sector, thus sidestepping the almost insoluble political issues that are involved in assigning differing priorities to major programs and programs. At the subprogram level, the Nordic delegations noted that, under the regulations, priorities are to be designated on the basis of three criteria: the importance of the objective to member states; the Organization's capacity to achieve it; and the usefulness of the results being achieved. They also concurred with a fourth criterion, proposed by the Secretary-General, that the objective should be such that international action is demonstrably important to its attainment. They suggested that all subprograms be classified as of high, medium, or low priority.

It was recognized by at least one speaker that a number of governmental bodies have had the same limited practical results with their medium-term planning as the United Nations. In some cases, these bodies have abandoned many of the planning, programming, and budgeting techniques that were introduced with such fanfare in the 1960s. At the same time, the discussion showed that most delegations were not yet ready to abandon medium-term planning but would prefer a presentation that is less detailed, that is couched in a less bureaucratic style, that contains more in the way of program analysis, and that features ideas for new activities and for weeding out obsolete ones. The Soviet delegate reminded his colleagues and the Secretariat that "the drastic changes in the international situation called for fresh and unorthodox approaches" [A/C.5/45/SR.19, p. 12]. Perhaps the possibility of an expanded introduction rather than a shortened plan should be considered, though that would fundamentally change the current practice of having a fully fleshed-out plan whose elements are then elaborated in successive program budgets. However, if the present comprehensive-type plan is maintained, the debate showed that the Secretariat must find some way to make it shorter and more readable.

In its resolution on this subject, the General Assembly adopted the plan with certain minor modifications. It reiterated the plan's role as a framework for the formulation of the biennial program budgets and endorsed the methodological conclusions and recommendations on the plan's format and content that had been made by the ACABQ and CPC. It pressed the various intergovernmental reviewing bodies to give more attention to their reviews and governments to participate more actively in the whole process. Meanwhile, the Secretary-General was instructed to pursue his efforts to achieve "greater concision, clarity, analytical rigor and prospective orientation of the plan." At the same time, the Assembly welcomed the plan's new simplified structure and urged that the plan's usefulness as a tool for managing the Organization's activities be enhanced [A/Res/45/253I].

Great importance had been attached to the plan's introduction, which was supposed to present the Secretary-General and his senior officials with an opportunity to come up with forward-looking program proposals. He submitted a document that attempted to walk the political tightrope required to satisfy delegations whose interests and priorities for international action differ greatly and are sometimes opposed. In this, the Secretary-General apparently succeeded quite well. In his introduction of its report in the Fifth Committee, the CPC Chairman noted the widespread feeling among the members of his Committee that "the plan's delicate balance should be maintained" [A/C.5/45/SR.12, pp. 7–8]. However, the CPC's discussion (at least as summarized in its report in A/45/16, pp. 10–12) seems to have been far from thought-provoking. Indeed, it underlined how hard it is to produce a report that will generate a give-and-take exchange of substantive views rather than a reiteration of well-known political positions. The introduction, which was designed to highlight the policy orientations and priorities of the United Nations for the next six years, did not seem to help very much the Committee's decision-making and, in the end, was merely "noted." Nor did it provoke any detailed discussion in the Fifth Committee. Yet, while the text may not have been as stimulating as it could have been, one has to wonder whether the CPC (or the Fifth Committee) would have been able to proceed much further, even if the Secretary-General had come forward with more ambitious and far-reaching suggestions.

Though it is a relatively new program planning device, some of the same doubts are being entertained with regard to the value of the outline that is now submitted almost a year ahead of the program budget itself. This outline sets the ceiling for the biennial expenditures; the broad program priorities; the growth rate in "real terms," after subtracting inflationary and exchange rate distortions; and the size of the contingency fund that provides leeway for adding new activities that cannot be paid for by discontinuing obsolete ones.

The short outline given to the Assembly in 1990 seems to have set the ceiling for expenditures in a rather mechanical way rather than on the basis of the likely costs of the programs themselves. This is a methodological question with strong political overtones. Developing countries hold that the level of U.N. expenditures should be based on needs rather than on arbitrary ceilings set by the major contributors to the U.N. regular budget. Nonetheless, the present system did produce a ceiling on which the major contributors and the membership as a whole, however reluctantly, were able to agree and thus created a financial framework within which this year's program budget could be prepared.

For reasons explained above, the authors of the outline did not really attempt to establish priorities among the various major programs and programs. The outline merely identified peacekeeping, development, the environment, drug control, and Africa—the lion's share of U.N. concerns—as the areas of main focus. At the same time, they did throw some indirect light on priorities by providing an interesting table of preliminary estimates of the widely differing amounts to be spent on each of the 11 major programs.

Finally, the outline projected the rate of real growth at zero percent, thereby going rather far in pleasing the major contributors, and suggested that the size of the contingency fund should remain at 0.75 percent of the budget [A/45/369].

Despite the dissatisfaction of a number of speakers with the so-called mechanical approach in setting the budget ceiling, it is not easy to see how the Secretary-General could have responsibly followed a different approach, at least as long as the Assembly espouses consensus-type financial decision-making, which means that the objections of the major contributors cannot be overridden readily. Even if voting were resumed, there is no assurance that the United States and other major contributors that cover three-quarters of U.N. costs would abide by the results. Delegations with opposing views on this issue reached an agreement that the methodology for producing the outline needs to be improved, and a study of what these improvements might be is being undertaken by the

ACABQ. But the main underlying problem, the impatience of developing countries with the no-growth policy of the major contributors, remains unresolved. The Assembly sought to meet this concern by calling attention to the program recommendations of the CPC and by requesting the Secretary-General to pay particular attention to them in preparing his program budget (and perhaps, correspondingly, less attention to the ceiling, although this was not spelled out) [A/Res/45/255].

As already indicated, the main task before the Fifth Committee and the Assembly in 1991 will be consideration and adoption of the program budget for 1992–93. At the time of writing, this program budget, which is issued in many separate installments, had only begun to appear. The highlights of the introduction are the following: The price tag given in the budget was $2,363 million, very close to the corrected figure that had been approved in December 1990. This represented a real growth rate of 0.9 percent, a modest concession to those who objected to a zero-growth rate. This includes 81 new posts to be added to the current total of 10,048 posts and the reclassification of 67 others to higher levels. The two program sectors benefiting most from this increase are human rights and humanitarian affairs (4.3 percent) and political affairs (1.9 percent).

The structure of the program budget has been slightly modified by redesignating the "program elements" as "activities." These activities have been grouped within each subprogram under the following headings: international cooperation; parliamentary services; published material; information materials and services; operational activities; coordination, harmonization, and liaison; conference services; and administrative support.

A steady effort has been made to meet the Assembly's wish that priorities be more clearly specified. Eighty of the 259 subprograms had already been designated in the medium-term plan as being of high priority. In the program budget, the "activities" for which the Secretariat is recommending high or low priority are also indicated; these represent, respectively, 10 percent and 20 percent of the resources requested for each program. As already indicated, the establishment of priorities in these two lower program echelons is much less likely to be politically controversial than in the case of major programs and programs. At the activity level, each one can be judged in terms of how well it meets the goals of the program it is intended to promote [A/46/6 (introduction)].

The effectiveness of the foregoing program planning machinery is jeopardized both by the several political and methodological obstacles already described and by still another obstacle that may be even more serious. A steadily increasing proportion of U.N. activities is being financed from extrabudgetary funds, which largely circumvent the program planning process. The voluntary funds likely to be available in the 1992–93 biennium are estimated at $3.1 billion, compared to the $2.4 billion requested by the Secretary-General in his program budget. To put matters in perspective, it must be added that these voluntary funds are heavily concentrated in a few program sectors. These include refugee operations ($1,781 million, up $25 million from the previous biennium); technical assistance ($228 million, down $53 million); the environment ($346 million, up $47 million); and international drug control ($182 million, up $59 million).

These funds finance, inter alia, some 4,087 posts, many of them for substantive Headquarters-type functions. These off-budget posts are, not surprisingly, concentrated in the same program sectors: refugee operations (1,989); technical cooperation (199); the environment (681); and international drug control (23). They also support regional activities in Asia and the Pacific (235), in Africa (175), and Latin America (62) [ibid., Tables 7 and 9].

A number of anomalies arise from this situation. Many of these funds are quite small, and some are financed mostly or wholly by a single government, which is likely to have an important say in how this money is spent. There is thus the suspicion that affluent members prefer to hold down regular-budget expenditures in order to be freer to make voluntary contributions to those program areas they wish to see strengthened. This leads to retaliatory pressures that program areas benefiting from such funds should receive less under the regular budget to offset their higher extrabudgetary receipts. Moreover, effective program planning would seem to require that planners and intergovernmental organs be able to review all the activities in each program sector regardless of their funding sources. This is a goal very difficult to achieve in practice because the level of extrabudgetary contributions cannot be known long in advance. Finally, the ACABQ has called attention to the fact that many of these small funds may have unnoticed overhead costs that burden the regular budget and that their expenditures should in any case be submitted to the same scrutiny and control as are those of the larger voluntary funds, such as UNDP, UNICEF, UNFPA, and WFP.

The Advisory Committee's 1990 report on these matters stimulated the Assembly to call upon the Secretary-General to produce a report "on all aspects of the role and use of extra-budgetary resources" in time for the Assembly's 46th Session [A/Res/45/254, para. 12].

If the Assembly was somewhat less than pleased by the medium-term plan and budget outline, it was even more unhappy with the performance reports submitted by the Secretary-General [A/45/218 and Add. 1]. They reported on the results achieved by U.N. program activities during the 1988–89 biennium in quantitative rather than qualitative terms (in other words, whether each program output was "completed" or not). The ACABQ complained that these reports were of little value in preparing subsequent plans and program budgets and urged that they be suspended until the underlying methodological difficulties could be resolved. The CPC stated that they should be improved in both their analytical content and scope. In its resolution on this subject, the Assembly endorsed the conclusions and recommendations of its subsidiary bodies and called upon the Secretary-General to submit, in time for its 46th Session, a report on the methodology for monitoring program performance [A/Res/45/253 II].

To sum up, the medium-term plan is probably an essential ingredient of effective program planning. However, if it is to open the way to timely priority adjustments and to greater efficiency and effectiveness in program performance, the Secretariat's capabilities for the central analysis of the program side of the program budgets need to be strengthened. At present, this remains the almost exclusive province of each individual program manager, and many complaints about the unevenness and unreadability of the plans and program budgets stem from this fact. Moreover, there needs to be greater involvement of senior officials in the "think-tank" aspects of program planning. For while most of the ideas may come from program managers, they have to be vetted, homogenized, and rendered into a coherent whole at a higher central level.

Finally, greater thought and effort must be focused on producing a plan that outsiders, such as government delegates, can absorb and use—a plan with fresh and unorthodox ideas that might even inspire the major contributors to be less tightfisted. For example, the Japanese delegate suggested that a broader range of efforts to advance cooperation for peace, encompassing the economic and social as well as the political aspects, should be elaborated. At the same time, the rather obvious weaknesses of the Committee for Program and Co-ordination as the Secretary-General's interlocutor for program planning suggest the need for structural change. The world community might be better served by a group of experts, as is the case with the ACABQ, sitting full-time in their personal capacities yet also reflecting the viewpoints of the parts of the world from which they come. And developing countries would surely benefit greatly if they had spokesmen who could articulate the kinds of services that are helping them the most.

3. Personnel and Staff Administration

The International Civil Service Commission and Its Comprehensive Review of Conditions of Service

Except for one or two minor loose ends, the first comprehensive review of the conditions of service of the professional staff of the United Nations and its specialized agencies (except the World Bank and the IMF) was completed by the **International Civil Service Commission (ICSC)** in August 1990. Inevitably, the expectations of radical and far-reaching reform of the present conditions of service—reform that would save money, maximize staff efficiency, and attract gifted people and highly qualified specialists to the several international services—proved too high.

When the Commission's report and recommendations reached the Assembly later in 1990, the response from many delegations was less than enthusiastic. The representative of Italy, speaking for the 12 members of the European Community, shared the Commission's obvious disappointment with "the rather meager results obtained after so much effort," and the Soviet delegate also spoke of "the very modest results" achieved. The U.S. representative complained that the system had been neither simplified nor provided with a sound methodological basis. The Australian delegate, speaking of the "confused discussion" in the Commission, was displeased that the Commission had settled for a "modified current system" rather than a "revised system." Only a group of developing-country speakers, including those from Bangladesh, Argentina, the Philippines, Cameroon, and India, supported the Commission's conclusions [A/C.5/45/SR.29–31, 34–36]. On the other side of the argument, the executive heads of the various U.N. organizations, speaking through their Administrative Committee on Co-ordination (ACC), grumbled that "our conditions of employment continue to be beset by instability, which leads to anxiety and insecurity; salary levels are still not competitive" [A/C.5/45/43].

It is easy for outsiders to underestimate the pitfalls and the difficulties of making fundamental changes in a system that has been evolving gradually over some 45 years, indeed over some 70 years if the League of Nations' earlier experience is taken into account. Even those who were most disappointed had no thought of changing the existing system fundamentally but, rather, of treating the cost of housing as a separate third component of remuneration rather than as one of many post adjustment factors.

In this context, the conclusion reached on this subject in *Issues Before the 45th General Assembly of the United Nations* remains valid:

> It seems highly unlikely that the existing system of staff conditions of service will be replaced or even drastically changed. What is occurring instead is a rather grudging admission that the founders of the present system built more soundly than had previously been acknowledged. The present exercise has mainly focused on how better to apply principles whose soundness has now been confirmed not only by long experience but also by the investigation of possible alternatives. The main importance of the rethinking process that has taken place rests in the fact that it has confirmed the fundamental wisdom, perhaps even the inevitability, of approaches long followed. At the same time, it has called forth the ingenuity of administrators and staff within and outside the commission to adjust and modernize the vastly complex machinery, which was beginning to creak a little, through which these principles and approaches are put into practice [pp. 258–59].

Thus, as it has turned out, the Commission's task has not been one of introducing new grand designs for the international civil service but, rather, of readapting existing designs to rapidly changing external conditions. Doing this has not been an easy task, nor one that has any specific sign-off point. The comprehensive review as such is now over, but the follow-up of the conclusions and adjustments produced by it is just beginning and will go on for many years to come.

Housing and Remuneration Structures

Housing is undoubtedly the wild card in any effort to establish equal and equitable remuneration for professional staff working in more than a hundred countries across the globe. The highly educated and technically qualified personnel required by international organizations to carry out their many complex activities arrive in their duty stations with widely varying expectations and needs for their homes away from home. The housing stocks in each of these duty stations vary equally widely in their capacity to meet these expectations and needs. An effort has to be made to compare the relative costs of the kind of housing required by international staff at all of these duty stations. This has to be done in spite of the fact that housing stocks even in developed-country cities are far from easy to compare; in developing countries each housing stock suitable for foreigners is *sui generis* and usually costly even in cities where the cost of living is otherwise very low.

In almost all cities, **housing** tends to be the largest and most volatile factor in the cost of living. From one duty station to another, these costs vary over a range of 300 percent, as compared with 50 to 60 percent for other cost-of-living factors. It is also necessary but not very easy to measure movements in housing costs at each duty station over time—for example, as between times when the kinds of housing required by international officials is in short supply and times when such housing may be going begging. Such measurements must be made, keeping in mind the disparate needs and situations of renters and home owners, of newcomers and longtime residents, and of Asian, African, and Eastern European staff and those from the Americas and Western Europe, all living in cities where they may not be equally welcome or secure.

These are just some of the complexities faced by international organizations in their effort to quantify what should be the housing component in a remuneration equitable to international staff. It is easy to see from this why it was tempting to separate housing from the other cost-of-living factors and make it a separate component in the remuneration structure.

However, adding housing as a separate component to base salary and post adjustment creates a consequential problem, for which the ICSC could ultimately find no widely acceptable answer. One of the principal conditions imposed on the comprehensive review was that any new system "should, as far as possible, be comparable to the costs of the current remuneration system" [A/Res/44/198]. This condition stems from the widespread conviction of many governments that the present level of remuneration errs, if in anything, in being overgenerous to international staff. Under the existing system, such staff already receive a remuneration that is 10 to 20 percent higher than that of the highest-paid national civil service (that of the United States). This differential is known as the "margin," and almost no one argues that this margin should be greater than 20 percent. It proved difficult to find ways of treating housing separately without in effect having overall remuneration exceed that margin. One of the staff representatives put the matter very plainly when she stated that the choice "was between a structure excluding housing from post adjustment and margin control, and the current structure" [A/45/30, para. 66]. Since no one expected that governments would agree to the first alternative, the current structure had to be maintained.

Nonetheless, the Commission sought, within generally recognized financial constraints, to introduce greater fairness in the housing component of post adjustment. It sought, in fact, to distinguish between duty stations where housing could be readily fitted within the post adjustment system and some others where special arrangements outside that system were required. Among the former, housing comparisons could be made, according to the Commission, "without serious difficulty." These included U.N. Headquarters in New York, as well as North American, European, and many field duty stations. The duty stations requiring special arrangements were mainly those with small numbers of staff and high staff turnover where there was government-provided housing and/or widely disparate housing costs. Because of the relatively small numbers of professional career staff working at those duty stations, these arrangements would not constitute a significant departure from the overall system.

Even at the first group of duty stations, however, some professional staff have been benefiting from temporary housing allowances above and beyond what is included in post adjustment. Such allowances are not considered part of their permanent remuneration and thus do not form part of the margin calculations. Current recipients are mainly newcomers whose housing expenses tend to be higher than normal, and the allowance is limited to five years, with the amount decreasing by 20 percent for each year.

The Commission proposed that this "regressive reimbursement formula" be replaced by a uniform 80 percent reimbursement rate that would remain in place until the rent/income ratio attained an acceptable level within housing standards regarded as reasonable for the staff member and his or her family. The subsidy payments would be subject to "maximum reasonable rents" set at a point equivalent to three-quarters of the range of rents at the duty station concerned. These arrangements would apply not only to newcomers but also to those having to seek larger apartments because of changes in family size and to those forced to move for other reasons, such as eviction or a deterioration of security in their living area. The Commission estimated "on the basis of the best available information" that these changes might cost about $3.8 million per annum.

Many delegates saw this proposal as overgenerous to the staff, and some urged that its costs be absorbed within existing budgetary appropriations. According to some speakers, the Commission's scheme would make the rental subsidy scheme "more cumbersome" and would jeopardize the unified treatment of the post adjustment system. One delegate argued that the removal of regressive reimbursement and of the five-year limit would transform the allowance into a simple salary supplement. Some other delegates defended these same changes as "a serious effort to correct the inequities of the past" [A/C.5/45/SR.29–31, 34–36].

The Assembly nonetheless liberalized the provisions of the housing allowance at Heaquarters duty stations, extending it from five to seven years and increasing to three years the period during which it would be paid at a high rate. At the same time, it asked the Commission to review its proposals for the rental subsidy scheme, concentrating on its goals of facilitating the resettlement of staff and of encouraging mobility within the common system, and to present its conclusions and recommendations to the forthcoming 46th Assembly.

As regards the second group of field duty stations for which ordinary post adjustments do not work very well, the Assembly called for a pilot project simulating the operation of the Commission's scheme in a limited number of duty stations and asked that the results of the project be made available by autumn 1991 [A/Res/45/241, III]. For a number of reasons, the Commission reached the conclusion in March 1991 that it could not submit the reports requested of it until the Assembly's 1992 session.

Net Remuneration and Maintaining the Margin

Under the post adjustment system, international officials are supposed to be fully compensated for upward movements in the cost of living at each duty station, whereas there is no such requirement for national officials in the comparator service, that of the United States. In recent years, because of that country's budgetary squeeze, the remuneration of U.S. officials has been steadily declining in terms of purchasing power.

This has meant that for international professional staff in the common system of salaries and allowances, either movements in the cost of living or margin requirements would have to be ignored. On the whole, the dilemma has been resolved by honoring margin requirements. According to figures offered by the ICSC, net remuneration, between January 1985 and July 1990, dropped 5.1 percent in New York, 5 percent in Rome, 13.2 percent in Geneva, 16.4 percent in Paris, 17 percent in Vienna, and 19.6 percent in London, all cities in which the U.N. organizations have substantial numbers of professional staff [A/45/30, para. 175].

In 1989 the Assembly imposed a further condition. While accepting the idea of a flexible margin under which the differential between U.N. and U.S. remuneration levels might vary between 10 and 20 percent, it insisted that by the end of a five-year period the average of successive annual margins should be near the midpoint of 15 percent [A/Res/44/198C]. Consequently, if the margin in the earlier years has been higher than 15 percent, in the later years it must be correspondingly lower. In the first year of the quinquennium 1990–94, the figure stood at 117.4, and for 1991, according to current predictions, it could reach the 120 level. The Commission

> considered that in the present circumstances the Assembly's request to maintain the average net remuneration margin over a five-year period around the mid-point of the range was unworkable. Bearing in mind the projected margins for 1990 and 1991, it was apparent that the five-year averaging arrangement would require the maintenance of the margin at around 112.5 . . . during 1992–1994. This could be achieved only if remuneration in New York were to remain frozen for the next three years. . . . Freezing the remuneration in New York over extended periods of time would have undesirable consequences not only in New York but also in other duty stations, some of which had not yet received a normal post adjustment increase as a result of the freeze imposed in 1984 . . . since relativities would be maintained with other duty stations, the effect would be to freeze all duty stations [A/45/30, paras, 186–87].

The Commission therefore asked the Assembly to reconsider its request that the margin should be managed so as to keep the five-year average at the midpoint of the range. The ACC sent the Assembly a special report, in which the executive heads urged that staff salaries not be frozen again and that the ICSC devise some way of ensuring that the purchasing power of these salaries is maintained [A/C.5/45/43].

These appeals evoked a sympathetic response from the Nordic countries and a number of developing countries, a guarded response from the representative of the European Community, and an initially negative response from the U.S., Australian, Japanese, and Soviet delegates. The Soviet delegate argued that acceptance of the Commission's recommendation would deny the Assembly its last mechanism for monitoring the margin. In view of these differing member state positions, the Assembly postponed taking any hard-and-fast position, asking the ICSC to continue to monitor the evolution of the margin and also the impact of potential changes in U.S. federal civil service pay levels. However, the fact that it decided to return to the Commission's recommendations at the 1991 Assembly "with a view to avoiding a future prolonged freeze of post adjustment within the five-year period beginning in 1990" seemed to reflect a certain reluctance to confront the Commission's judgment on this issue [A/Res/45/241 VII].

This wait-and-see attitude may have been induced by indications that major changes are on the horizon for U.S. federal civil service pay arrangements. It now looks as if, beginning in 1992, federal salary scales will be tied more closely to salaries paid in private industry. Also, cost-of-living differentials within the country, until now largely ignored, will in the future probably be reflected by linking a portion of workers' annual raises to local labor markets. It remains to be seen how these changes will play out in the comparisons between U.S. and U.N. salary levels, but they should help in easing margin problems.

However, the immediate problem remains. When it met in March 1991, the Commission learned that, on the basis of current and projected data, the 1991 margin was expected to reach 120.3, slightly exceeding the range ceiling. This meant that later this year the professional staff could face another salary freeze. The Commission asked its secretariat to review alternative freeze methodologies and salary adjustment mechanisms so as to enable it to respond to the Assembly's injunction to find ways around any prolonged freeze. At its August 1991 session, it will also study a proposal being worked out by the organizations (that is, the secretariats of the United Nations and its specialized agencies) that would mitigate somewhat the worldwide adverse effects of such freezes on staff. These effects often perversely linger longer in duty stations outside the dollar area than in the New York Headquarters where they are first felt. Still, correcting this problem should not jeopardize the principle of maintaining equal purchasing power for staff at all duty stations.

A number of Commission members are concerned over this pattern of rapid salary increases followed by freezes, which is having an adverse effect on staff/management relations. One solution might be to have the base of the system depend on the cost of labor rather than on the cost of living. This might make it easier for it to move in concert with the pay scales of the comparator service. Other duty stations would then be adjusted by the local cost-of-living index, modified by a factor taking account of differences between the cost of living and the cost of labor at the base. This idea will be explored further at the Commission's August session.

Back in 1990 the Commission also proposed to the Assembly that the base salary scale for professional staff be increased by 8.5 percent, by incorporation within it of an equivalent amount of post adjustment on a no-gain no-loss basis. This would place it in line with an annual increase in U.S. civil service base salaries and U.S. income tax changes. The Assembly approved only a 5 percent increase on the same basis [A/Res/45/ 241 VIII].

The steady erosion of U.S. federal civil service pay levels in terms of purchasing power led the Japanese and European Community representatives to encourage the Commission to develop a suitable methodology for determining whether the United States remained the highest paid national civil service. The Commission had already asked its secretariat to provide it with a methodology for identifying the highest-paid national civil service by March 1991. It envisaged that an initial study would identify potential comparators, with a more refined comparison being undertaken only if and when it appeared that a potential comparator had overtaken the present comparator service. However, since initial inquiries seem to indicate that no other civil service comes close to equaling the remuneration offered its civil servants by the U.S. government, the ICSC has decided to give priority to other, more pressing tasks.

Usually the setting of salaries for locally recruited staff is a routine process. The Commission conducts technical surveys of the best prevailing local remuneration levels and makes recommendations to the U.N. organizations on a city-by-city basis. The executive heads usually accept and implement these recommendations, though they may occasionally question them on administrative or practical grounds. These arrangements cover more than half of the staff hired, including security services, trades and crafts, and a very large group of secretarial and housekeeping staff known in U.N. parlance as "general service." What is usually routine, however, ended up last year in a far-from-routine confrontation between the Commission and the U.N. administration in New York, when the latter rejected the Commission's recommendation regarding locally based salaries.

The dispute centered on a survey conducted in the fall of 1989. The U.N. administration was unhappy with the results of that survey and requested that the results be set aside until July 1990. Meanwhile, the Commission reviewed its own findings and concluded that they had been obtained in a technically competent manner and that there was no reason to cast doubt on them. The Secretary-General simultaneously conducted his own review with the participation of the other organizations headquartered in New York (UNDP, UNICEF). He ultimately accepted the Commission's results in setting the salaries for staff in the trades and crafts and security service sectors, but for the general service category he applied a higher scale based on an interim adjustment procedure used by the Commission in 1984. This was regarded by the Commission as a challenge to the technical basis of its recommendations, a realm in which it is supposed to have the final say. In justifying this step, the Secretary-General's representatives argued that other groups had recently benefited from salary increases, that many of those concerned had seen arduous service in Namibia, and that the advisory committee convened by him had been assisted in its work by the Commission's own secretariat.

The Commission believed that the action of the Secretary-General created an unfortunate precedent. Any recommendation of the Commission, regardless of its technical validity, might henceforth generate intense pressure from staff on executive heads to take contrary actions, thus posing grave risks to the common system. In particular, the Commission complained that the technical reasons given for rejecting the survey did not appear to be well founded [A/45/30, paras. 289–306].

While appreciating the "broader managerial considerations involved," the Assembly, on the whole, sided with the Commission. It decided that the offending salary scale should not constitute a precedent for future surveys and requested the Secretary-General to adjust the salaries of the staff concerned to levels consistent with the best prevailing rates of local remuneration as determined by the Commission so that there would be no disparity by the time of the next survey. It also asked him to propose procedures whereby executive heads disagreeing with the Commission's recommendations on general service salary scales could set different scales only after consultations with intergovernmental bodies and with the Commission itself. The problem may resurface at the 1991 Assembly [A/Res/45/241 XIII].

Cost-of-Living Adjustments

The nitty-gritty of establishing equitable remuneration is nowhere more in evidence than in the highly abstruse realm of post adjustments reflecting cost-of-living differences. In light of earlier decisions, new cost-of-living surveys, based on a greatly simplified methodology, are being conducted at all duty stations. These have now been completed for all of the main duty stations, and the results reveal that (except in Tokyo, where no survey has yet been made) the discrepancies between the level of post adjustment called for under the old and new systems are minimal. This seems to confirm that the U.N. system of post adjustments provides a pretty good gauge of cost-of-living differences.

Comprehensive Review of Allowances

In addition to base pay and post adjustment, there is a third major element of remuneration, that of allowances. These include the education grant, allowances for spouses, children, and secondary dependents, separation payments, and travel entitlements. The Assembly had been unconvinced of the thoroughness of the Commission's review in this area and had requested an "overview of the package of common allowances" together with the package of common allowances provided by the U.S. federal civil service. This overview was duly prepared and submitted to the Assembly [A/45/30, Annex VII]. The review itself could not be completed in the absence of information on U.S. tax practices with regard to dependents, and the Assembly is expecting a further report on this matter at its 46th Session [A/Res/45/241 IV].

The Assembly also received important proposals from the ICSC with regard to the education allowance. Expatriate staff with children face special problems in securing for their children an education that will equip them to the same extent as their peers who stay at home for later life in their home countries or elsewhere. This goal is achieved by sending them home to boarding school or to special schools in countries where their parents are serving. The ICSC's proposals were aimed at updating the financial entitlements that make this process possible.

Last year the ceiling on allowable costs stood at $9,000, with 8.2 percent of parents' actual expenses exceeding that figure. Determining a single amount that would be adequate for all duty stations and home countries is hard because the ceiling is expressed in U.S. dollars, while most of the school fees and other expenses have to be paid in currencies whose relationship to the dollar is continually varying. Also, such fees and expenses are affected by widely different rates of inflation. Under the system previously in force, currency relationships were taken into account while inflation was not, which penalized parents with children in schools in low-inflation countries where inflation was not largely factored into currency devaluations vis-à-vis the dollar.

In order to bring greater fairness to the system, the ICSC suggested that the ceiling be kept unchanged at $9,000 for most currency areas but be increased slightly for fees and expenses paid for in British, German, Italian, Spanish, and U.S. currencies. The Assembly approved this suggestion as an interim measure on the understanding that the Commission would conduct a full study in 1991 of the whole process for setting education grant levels [A/45/30, paras. 240–53, A/Res/45/241 X].

In March 1991 the Commission returned to this technically thorny and emotionally charged subject. The organizations felt that the implications of the shift from a "countries" to a "currencies" base needed further consideration. School prices would need to be checked against parents' expenditure reports. The Commission plans to revert to this matter in August 1991 on the basis of a paper refining the methodology now in use.

Pension Matters

Pension entitlements might be regarded as a fourth element of staff remuneration. In view of the U.N.'s compulsory early retirement age— formerly 60, now 62—its career staff are naturally concerned that they could suffer financial hardships during a period of retirement that now averages about 17 years. The early retirement age and the increasing longevity of both men and women make it more and more expensive to finance the U.N. Pension Fund on an actuarially sound basis. For each dollar of staff remuneration, nearly 24 cents has to be paid into the Fund, with one-third deducted from staff paychecks and two-thirds added to the assessments imposed on governments.

A comprehensive review of pension arrangements was also called for as long ago as 1986, but could not be completed until after other conditions of service had been reviewed. Had the Commission decided to alter the basic structure of remuneration by separating out housing from post adjustments, this would have necessitated a rethinking of the way in which pensionable remuneration is calculated. The technical complexities that this would have involved were one of several factors militating against making that change.

The General Assembly has two subsidiary bodies that deal with pensions: the ICSC, composed exclusively of independent experts appointed by it, and the Joint Staff Pension Board, composed of representatives of governments, U.N. administrations, and staff. The relative roles and pecking-order positions of the two bodies have been somewhat murky in the past, but the Assembly reaffirmed "the central role of the ICSC in the regulation and co-ordination of conditions of service, *including pensionable remuneration of all graded and ungraded staff*, of the U.N. common system" (emphasis added) [A/Res/45/241]. The Board retains its primacy in other pension areas (such as investments and pensioners' payment entitlements), and its views on pensionable remuneration continue to be taken into account by the Commission and the Assembly.

Paralleling the margin problems between U.N. salary levels and comparator salary levels are similar margin problems between U.N. pensions and pensions received by retired U.S. civil servants. If the margin between the two widens, voices are raised to complain that it has become excessive. At the same time, international staff feel that they have a right to expect that their after-service remuneration in their home countries will not be attenuated to conform with the eccentric movements of the pension levels of one set of national officials or the exigencies of successive U.S. budgetary crunches.

In its 1990 discussions, some members of the Pension Board continued to oppose the introduction of a margin range. They feared that, if introduced, it would probably lead to the same 110 to 120 range restrictions on pension movements that governed other forms of remuneration. They felt that staff pensions, which were supposed to be set at a pre-agreed percentage of the remuneration they enjoyed while serving the Organization (an approach known as "income replacement"), should not be made subject to margin considerations. They pointed out that this was unnecessary since pensionable remuneration already derived directly from net remuneration, which was in its turn controlled by the 110 to 120 margin range [A/45/9, para. 51].

The Commission agreed that there was a need for stability of pensionable remuneration and pensions and that income replacement should remain the cornerstone for determining their levels. On the other hand, it felt that controlling pensionable remuneration by merely monitoring it without a clearly defined and approved margin range was not sufficient. It saw a need to agree on what constituted maximum and minimum margin levels; at the same time, it believed that the levels at which action would be required should be left open-ended and decided on a case-by-case basis. With that understanding, there was wide support within the Commission for the establishment of a margin range for pensionable remuneration, and a range of 110 to 120 was actually recommended. There was hope that the coming changes in U.S. federal salary arrangements mentioned earlier would ultimately help minimize margin problems in pensionable remuneration [A/45/30, paras. 20–38]. However that may be, the Assembly contented itself with calling for income replacement ratios to be calculated at the end of each year for both the U.N. system and the comparator and for the Commission and the Board to continue to submit their recommendations thereon to the Assembly [A/45/Res/242I].

More vexing are the problems with regard to the establishment of pensionable remuneration and pension levels for locally recruited staff. There are more than 150 separate scales for this category of staff based on the best prevailing wages at each local duty station throughout the world. At present, the full gross salaries received by locally recruited staff are used in calculating their pension entitlements. This approach has been criticized as being overgenerous and out of line with pensions being paid to professional retirees.

In March 1991, in addressing this problem, the Commission pointed out that logic suggested that pensions, as well as salaries, should be based on the best prevailing local conditions. The problem that this approach might leave some local staff without any (or very low) pensions might be remedied by offering a generous minimum pension. The Commission also noted that the obstacles to this approach had been identified prior to 1980 and that a fresh effort was needed to assess whether it could and should now be pursued. If the needed documentation is ready by the time the Commission meets in August 1991, the 46th Assembly may have before it the Commission's proposals for revamping the basis on which this large category of pensions is calculated.

Maintaining the Integrity of the Common System of Salaries and Allowances

Organizations and governments, like individuals, dislike having to adhere to common procedures that they deem contrary to their best interests. There is, accordingly, always pressure for variances. For example, it is argued that doctors and atomic scientists cannot be recruited at pay scales suitable for administrators. Sometimes these variances are not requested but simply adopted without permission being sought. Such actions place the Commission in an adversarial relationship with the various Secretariat executive heads, and the Assembly at loggerheads with the governing organs of the specialized agencies or even with individual governments. Two further instances of such coordination problems occurred during the past year: **supplementary payments by some governments** to their own nationals on international organization payrolls and the **granting of extra longevity steps** to staff by some organizations.

The problem of governments persuading national officials to join international secretariats by sweetening their pay packages (sometimes by promising payments after they leave these secretariats) is an old one. The several administrations and staff unions are united in their opposition to these practices. Governments engaging in them violate the principle of equal pay for equal work and jeopardize the independence of their nationals working in the various secretariats, who could not escape the suspicion of being beholden to the sources of their additional income. It may be noted that in Article 100 of the Charter, governments have promised "not to seek to influence them in the discharge of their responsibilities." In the past, governments had been asked to report on their involvement in such unacceptable practices, but some may have evaded the matter by simply failing to reply. Others, such as Germany,

306 • A Global Agenda: Issues Before the 46th General Assembly

Japan, and the United States, have openly acknowledged that they engage in them.

In 1990, the increasingly frustrated Commission weighed the possibility of instituting disciplinary procedures against staff members in receipt of such payments and even of asking staff to attest to the fact that they did not receive them. It decided against taking this course, which would have infringed upon the privacy of the overwhelming majority of staff who were not involved. It did report to the Assembly that 51 states had not replied to the questionnaire, including four of the permanent members of the Security Council (Britain, China, France, and the Soviet Union). It reaffirmed that "such arrangements were unnecessary, inappropriate and undesirable and, moreover, inconsistent with the provisions of the staff regulations of the organizations and as such must stop" [A/45/30, paras. 209–20].

The Assembly continued to support the Commission's position, noting the efforts of some governments to reduce these practices and inviting others to reply to the Commission's questionnaire. It also requested the executive heads of U.N. organizations and the Commission to do what they could to resolve this problem. It failed, however, to single out and criticize the governments that persisted in creating the problem [A/Res/45/241 IX].

Another issue, this one involving organizations more than governments, is raised by what are called **longevity steps.** Under the base salary scales set by the Assembly, there are both "grades," reflecting functions of differing importance and responsibility, and in-grade "steps," reflecting growing experience and satisfactory service in carrying out the same functions. Promotions to a higher grade usually take place at fairly long intervals. In the meantime, each year, or two years in some cases, staff receive small increases in their base salaries that recognize increasing length of satisfactory in-grade service. However, the number of such steps is limited, and many staff reach the top step, after which their pay is frozen (except for cost-of-living increases). It follows that the number of steps in each grade is of importance to staff, and that variations in these numbers among organizations—for example, by having more steps in a particular grade—threaten the impartial administration of the common system of salaries and allowances as a whole.

The ILO has two additional steps and the WHO has six (in some cases seven) additional steps for each grade beyond the number approved by the Assembly. The concern that this creates is heightened by the fact that appointments are not always made at the lowest step of a grade; candidates may be hired at a mid-step or even a high step. Putting all this together, the pay scales offered by these organizations are appreciably more generous than those of other U.N. organizations.

Again, the problem is not a new one; the WHO arrangements date back to 1948. In 1990 the representative of WHO, speaking to the Commission, insisted that theirs is a merit scheme, not a longevity scheme, which was installed and continues to be supported by its governing organs. The ILO representative, citing similar arguments, informed the Commission that its Director-General had on two occasions informed the Organization's Governing Body of the ICSC's recommendation to abolish the system and of his intention to maintain it. On neither occasion had the Governing Body raised any objection to this course. The WHO sometimes argues that it is difficult to recruit doctors at pay levels sufficient to attract other professional categories of staff. The ILO, because of its association with labor and workers' rights, regards itself as occupying a somewhat special position in matters of this kind.

The Commission pointed out that only ILO and WHO had granted both their professional and general service staff extra longevity steps. The morale problem of having too many staff at the top level of their grade had been addressed by the Commission in the context of the general review, and extra steps had been added to most grades. The Commission also said that merit as well as long service were already implicit in this lengthening of horizontal steps. Other ways of rewarding merit had also been suggested in its earlier report (see *Issues/45*, pp. 253–54 for details). The Commission added that the variances in the ILO and WHO pay scales meant that their staff would receive pensions as much as 16 percent higher than their colleagues in other U.N. agencies and organizations.

The Commission once again asked the Directors-General of ILO and WHO to bring this matter to the attention of their legislative bodies; it suggested that the changeover be sweetened by the payment of one-time nonpensionable cash awards to the staff who would be adversely affected; and it asked them to report back in 1992 [A/45/30, paras. 143–63]. In its turn, the Assembly stressed the importance of agency governing bodies taking common positions on matters of concern for the U.N. common system and, in particular, urged the governing bodies of the ILO and WHO "to bring their salary scales into line with those of other U.N. organizations." It went on to urge member states to ensure that their representatives attending meetings of the agency governing organs are informed of these positions taken by the Commission and the Assembly. Judging from the tenure of the debate, the representative of the Philippines was speaking for almost all members when he said "that all measures to improve the working conditions of the staff should be uniformly and universally applied. The decisions of certain U.N. agencies to make individual adjustments defeated the very idea of a common system" [A/C.5/45/SR.31, p. 5; A/Res/45/241 VI].

The General Assembly has now largely completed its action on the ICSC's general review, and the Commission will henceforth be mainly involved in seeing that organizations carry out the changes in conditions of service that have been approved. Despite the disappointment expressed by a number of delegations over the extent of the reforms achieved, it would appear that the Commission has done as well as it could given the constant pressure (maintained by the 45th Assembly) that any and all additional costs should somehow be absorbed [A/Res/45/241I, para. 3].

Review of the Commission's Functioning

For several years now questions have been raised in the Assembly and elsewhere as to whether the Commission is functioning as well as it should be. In December 1989 the Assembly asked the Secretary-General to consult the executive heads of the U.N. system in the Administrative Committee on Coordination (ACC) and the Commission itself and to submit his views and suggestions on this subject.

At its March 1991 session the Commission was consulted on a draft paper prepared by the system's administrators for their bosses in the ACC, which inter alia visualized the possibility of transforming the Commission into a tripartite body like the Pension Board, composed of representatives of governments, organizations, and staff. It also addressed a staff proposal that decisions emanating from the Commission should be a negotiated set of decisions. Members felt that such a working arrangement would be contrary to the existing statute and incompatible with the independent role that an impartial body of experts advisory to the General Assembly should exercise. They also expressed the view that the employers of international staff were those who financed the organizations—that is to say, member states and their governments, rather than executive heads. The Commission plans to return to these politically charged questions at its August 1991 session and to present its views on them to the Assembly in its annual report.

Other Personnel Questions: Secondment of National Civil Servants

The Soviet Union and a number of other governments had long insisted that their nationals could serve in the U.N. Secretariat only as "seconded staff" loaned to the Organization for a fixed term of years and subject to recall when they were needed at home. Many of these governments have now revised this policy to allow their nationals to join the international career service in the usual way. The Soviet representative signified his government's change of policy with the following statement in the Fifth Committee:

> The Soviet Union had made its own contribution to [improving the functioning of the U.N. executive machinery] by discarding obsolete approaches to personnel matters. Recognizing the need to ensure continuity and maintain a permanent core of highly qualified personnel, it has amended its recruitment criteria; henceforth, Soviet specialists would serve in the Secretariat so long as the Organization required. Some of them had received career appointments and the number was increasing. The Soviet Union intended to comply fully with the international norms and standards for practices associated with the service of Soviet citizens in international organizations" [A/C.5/45/SR.15, p. 7].

Traditionally, secondment is the practice by which an official is posted to another service for a specified period, under defined terms and conditions, with the expectation that at the end of that period he or she will return to the service of origin. As of July 1990, seven member states had approximately 430 nationals on secondment to the U.N. Secretariat who served without having severed their legal relationship with their own governments.

In his report to the Assembly [A/C.5/45/12], the Secretary-General explained that secondment has advantages and disadvantages. Among the former is its value in obtaining skilled and experienced staff unavailable on any other basis and in helping maintain an appropriate balance latterbetween fixed-term and career staff. Among the disadvantages of secondment are that it undermines the impression of a truly independent international civil service responsible only to the Secretary-General and involves a more frequent rotation of staff members, with attendant higher costs in money and efficiency. He concluded that while secondment might be beneficial on a limited scale, it could, under certain circumstances, undermine the independence and efficiency of the Secretariat.

More serious problems have arisen when seconded staff have asked to join the U.N. career service. When turned down, some of these staff have appealed to the **Administrative Tribunal,** which has on a number of occasions reviewed aspects of the practice of secondment. In a judgment handed down on May 25, 1990, the Tribunal held that the arrangements to which the applicants were parties had not constituted genuine secondment because their status had not been defined in writing to specify the conditions and duration of the secondment. It also held that the refusal to grant the applicants career appointments after five years of good service on fixed-term appointments was a violation of Article 100 of the Charter and of the 37th General Assembly's Resolution 126.

The Secretary-General explained to the Assembly that while the judgment maintained the institution of secondment, it would be necessary to introduce more formal procedures to ensure that all parties were left in no doubt about the nature of the particular contract. It also meant that all staff, including those on secondment, would be entitled to "every reasonable consideration for career appointment after five or more years of continuing good service." However, in deciding whether to grant such appointments, the Secretary-General would be guided by what he deemed to be in the best interests of the Organization.

In the debate in the Fifth Committee, only the Chinese delegation supported the old system and expressed disappointment with the Tribunal's decision. The Assembly endorsed the basic approach outlined above and requested the Secretary-General to review the procedures for future secondments from government service, taking into account the legitimate interests of the Organization, the government service, and the individual concerned. It also asked him to submit appropriate amendments to the staff regulations to the Assembly's 1991 session; such amendments are now in preparation [A/Res/45/239 II].

Women in the Secretariat

The United Nations' long campaign to increase the proportion of women staff members in the Secretariat's professional posts subject to geographical distribution continued to make progress but failed at year-end 1990 to attain its target of 30 percent. As of April 1991 the figure had finally moved above 29 percent, a level only about 0.7 percent higher than in mid-1990. At the same time, if language posts not subject to geographical distribution are included, the goal was attained in mid-1990, the overall figure having been 30.14 percent. This is because nearly 35 percent of the staff in this latter category are women. In assessing these results, it must be borne in mind that between 1986 and 1990 the number of professional posts subject to geographical distribution shrank from 2,710 to 2,541, or 6.24 percent, reducing by that much the number of posts for which women could be hired.

Certain regions continue to lag far behind others in this campaign, as the following figures for the end of February 1991 reveal:

Region	*Proportion of Women Staff*
Africa	15.79%
Asia and the Pacific	34.00%
Eastern Europe	9.77%
Latin America	32.42%
Middle East	18.94%
Western Europe	32.66%
North America and the Caribbean	42.32%

[Source: U.N. Secretariat]

Rapid further progress seems unlikely so long as the three laggard regions remain so far behind the other four. On the positive side, authorities in the Soviet Union and other Eastern European countries are now actively involved in improving their region's record.

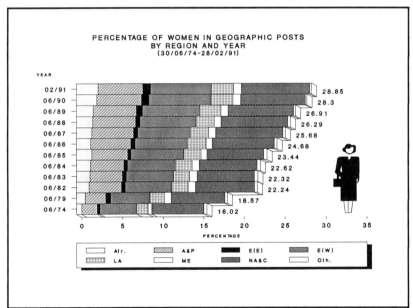

The situation at the higher levels of the Secretariat remains very unsatisfactory, as the following figures for the end of February 1991 show:

Level	No. of Posts	No. of Posts Occupied by Women	Proportion Occupied by Women
Under-Secretary-General	26	2	7.7%
Asst. Secretary-General	19	0	0
D-2	84	10	11.9%
D-1	234	15	6.4%
Total:	363	27	7.4%

[Source: U.N. Secretariat]

The table shows the extent to which women continue to be underrepresented in U.N. policy-making posts. Even more than in the case of the overall figures, this may be attributed to the deliberate shrinkage of the number of these posts during the recent downscaling of the Secretariat, which hit the highest-level posts hardest. The disparity also reflects the intense interest that governments have in who among their nationals occupies the few high posts available to them and the keen competition between governments and regions for such posts, particularly for the top ones. These realities limit the extent to which the Secretary-General and his human resources chief can guide the recruitment process in favor of women candidates.

The ICSC has long been involved in this effort on behalf of women staff members. In 1990 it sought to clarify the situation regarding the employment of spouses. It has long been recognized that when the recruit is a married woman, her husband will often be unwilling to join her unless he can find appropriate employment at her duty station, which is often impossible because of the rules and attitudes of national authorities. One solution to this problem is that he, too, should find work with the international organization, assuming that he is qualified to fill a post that happens to be vacant.

The Commission noted that while no organization absolutely prohibited the employment of spouses, it was not usually encouraged for obvious reasons. In some organizations, spouses could be hired subject to certain conditions (for example, that there would be no direct hierarchical relationship in the work place); in others it was not normally permitted, but exceptions were occasionally made; while in very small organizations it was simply not feasible. Recognizing the delicacy of this question, the Commission limited itself to recommending that organizations rescind any staff rule they might have prohibiting the employment of spouses and intensify their efforts "to facilitate as appropriate the employment of staff members' spouses."

The Commission also blamed "traditional attitudes" for the slow progress of the campaign. While agreeing that qualifications had to be "the main and indeed the sole criterion" in the recruitment and promotion of men and women, most members held that affirmative action programs favoring women were a necessity until the organizations had attained the targets set by them. To this end, organizations should inform those national administrations that still require their candidates to be sponsored of the importance they attach to submitting the names of women candidates. The Commission also urged the highly technical organizations that had the most trouble recruiting women to consider outreach training programs along the lines of the one already developed by the International Maritime Organization. Finally, it invited all the organizations in the U.N. system to intensify their efforts to increase the proportion of women in their decision-making and policy-shaping posts [A/45/30, paras. 271–80].

Returning now to the situation in the United Nations itself, in 1990 the Secretary-General submitted his usual report on improving the status of women in the Secretariat [A/45/548]. As in past years, attention has centered on recruitment and promotion policies for women. With regard to recruitment, over half the women entering the Secretariat have been appointed on the basis of their performance in competitive examinations. As in the past, full use has been made of staff on official missions to address meetings of national professional women's groups in order to spread information about employment opportunities at the United Nations and to encourage women to take part in the various competitive examinations. Sixty-one permanent missions in New York have nominated one of their staff members to serve as "focal point" and have received kits with information on the proportion of women in their country's contingent in the Secretariat, together with a note on how to find vacancy announcements and on how to apply for the vacant posts. They are also urged to establish rosters of their qualified women who might be available for international service.

Career development is another realm in which the situation of women requires monitoring and improvement. Almost all posts should be open to women on an equal basis with men, and the increasing service of women on missions and at hardship posts indicates that more can be done to achieve this equality in practice. For example, women made up 50 percent of the U.N. Assistance Group in Namibia. It is of even greater importance that their progress up the career ladder be at least as rapid as that of their male colleagues. In the promotions to grades P-3, P-4, and P-5 that took place between mid-1989 and mid-1990, this goal was achieved, but there were only three promotions of women to the D-1 level, representing a mere 11 percent of the total. Still, in years to come the presence of 72 and 197 women in the P-5 and P-4 pools, respectively, should make it easier to find suitable candidates for policy-making posts at the higher levels.

The institutional arrangements for achieving these goals remain the same: a Steering Committee for the Improvement of the Status of Women in the Secretariat and a focal point for women in the Office of the Assistant Secretary-General for Human Resources Management. The Steering Committee meets regularly and has so far come up with some 50 recommendations that either have been implemented or are in the process of being implemented. The focal point maintains ties not only with the permanent governmental missions in New York but with persons designated by each of the departments and offices within the Secretariat, thus creating a double network to facilitate forward movement in this area. The main obstacles to such progress continue to be the lack of commitment on the part of some senior officials, a still inadequate cumulative base of experienced female professional staff, and what is perceived as the usual male networking.

At the 45th Assembly almost all speakers paid at least lip service to the goal of increasing the proportion of women professionals in posts subject to geographical distribution. Some of them went a good deal further than that. The representative of Australia, speaking on behalf of Canada and New Zealand as well, complained that none of the 19 persons appointed to posts at the P-5 level and above in the year ending June 30, 1990, had been a woman. He went on to say:

> It could not, moreover, be assumed that women at the lower levels of the Secretariat would eventually rise to the top. Even if some did so, there remained barriers—sometimes referred to as the "glass ceiling"— which prevented women from rising to senior posts; in its evaluation, the Secretariat should identify such barriers and develop an action plan to remove them. Women were needed in senior posts not only as a matter of social justice, but also because they brought distinctive management styles with them, including open dialogue with employees, the sharing of information, an ability to listen and to build consensus, and an emphasis on participation and teamwork [A/C.5/45/SR.19, p. 6].

In its resolution on this subject, the General Assembly for the first time set a new target—35 percent by 1995—for the proportion of professional staff subject to geographical distribution that should be women. At the same time, it indicated that this target should be achieved without affecting standards of efficiency, competence, and integrity or violating the principle of equitable geographical distribution. It also set a target of 25 percent for the proportion of women to be in posts at the D-1 level or higher by 1995. The Secretary-General was asked to make every effort to increase the number of women from developing countries, particularly at the higher levels. He was also asked to develop an action program in this area that would include an analysis of the main obstacles, his ideas on how they could best be overcome, and a detailed program of activities accompanied by monitoring procedures and a timetable for their completion. Finally, member states were requested to nominate more women candidates, particularly for higher posts, and to set up rosters of such candidates that they would share with the personnel offices of the various U.N. organizations [A/Res/45/239C].

In March 1991 the Secretary-General established the following new policy to meet the targets just established by the Assembly for 1995:

> In departments and offices with less than 35 percent of women overall and in those with less than 25 percent women at levels P-5 and above, vacancies overall and in the latter group, respectively, shall be filled, when there are one or more female candidates whose qualifications match all the requirements for a vacant post, by one of those female candidates.

Also, he ordered that the same policy apply to posts being filled by outside recruitment, except when competitive examinations had been scheduled for this purpose or 18 months had passed without a qualified woman candidate being found [ST/SGB/237].

Composition of the Secretariat

This old war-horse issue aroused less delegation interest than usual last year because fewer member states can now claim to be unrepresented (only 11 remain) or underrepresented (in the last year the number fell from 26 to 19) in the Secretariat. The unrepresented states are Albania, the Bahamas, Brunei, Djibouti, Dominica, Kuwait, the Maldives, Mozambique, Sao Tome and Principe, the Solomon Islands, and Vanuatu, many of them ministates not very active in U.N. affairs. On the other hand, the underrepresented states include major countries, such as China, Indonesia, Italy, Japan, Portugal, Romania, and Vietnam, as well as very small states, such as Cape Verde, Qatar, and St. Vincent and the Grenadines. While most of the oil-rich Gulf states, including Saudi Arabia and the United Arab Emirates, are appreciably underrepresented, the most glaring example is that of Japan, which should have between 152 and 206 staff members and actually has only 91. Because these unrepresented and underrepresented countries are not concentrated in any single region and include both developed and developing countries, the issue no longer creates a general stir, apart from the feeling among many developing countries that their claims have been insufficiently met. At the same time, expressions of indignation on the part of those most affected seem to evoke little general response.

However, in addition to the matter of the sex ratio, three main issues remain: the distribution of higher-level posts; the question of the entitlement formulas that determine for each member the so-called desirable range that governs the number of posts allocated to it; and finally the question of whether more posts should be brought within the scope of those subject to geographical distribution. Not surprisingly, the competition for higher-level posts (D-2 and above) has grown in intensity since their number was reduced from 143 in 1986 to 123 in 1990. The Secretary-General's report on the composition of staff [A/45/541, Table D] revealed that six of the seven regional groups now had fewer nationals serving at these higher levels, while the seventh, Western Europe, had seen its number increase from 29 to 32. The decreases for other regions had been as follows: Africa (1), Asia and the Pacific (9), Eastern Europe (3), Latin America (3), Middle East (4), and North America and the Caribbean (3). Several speakers complained of this, and the General Assembly requested the Secretary-General "to take every available measure to ensure, at the senior and policy-formulating levels of the Secretariat, the equitable representation of Member states, in particular of developing countries and Member states with inadequate representation at those levels. . . ." It approached the problem from other angles by insisting that no Assistant Secretary-General or Under-Secretary-General should serve for more than ten years and that no such post should be considered the "exclusive preserve" of any member state [A/Res/45/239, paras. 6–8].

Pressure is building for taking a new look at the entitlement formulas for "desirable ranges." The present formula is 40 percent for equal division among all members, large or small (the "membership factor"); 5 percent to be based on the population factor; and 55 percent to reflect the level of regular-budget assessment. The membership factor entitles each member to a desirable range of at least 2 to 14 posts without reference to their population and assessment levels. Some countries would like to have this range widened to 15 or 16 posts and to increase the proportion of posts allocated under this factor upward from 40 percent of the total. Some of these are smaller developing countries, either already overrepresented or near their ceilings under the existing system. Developed countries with high assessments may be expected to oppose such changes. The Secretary-General has been asked to prepare a report for the forthcoming session of the Assembly on alternative options, including other possible methods of distributing posts subject to geographical distribution. The Assembly also resolved to decide this matter then "on a priority basis" [A/Res/45/239 III].

Another way of resolving this problem would be to enlarge the pool of posts subject to geographical distribution, an approach advocated by some speakers in the Fifth Committee. Yet it is hard to see how this could be done without raising further problems. If posts financed from extrabudgetary sources, such as voluntary contributions to UNDP and UNICEF, were included, it might affect the level of those contributions. If posts excluded on grounds of special language requirements (translators, interpreters) were added, there would be loud complaints from those countries, a large and influential group, that now furnish most of this category of staff. If locally recruited staff were included, as one delegate suggested, their concentration at large duty stations would distort the entitlements of the host countries. However, in spite of these obstacles, some enlargement of the pool should not be entirely ruled out.

Promotion of Serving Staff

In 1989 the General Assembly asked the Secretary-General to submit a report on (a) the rules, regulations, and criteria that were being used for the promotion of serving staff; (b) the work of appointment and promotion bodies; and (c) the possibility of including in the vacancy management program effective appeal and recourse mechanisms [A/Res/44/185A]. He had not been able to prepare this report in time for the Assembly's 45th Session, which asked him to submit it in 1991. The Assistant Secretary-General for Human Resources Management nonetheless raised the promotion question in his opening statement:

> There was a growing malaise among staff members, who now had fewer opportunities for advancement because of the retrenchment exercise and because of the rigidity of the job classification system that led to the blocking of staff members at the same level whatever their experience or the quality of their work. One way to improve the morale and motivation of the staff while at the same time maintaining

the integrity of the job classification system would be, in the case of the entry and middle levels (G-1 to G-5 and P-2 to P-4), to base the promotion of staff members on merit and seniority whether posts existed or not. For staff at the higher levels, the availability of posts classified at the higher level would still remain a prerequisite for promotion. Those ideas required further reflection [A/C.5/45/SR.15, p. 4].

The Assembly agreed that the Secretary-General should pursue his efforts toward the establishment of a comprehensive career development system for all categories of staff. He was also asked to further refine the present staff classification and evaluation systems and promotion proce- dures as an integral part of the vacancy management system. However, there was a division of opinion on the merits of the personal promotion proposal. On this the Assembly as a whole took no position, pending its receipt of the Secretary-General's report on this subject later in 1991 [A/Res/45/239A].

Safety and Security of International Officials

The U.N. World Food Programme (WFP) put its finger on an ugly reality of some forms of international service: In times of civil war and other disturbances, operational requirements may compel its officials to take certain risks that place them in personal jeopardy. Nonetheless, governments have the duty, under the terms of multilateral treaties adopted for the safety and protection of international staff in carrying out whatever functions they may be assigned, to minimize such occa- sions. Above all, governments themselves should not interfere with staff when they are carrying out functions legally assigned to them.

These concerns are far from being merely academic. As the Secre- tary-General reported, three staff members were killed and another was brutally attacked during the period between mid-year 1989 and mid-year 1990. In Lebanon a UNICEF official driving home from the office was dragged from her car and then shot and killed. In Uganda three WFP employees were ambushed, with one of them killed and another suffering bullet wounds. Another WFP staff member was killed when a light plane flying over southern Sudan was deliberately shot down. Other examples of similar misbehavior could be cited. There has been a proposal that an international fund be set up to support the families of those who lose their lives in the line of duty.

The Middle East continues to be the region in which the arrest, detention, and abduction of officials is most common. For example, during the reporting period, 160 staff members of the U.N. Relief and

Works Agency for Palestine Refugees in the Near East (UNRWA) were arrested or detained, mostly by Israeli security forces; of these, some 100 were released without being charged or tried (2 in Jordan, 39 in the Gaza Strip, 53 in the West Bank, and 6 in Lebanon). In no case did UNRWA receive adequate and timely information on the reasons for these arrests and detentions. It did have access to 13 detained staff members from the West Bank and 47 from the Gaza Strip, while it learned that several others were being held in Israeli prisons. UNRWA also reports that unauthorized intrusions into its premises have resulted at times in injuries to its staff. In two such incidents, two UNRWA international staff members and one local staff member were arrested and force was used against them. Of those remaining in detention at the end of the reporting period, one was being held in Lebanon by the Syrian armed forces; one was in Syria; and the other 49 were being held in the Gaza Strip or the West Bank. In addition, 43 persons involved in earlier incidents were still being held in one or another of these places [A/C.5/45/10].

The Legal Counsel, in presenting the Secretary-General's report to the Fifth Committee, pointed out that the problem of staff security was growing now that the United Nations was more operationally oriented and had more staff serving in troubled areas; sometimes it also involved their families, including children. He cited one troubling example, that of Guenet Mabrahtu, a WHO staff member arrested by the Ethiopian security forces in June 1989 who was still being held in custody without formal explanation 16 months later. The representative of Ethiopia informed the Fifth Committee a few days later that Mrs. Mabrahtu had been arrested "for activities inconsistent with her responsibilities as an international civil servant" and that upon completion of the investigation she would be brought to trial in accordance with Ethiopian laws. He added that every effort was being made to ensure her well-being and that her WHO supervisor had been allowed to visit her. The Legal Counsel replied that the rather general allegations brought against Mrs. Mabrahtu did not seem to justify her continued detention and appealed for her release [A/C.5/45/SR.15, 26, 28].

Many speakers in the debate on personnel matters stressed the great importance that their governments attached to the protection and safety of international staff in the performance of their official duties. In its resolution on this subject, the Assembly urged member states and others responsible for the illegal detention of U.N. staff members to release them immediately. It called upon member states holding officials under arrest or detention to allow officials from their organizations to have immediate access to them. It also asked that they be provided, as necessary, with medical care and treatment, in some cases by independent medical teams. At the same time, it reminded international officials of their duty to observe both the laws and regulations of member states and of their responsibilities to the organizations they serve [A/Res/45/240].

Role of the Staff Union

Questions were raised in the Fifth Committee on the role of the Staff Union in decisions on pay and benefits and on the threat of job actions. It was held that the practice of financing Union activities from the Organization's budget was difficult to justify, and the Secretary-General was asked to provide information concerning such expenditures in his program budget, which will be before the Assembly at its 1991 session [A/Res/45/239, para. 21].

Appendix

The United Nations at a Glance

THE
UNITED
NATIONS
AT A GLANCE

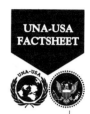

UNA-USA
FACTSHEET

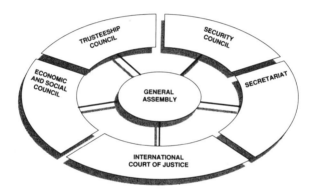

I. GENERAL ASSEMBLY

The General Assembly is composed of the U.N.'s 159 members, and each has one vote. It controls the U.N.'s finances, makes nonbinding recommendations on a variety of issues, and oversees and elects some members of other U.N. organs. By tradition, the Assembly meets in plenary session from the third Tuesday in September through mid-December, but with the growth of its agenda in recent years it has tended to resume the plenary shortly after January 1 to extend the session for a few weeks. The Assembly can also meet in emergency session to address an immediate threat to international peace and security—as it has done on nine occasions (most recently in 1982)—and in special sessions—as it has done on 18 occasions (most recently in April 1990 on International Economic Cooperation).

Major Committees of the General Assembly

President of the 45th General Assembly .... H.E. Guido de Marco (Malta)

Committees	Chairpersons
First Committee (Political and Security)	H.E. Jai Pratap Rana (Nepal)
Special Political Committee (Other political issues, including most disarmament issues)	H.E. Perezi Karukubiro-Kamunanwire (Uganda)
Second Committee (Economic and Financial)	H.E. George Papadatos (Greece)
Third Committee (Social, Humanitarian and Cultural)	H.E. Juan O. Somavia (Chile)
Fourth Committee (Decolonization)	H.E. Martin Adouki (Congo)
Fifth Committee (Administrative and Budgetary)	H.E. Ernest Besley Maycock (Barbados)
Sixth Committee (Legal)	H.E. Vaclav Mikulka (Czechoslovakia)

Housekeeping committees make recommendations on the adoption of the agenda, the allocation of items, and the organization of work. Some housekeeping committees:

1. General Committee
2. Credentials Committee
3. Committee on Relations with the Host Country
4. Committee on Conferences
5. Committee on Contributions
6. Committee for Programme and Coordination

Other bodies include:

1. Board of Auditors
2. International Civil Service Commission
3. Joint Inspection Unit
4. Panel of External Auditors of the United Nations, the Specialized Agencies, and the International Atomic Energy Agency
5. Administrative Tribunal
6. United Nations Joint Staff Pension Board
7. United Nations Staff Pension Committee
8. Investments Committee
9. Advisory Committee on Administrative and Budgetary Questions

Special Committees that Report on Special Issues

There are some 75 such subsidiary organs, among them:

1. Special Committee on the Situation with regard to the Implementation of the Declaration on the Granting of Independence to Colonial Countries and Peoples
2. Committee on the Exercise of the Inalienable Rights of the Palestinian People
3. Special Committee against Apartheid
4. Ad Hoc Committee on the Drafting of an International Convention against Apartheid in Sports
5. Committee on the Peaceful Uses of Outer Space
6. Special Committee on Peacekeeping Operations
7. United Nations Scientific Committee on the Effects of Atomic Radiation
8. Ad Hoc Committee on International Terrorism

Commissions

Three major commissions report to the General Assembly:

1. *International Law Commission*, established in 1947 to promote the development and codification of international law. The Commission, which is made up of 25 experts elected by the Assembly for five-year terms, meets every year in Geneva to prepare drafts on topics of its own choice and on topics referred to it by the Assembly and by the Economic and Social Council.

2. *United Nations Commission on International Trade*, established in 1966 to promote the harmonization of international trade law and to draft international trade conventions. The 36-country body also provides developing countries with training and assistance in international trade law.

3. *Disarmament Commission*, a deliberative body established by the General Assembly in 1952. Reporting annually to the Assembly, it makes recommendations on various problems in the field of disarmament to be submitted as recommendations to the Assembly and, through it, to the negotiating body—the Conference of the Committee on Disarmament.

Other Organizations Created by and Reporting to the General Assembly:

■ **Office of the United Nations Disaster Relief Coordinator (UN-DRO)**—clearinghouse for information on relief needs and assistance, and mobilizer and co-ordinator of emergency assistance.

■ **Office of the United Nations High Commissioner for Refugees (UNHCR)**—extends international protection and material assistance to refugees and negotiates with governments to resettle or repatriate refugees.

■ **United Nations Centre for Human Settlements (Habitat)**—deals with the housing problems of the urban and rural poor in developing countries, providing technical assistance and training, organizing meetings, and disseminating information.

■ **United Nations Children's Fund (UNICEF)**—provides technical and financial assistance to developing countries for programs benefiting children and also provides emergency relief to mothers and children. It is financed by voluntary contributions.

■ **United Nations Conference on Trade and Development (UNCTAD)**—works to establish agreements on commodity stabilization and to codify principles of international trade that are conducive to development.

■ **United Nations Development Fund for Women (UNIFEM)**—an autonomous agency associated with the U.N. Development Programme that supports projects benefiting women in developing countries. It is financed by voluntary contributions.

■ **United Nations Development Programme (UNDP)**—coordinates the development work of all U.N. and related agencies. The world's largest multilateral technical assistance program (UNDP currently supports more than 5,000 projects around the world), it is financed by voluntary contributions.

■ **United Nations Environment Programme (UNEP)**—monitors environmental conditions, implements environmental projects, develops recommended standards, promotes technical assistance and training, and supports the development of alternative energy sources.

■ **United Nations Population Fund (UNFPA)**—helps countries to gather demographic information and to plan population projects. Its governing body is the Governing Council of UNDP, and it is financed by the voluntary contributions of governments.

■ **United Nations Institute for Training and Research (UNITAR)**—an autonomous organization within the U.N. that provides training to government and U.N. officials and conducts research on a variety of international issues.

■ United Nations Relief and Works Agency for Palestine Refugees in the Near East (UNRWA)—provides education, health, and relief services to Palestinian refugees.

■ United Nations University (UNU)—an autonomous academic institution chartered by the General Assembly. It has a worldwide network of associated institutions, research units, individual scholars, and UNU fellows, coordinated through the UNU center in Tokyo, but no faculty or degree students.

■ United Nations International Research and Training Institute (INSTRAW)—an autonomous, voluntarily funded body that conducts research, training, and information activities to integrate women in development.

■ World Food Council (WFC)—a 36-nation body that meets annually at the ministerial level to review major issues affecting the world food situation.

■ World Food Programme (WFP)—jointly sponsored by the U.N. and the Food and Agriculture Organization, supplies both emergency food relief and food aid to support development projects.

II. SECURITY COUNCIL

The Security Council has primary responsibility within the U.N. system for maintaining international peace and security. It may determine the existence of any threat to international peace, make recommendations or take enforcement measures to resolve the problem, and establish U.N. peacekeeping forces. The Security Council has 15 members: 5 permanent members designated by the U.N. Charter and 10 nonpermanent members nominated by informal regional caucuses and elected for two-year terms; five are elected each year. Decisions on substantive matters require nine votes; a negative vote by any permanent member is sufficient to defeat the motion. Security Council resolutions are binding on all U.N. member states.

Permanent Members	Term Ending Dec. 31, 1991	Term Ending Dec. 31, 1992
China	Côte d'Ivoire	Austria
France	Cuba	Belgium
USSR	Romania	Ecuador
United Kingdom	Yemen	India
United States	Zaire	Zimbabwe

III. ECONOMIC AND SOCIAL COUNCIL (ECOSOC)

Under the authority of the General Assembly, ECOSOC coordinates the economic and social work of the U.N. and its large family of specialized and affiliated institutions. ECOSOC meets in plenary session twice a year for a month at a time, once in New York and once in Geneva. The 54 members of ECOSOC are elected by the General Assembly for three-year terms; 18 are elected each year.

Term Expires Dec. 31, 1991	Term Expires Dec. 31, 1992	Term Expires Dec. 31, 1993
Bahamas	Algeria	Argentina
Brazil	Bahrain	Austria
Cameroon	Bulgaria	Botswana
Czechoslovakia	Burkina Faso	Chile
Indonesia	Canada	France
Iraq	China	Germany
Italy	Ecuador	Guinea
Jordan	Finland	Japan
Kenya	Iran (Islamic	Malaysia
Netherlands	Republic of)	Morocco
New Zealand	Jamaica	Peru
Nicaragua	Mexico	Somalia
Niger	Pakistan	Spain
Thailand	Romania	Syrian Arab
Tunisia	Rwanda	Republic
Ukrainian Soviet	Sweden	Trinidad & Tobago
Socialist Republic	Union of Soviet	Togo
United States of	Socialist Republics	Turkey
America	United Kingdom of	Yugoslavia
Zambia	Great Britain and	
	Northern Ireland	
	Zaire	

IV. TRUSTEESHIP COUNCIL

The five members of the Trusteeship Council—China, France, the USSR, the U.K., and the U.S.—are also the five permanent members of the Security Council. Only the U.S. still administers a trust territory—the strategic Trust Territory of the Pacific Islands (Micronesia). At birth, the Trusteeship Council had more members and administered 11 trust territories, but as the latter achieved independence or joined neighboring independent countries, the membership of the Council was reduced.

ORGANIZATION OF THE ECONOMIC AND SOCIAL COUNCIL

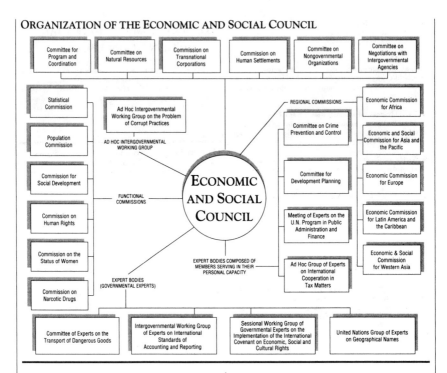

V. INTERNATIONAL COURT OF JUSTICE (WORLD COURT)

The International Court of Justice hears cases referred to it by the states involved and provides advisory opinions to the General Assembly and the Security Council at their request. It is made up of 15 members, who are elected by an absolute majority of both the Security Council and the General Assembly for nine-year terms; five judges are elected every three years.

Term Expires Feb. 5, 1994	Term Expires Feb. 5, 1997
Taslim Olawale Elias (Nigeria)	Roberto Ago (Italy)
Jens Evensen (Norway)	Mohammed Bedjaoui (Algeria)
Manfred Lachs (Poland)	Stephen M. Schwebel (U.S.)
Ni Zhengyu (China)	MohamedShahabuddeen(Guyana)
Shigeru Oda (Japan)	Nikolai Konstantinovich Tarassov
	(USSR)

Term Expires Feb. 5, 2000
Andres Aguilar Mawdsley (Venezuela)
Gilbert Guillaume (France)
Robert Jennings (United Kingdom)
Christopher Gregory Weeramantry (Sri Lanka)
Raymond Rangeva (Madagascar)

VI. SECRETARIAT

The Secretariat administers the programs and policies established by the other U.N. organs. It is headed by the Secretary-General (currently Javier Pérez de Cuéllar of Peru), who is elected by the General Assembly on the recommendation of the Security Council for a five-year term. The Secretary-General is authorized by the U.N. Charter to bring to the attention of the Security Council any matter that he believes may threaten international peace and security (Article 99) and may use his good offices to attempt to resolve international disputes. Under the Secretary-General are the Director-General for Development and International Economic Co-operation (currently Antoine Blanca of France), 26 Under-Secretaries-General, and 26 Assistant Secretaries-General. Carrying out the day-to-day activities delegated to the Secretary-General is an international civil service staff of 14,000 (5,000 in New York, 9,000 elsewhere). Numbered among these are the technical experts and economic advisors who, working in the field, oversee economic and peacekeeping projects. Article 100 of the Charter calls upon the Secretary-General and the staff to maintain their independence from governmental or other authority external to the Organization and calls upon member states to recognize and respect "the exclusively international character of the responsibilities of the Secretary-General and the staff."

VII. SPECIALIZED AGENCIES

The specialized agencies are autonomous intergovernmental organizations related to the U.N. by special agreements. They report annually to the Economic and Social Council.

■ **Food and Agriculture Organization of the United Nations (FAO)** works to increase food production, raise rural standards of living, and help countries cope with emergency food situations.

Edouard Saouma (Lebanon), Director-General
Via delle Terme de Caracalla
Rome 00100, Italy

Washington, D.C. Office:
1776 F Street, N.W.
Washington, D.C. 20437

■ **International Civil Aviation Organization (ICAO)** works to facilitate and promote safe international air transportation by setting binding international standards and by recommending efficient practices. ICAO regulations govern international flights.

Shivinder Singh Sidhu (India), Secretary-General
1000 Sherbrooke Street W.
Montreal, Quebec H3A 2R2
Canada

■ **International Fund for Agricultural Development (IFAD)** lends money on concessional terms for agricultural development projects, primarily to increase food production for the poorest rural populations.

Idriss Jazairy (Algeria), President
Via Del Serafico 107
Rome 00142, Italy

■ **International Labour Organisation (ILO)** formulates international labor standards and provides technical assistance training to governments.

Michel Hansenne (Belgium), Director-General
4 Route des Morillons, CH-1211
Geneva 22, Switzerland

■ **International Maritime Organization (IMO)** promotes international cooperation on technical matters related to shipping and provides a forum to discuss and to adopt conventions and recommendations on such matters as safety at sea and pollution control.

C.P. Srivastava (India), Secretary-General
4 Albert Embankment
London, SEI 7SR, England

■ **International Monetary Fund (IMF)** provides technical assistance and financing to countries that are experiencing balance of payments difficulties.

Michel Camdessus (France), Managing Director
700 19th Street, N.W.
Washington, D.C. 20431

■ **International Telecommunication Union (ITU)** promotes international cooperation in telecommunications, allocates the radio-frequency spectrum, and collects and disseminates telecommunications information for its members.

Pekka J. Tarjanne (Finland), Secretary-General
Place Des Nations
1211 Geneva 20, Switzerland

■ **United Nations Educational, Scientific and Cultural Organization (UNESCO)** pursues international intellectual cooperation in education, science, culture, and communications and promotes development by means of social, cultural, and economic projects.

Federico Zaragoza Mayor (Spain), Director-General
UNESCO House
7, place de Fontenoy
75007 Paris, France

■ **United Nations Industrial Development Organization (UNIDO)**—to date, the only U.N. organ ever to be converted into an independent, specialized agency—serves as intermediary between developing and developed countries in the field of industry and as a forum for contacts, consultations, and negotiations to aid the process of industrialization.

Domingo L. Siazon, Jr. (Philippines), Director-General
Wagramerstrasse 5
Vienna XXII, Austria

■ **Universal Postal Union (UPU)** sets international postal standards and provides technical assistance to developing countries.

Adwaldo Cardoso Botto de Barros (Egypt), Director-General
Weltpoststrasse 4
Berne 1, Switzerland

■ **The World Bank** is actually three institutions: the **International Bank for Reconstruction and Development (IBRD)**; the **International Finance Corporation (IFC)**; and the **International Development Association (IDA)**. IBRD lends funds to governments (or to private enterprises, if the government guarantees repayment), usually for specific, productive projects. IFC lends to private corporations without government guarantees. IDA provides interest-free "credits" to the world's poorest countries for a period of 50 years, with a ten-year grace period.

Barber B. Conable (United States), President
1818 H Street, N.W.
Washington, D.C. 20433

New York Office:
737 Third Avenue, 26th Floor
New York, N.Y. 10017

■ **World Health Organization (WHO)** conducts immunization campaigns, promotes and coordinates research, and provides technical assistance to countries that are improving their health systems. It is currently coordinating a major effort to control and cure acquired immune deficiency syndrome—AIDS.

Dr. Hiroshi Nakajima (Japan), Director-General
20, avenue Appia
1211 Geneva 27, Switzerland

■ **World Intellectual Property Organization (WIPO)** promotes the protection of intellectual property (e.g., patents and copyrights). It encourages adherence to relevant treaties, provides legal and technical assistance to developing countries, encourages technology transfers, and administers the International Union for the Protection of Industrial Property and the International Union for the Protection of Literary and Artistic Works.

Dr. Arpad Bogsch (United States), Director-General
34 chemin des Colombettes
1211 Geneva 20, Switzerland

■ **World Meteorological Organization (WMO)** promotes the exchange and standardization of meteorological information through its World Weather Watch and conducts research and training programs.

G.O.P. Obasi (Nigeria), Secretary-General
41, avenue Giuseppe-Motta
1211 Geneva 20, Switzerland

Other Autonomous Affiliated Organizations

■ **General Agreement on Tariffs and Trade (GATT)** is a multilateral regime that sets out norms and rules for international trade and provides a forum for their further elaboration.

Arthur Dunkel (Switzerland), Director-General
Centre William Rappard
154, rue de Lausanne
1211 Geneva 21, Switzerland

■ **International Atomic Energy Agency (IAEA)** was established under U.N. auspices but is autonomous and not formally a specialized agency. It promotes the peaceful uses of nuclear energy; establishes standards for nuclear safety and environmental protection; and, by agreement with parties to the Non-Proliferation Treaty, carries out inspections to safeguard against diversion of nuclear materials to military uses.

Dr. Hans Blix (Sweden), Director-General
Vienna International Centre
P.O. Box 100
A-1400 Vienna, Austria

U.N. MEMBER STATES

Membership in the United Nations has more than tripled since the Organization's founding in 1945. There were 51 original member states; today there are 159 members, representing the majority of the world's nations.

Afghanistan, Democratic Republic of
Albania, Socialist Republic of
Algeria, Democratic and Popular Republic of
Angola, People's Republic of
Antigua and Barbuda
Argentina, Republic of
Australia, Commonwealth of
Austria, Republic of
Bahamas, Commonwealth of The
Bahrain, State of
Bangladesh, People's Republic of
Barbados
Belgium, Kingdom of
Belize
Benin, The People's Republic of
Bhutan, Kingdom of
Bolivia, Republic of
Botswana, Republic of
Brazil, Federative Republic of
Brunei (Brunei Darussalam)
Bulgaria, People's Republic of
Burkina-Faso (formerly Upper Volta)
Burma, Socialist Republic of the Union of
Burundi, Republic of
Byelorussia (Byelorussian Soviet Socialist Republic)
Cambodia
Cameroon, United Republic of
Canada
Cape Verde, Republic of
Central African Republic
Chad, Republic of
Chile, Republic of
China, People's Republic of
Colombia, Republic of
Comoros, Federal Islamic Republic of the
Congo, People's Republic of
Costa Rica, Republic of
Côte d'Ivoire
Cuba, Republic of
Cyprus, Republic of
Czechoslovakia (Czech & Slovak Federal Republic)
Denmark, Kingdom of
Djibouti, Republic of

Dominica, Commonwealth of
Dominican Republic
Ecuador, Republic of
Egypt, Arab Republic of
El Salvador, Republic of
Equatorial Guinea, Republic of
Ethiopia, Socialist
Fiji
Finland, Republic of
France (French Republic)
Gabon (Gabonese Republic)
Gambia, Republic of the
Germany
Ghana, Republic of
Greece (Hellenic Republic)
Grenada
Guatemala, Republic of
Guinea, People's Revolutionary Republic of
Guinea-Bissau, Republic of
Guyana, Cooperative Republic of
Haiti, Republic of
Honduras, Republic of
Hungary, Republic of
Iceland, Republic of
India, Republic of
Indonesia, Republic of
Iran, Islamic Republic of
Iraq, Republic of
Ireland
Israel, State of
Italy (Italian Republic)
Jamaica
Japan
Jordan, Hashemite Kingdom of
Kenya, Republic of
Kuwait, State of
Laos (Lao People's Democratic Republic)
Lebanon, Republic of
Lesotho, Kingdom of
Liberia, Republic of
Libya (Socialist People's Libyan Arab Jamahiriya)
Liechtenstein, Principality of
Luxembourg, Grand Duchy of
Madagascar, Democratic Republic of
Malawi
Malaysia
Maldives, Republic of
Mali, Republic of
Malta
Mauritania, Islamic Republic of

Mauritius
Mexico (The United Mexican States)
Mongolia (Mongolian People's Republic)
Morocco, Kingdom of
Mozambique, People's Republic of
Namibia, Republic of
Nepal, Kingdom of
Netherlands, Kingdom of the
New Zealand
Nicaragua, Republic of
Niger, Republic of
Nigeria, Federal Republic of
Norway, Kingdom of
Oman, Sultanate of
Pakistan, Islamic Republic of
Panama, Republic of
Papua New Guinea
Paraguay, Republic of
Peru, Republic of
Philippines, Republic of the
Poland, Republic of
Portugal, Republic of
Qatar, State of
Romania, Socialist Republic of
Rwanda, Republic of
St. Christopher-Nevis
St. Lucia
St. Vincent and the Grenadines
Samoa, Independent State of Western
Sao Tome and Principe, Democratic Republic of
Saudi Arabia
Senegal
Seychelles, Republic of
Sierra Leone, Republic of
Singapore, Republic of
Solomon Islands
Somalia (Somal Democratic Republic)
South Africa, Republic of
Spain (Spanish State)
Sri Lanka, Democratic Socialist Republic of
Sudan, Democratic Republic of
Suriname, Republic of
Swaziland, Kingdom of
Sweden, Kingdom of
Syria (Syrian Arab Republic)
Tanzania, United Republic of
Thailand, Kingdom of
Togo, Republic of
Trinidad and Tobago, Republic of

Tunisia, Republic of
Turkey, Republic of
Uganda, Republic of
Ukraine (Ukrainian Soviet Socialist Republic)
Union of Soviet Socialist Republics
United Arab Emirates
United Kingdom of Great Britain and Northern Ireland
United States of America
Uruguay
Vanuatu, Republic of
Venezuela, Republic of
Vietnam, Socialist Republic of
Yemen, Republic of
Yugoslavia, Socialist Federal Republic of
Zaire, Republic of
Zambia, Republic of
Zimbabwe

The following maintain Permanent Observer Missions to the U.N.:

Holy See
Korea, Democratic People's Republic of (North Korea)
Korea, Republic of (South Korea)
Monaco, Principality of
San Marino
Switzerland (Swiss Confederation)

Prepared as a public information service by the United Nations Association of the United States of America (UNA-USA), an independent, nonpartisan, nationwide membership organization. Through its programs of research and education, UNA-USA seeks to strengthen public knowledge about the United Nations, to increase the effectiveness of international organizations, and to promote constructive U.S. policies on matters of global concern.

United Nations Association of the United States of America

485 Fifth Avenue
New York, N.Y. 10017
(212) 697-3232
FAX (212) 682-9185

Washington Office:
1010 Vermont Avenue, N.W.
Suite 905
Washington, D.C. 20005
(202) 347-5004
FAX (202) 628-5945

Index

Abortion, 141, 143, 144

Accelerated Development in Sub-Saharan Africa: An Agenda for Action (AD), 30, 31, 32

Accounting standards, 124–25

Acquired immune deficiency syndrome (AIDS), 205, 208, 209, 221, 224

Affirmative action programs, 313

Afghanistan: civil war and, 48–51; elections, 50, 187, 188; human rights abuses, 51, 52, 187–89; Soviet withdrawal of, 1, 48, 187

Africa, 168, 169; denuclearization of, 88; development aid to, 103; discrimination against women, 221; economics, 29–34, 101, 102, 115; food issues, 33–34, 130, 133; fuel demands, 138; industrial development, 30–31; population, 135, 136; water supplies, 138; *see also names of specific countries;* South Africa; Sub-Saharan Africa

African Charter, 33

African National Congress (ANC), 35–36, 37, 38, 41, 198

Afrikaner Resistance Movement, 38

Agenda 21: 139, 148

Aging, 228–29

Agriculture, 128; Africa, 30; World Food Council and, 127–28, 131, 132

Ahmed, Rafeeuddin, 53, 57, 58, 61

Albania, 199; human rights abuses, 186; nuclear-free zones and, 86; Secretariat and, 315

Algeria, 69, 192, 194; Arab-Israeli conflict and, 23; Morocco and, 69

Amazon region: deforestation, 136; oil spills, 153

American Samoa, 72

Angola, 199; Cuban troops in, 39, 42; economic rehabilitation of, 43; food relief and, 34; hunger issues, 129; Namibia and, 39

Anguilla, 72

Antarctic and Southern Ocean Coalition (ASOC), 164

Antarctic Treaty, 35, 162–66

Aoun, Michel, 23–24

Apartheid, 34–38, 40, 162, 198, 221, 248, 271

Arab League, 10, 23

Arab Tripartite Commission, 23

Arab-Israeli conflict, 2, 3, 14, 17–22, 26

Arafat, Yasser, 7, 22, 25

Argentina, 191; economic growth rate, 100–101; ICSC review and, 291; inflation, 102; U.N. debt, 271

Armenia, 68

Arms control and disarmament, 46, 50, 77, 78–79, 81–82, 91–92, 224, 239; outer space, 265

Asia, 167, 168; economics, 114; food issues, 130; Green Revolution, 132–33; Nuclear Weapon-Free Zone, 88; population, 135, 136; water supply, 138

Association of Southest Asian Nations (ASEAN), 54, 56, 85

Australia, 65, 143, 277; carbon emissions, 146; dispute with Nauru, 268; East Timor and, 70–71, 268–69; population-environment linkage, 140

329

An invitation from thousands of your fellow citizens

Do you feel powerless to deal with terrorism, AIDS, hunger, human rights violations, drug abuse? Do you wish there was a way you, as an individual, could help international efforts to address these global problems?

There is a way! Join with thousands of your fellow citizens in an effort to make the United Nations even more effective. Join the United Nations Association.

UNA-USA is a nonpartisan, nonprofit organization working in Washington, at U.N. Headquarters in New York, and in thousands of communities across America to build public understanding of, and support for, international cooperation through the United Nations.

■ *Get the inside story*

Founded a quarter-century ago, UNA boasts a membership of more than 20,000 Americans—citizens who want to get beyond the headlines of the popular media.

As a UNA member you will receive the Association's acclaimed news journal, *The InterDependent*, with expert analysis of the global issues that affect our lives. You will learn from UNA's Policy Studies reports the latest in Soviet policy toward the United Nations, the newest thinking on Third World debt, and the future of U.N. reform as the world body prepares to enter the 21st century.

■ *Be a part of it all*

You are invited to participate in your local UNA Chapter to whatever degree your schedule permits: planning U.N. Day observances (October 24); sponsoring Model U.N. conferences for local high school and college students; attending lectures and conferences, often with the participation of senior U.N. officials and representatives of U.N. member governments; and setting up seminars for educators, the media, and elected officials—all aimed at shaping a U.S. agenda for a stronger and more effective U.N.

■ *Sign up and receive . . .*

• One year's subscription to the *Inter-Dependent*.
• A membership kit, containing UNA Fact Sheets, *ABCs of the U.N.*, and other vital information on global issues.
• Discounts on all UNA materials.
• The opportunity to become active in your local UNA-USA Chapter.

$35 ☐ Individual	$20 ☐ Limited income (individual)	$500 ☐ Patron
$40 ☐ Family	$25 ☐ Limited income (family)	$1,000 ☐ Ambassador
$10 ☐ Student	$100 ☐ Sponsor	

☐ Additional contribution for my local chapter $_____
☐ Additional contribution for UNA's national programs $_____

Contributions are tax deductible.   **Total enclosed $_____**

Please make checks payable to UNA-USA.

Name_____

Address_____

City_____ State_____ Zip_____

Mail this form and check to: UNA-USA Membership Dept. 485 Fifth Avenue New York, N.Y. 10017